Spinal Osteotomy Orthopaedics

Huizhong Tian • Yuan Ma • Jingming Xie
Yingsong Wang
Editors

Spinal Osteotomy Orthopaedics

Deformity Correction

SPM SOUTHERN PUBLISHING AND MEDIA
GUANGDONG SCIENCE & TECHNOLOGY PRESS

Springer

Editors
Huizhong Tian
Spinal Surgery
The Sixth Affiliated Hospital
of Xinjiang Medical University
Urumqi, China

Yuan Ma
Spinal Surgery
The Sixth Affiliated Hospital
of Xinjiang Medical University
Urumqi, China

Jingming Xie
Department of Orthopedics
The 2nd Affiliated Hospital
of Kunming Medical University
Kunming, China

Yingsong Wang
Department of Orthopedics
The 2nd Affiliated Hospital
of Kunming Medical University
Kunming, China

Associate Editors
Shaoyu Liu
Department of Orthopedics
The seventh Affiliated Hospital of Sun Yat-sen University
Shenzhen, China

Weibin Sheng
Spine Surgery
The First Affiliated Hospital of Xinjiang Medical University
Urumqi, China

Yijiang Liang
Spine Surgery
Affiliated Hospital of Southwest Jiaotong University
Chengdu, China

Ying Zhang
Department of Orthopedics
The 2nd Affiliated Hospital of Kunming Medical University
Kunming, China

Zhi Zhao
Department of Orthopedics
The 2nd Affiliated Hospital of Kunming Medical University
Kunming, China

Tao Li
Department of Orthopedics
The 2nd Affiliated Hospital of Kunming Medical University
Kunming, China

Yilihamu Tuoheti
Department of Orthopedics
The Seventh Affiliated Hospital of Xinjiang Medical University
Urumqi, China

Jiangtao Sui
Spine Surgery
The Sixth Affiliated Hospital of Xinjiang Medical University
Urumqi, China

Junjie Chen
Department of Orthopedics
Zhongshan People's Hospital
Zhongshan, China

Xia Lv
Spine Surgery
The Sixth Affiliated Hospital of Xinjiang Medical University
Urumqi, China

ISBN 978-981-16-1389-0 ISBN 978-981-16-1387-6 (eBook)
https://doi.org/10.1007/978-981-16-1387-6
Jointly published with Guangdong Science & Technology Press Co., Ltd

This Springer imprint is published by the registered company Springer Nature Singapore Pte Ltd.
The registered company address is: 152 Beach Road, #21-01/04 Gateway East, Singapore 189721, Singapore

Foreword

Spinal Osteotomy for Deformity Correction is a monograph on the research and introduction of spinal osteotomy. The content is focused and comprehensive, and the layout is unique. The expression and narration combined with graphics and text is concise, intuitive, and vivid. This monograph meets the current clinical practice needs, with reference value and teaching significance.

The publication of *Spinal Osteotomy Orthopaedics* further promotes osteotomy and orthopedics, further expands the scope of the treatment of osteotomy combined with internal fixation with instrumentation, and solves the problems that were difficult for treatment merely by instrumentation in the past. It has been further accepted by spine surgeons in the clinical application of spinal osteotomy in correcting spinal deformity. In recent years, various methods of spinal osteotomy have been reported and applied clinically, to name just a few, curetting (decancelous or eggshell surgery) or with a burr. However, still the use of a thin-blade osteotome for osteotomy is in the minority. As circular osteotomy surrounding the dural tube with thin-blade osteotome is technically demanding, this is a basic skill to be acquired by special training and long-term practice. This book *Spinal Osteotomy for Deformity Correction* is a tutorial for the young surgeons to master the thin-blade osteotome for spinal osteotomy.

This book emphasizes the importance of traction, osteotomy, and instrument correction for children's spinal curvature during development. After this golden age, it will bring difficulties to the correction of spinal deformity. It provides surgical strategies for congenital spine deformity, preventive osteotomy, and maneuver deformity correction.

A good book should be a handy tool dedicated to the reader. I believe that readers will benefit from it, and improve the ability toward a high grade of spinal osteotomy.

2016.3.10

Shibi Lu
Academician of the Chinese Academy of Engineering
Beijing, China
Beijing PLA General Hospital
Beijing, China

Foreword

In cases of ankylosing spondylitis kyphosis, spinal osteotomy is the only treatment, and it is impossible to correct this spinal deformity without osteotomy. Therefore, spinal osteotomy started from ankylosing spondylitis kyphosis. Spinal osteotomy was gradually applied to spinal curvature deformities due to other causes in the early 1980s. Spinal deformities such as congenital spinal deformity, idiopathic scoliosis, tuberculosis kyphosis, traumatic kyphosis, and degenerative scoliosis were corrected with spinal osteotomy combined with instrumentation, obtaining a better therapeutic effect than the conventional treatment by instrumentation only for correcting spinal deformity.

Tian Huizhong and his team started this work earlier in China. On the basis of treating kyphosis deformity of ankylosing spondylitis, they gradually developed the application of osteotomy for the treatment of spinal deformities caused by other causes. They designed and made the Tian's spine osteotome through the accumulation of a large number of clinical cases. They held the Tian's osteotome courses in China and Japan several times and trained a large number of young doctors using the Tian's spine osteotome for osteotomy, because the use of a thin-edged osteotome for osteotomy is a specialized technique that requires special training and long-term practice. The book of *Spinal Osteotomy for Deformity Correction* is a handy tool dedicated to readers. You will find the book a great help. You will understand tacitly and grasp the essentials of the operation with a thin-blade osteotome.

2016.3.18

John Chi-Yan Leong
Academician of Chinese Academy of Sciences
Beijing, China
Open University of Hong Kong
Ho Man Tin, Hong Kong

Original Introduction in Chinese Version

Smith Petersen (1945) was the first person to perform spinal osteotomy for ankylosing spondylitis kyphosis (ASK). He began to use laminectomy plus manipulation to correct ankylosing kyphosis. Meanwhile, Smith Petersen named simple laminectomy as "spinal osteotomy." Professor Tian Huizhong performed the first case of ASK osteotomy at the Xinjiang Institute of Spinal Surgery in 1961, which is the earliest case of spinal osteotomy in China. Since then, we have entered into the era of treating ASK with simple laminectomy. But our method is different from Smith Petersen's. We retain spinous process and lamina and use thin-blade osteotomy for osteotomy. The second part of this book first introduces various osteotomy correction techniques for kyphosis deformity of ASK (funded by the National Natural Science Foundation of China, project number 81360280). Spinal osteotomy is the only way to treat ankylosing spondylitis hump (ASK). Unfortunately, there is no alternative.

The internal fixation technology for scoliosis correction with simple instruments has developed rapidly, which has improved the treatment standard of spinal surgery and solved most cases in younger age groups with smaller curvature and better compliance since Harrington instruments were developed in the 1960s. However, it is difficult for rigid and structural severe scoliosis to be corrected by only instrumentation such as pedicle screw and rod system. Even the best quality instrumentation can hardly overcome the deforming force of scoliosis. In the end, the screw will be pulled out and the rod will be broken. This is the failure of correction as well as the source of complication. How to eliminate the deforming force of curved spine? Osteotomy is the best way to eliminate the deforming force of curved spine and lift the load of instrumentation. Therefore, the combination of spinal osteotomy and instrumentation is the best choice for the treatment of spinal deformity.

This book helps the readers when they find treating cases just with instrumentation is difficult and cases of early-onset deformity requiring osteotomy. It is only a remedy for the deficiency of instrumentation. Through clinical application and continuous summary of experience, the surgical methods of instrumentation and treatment scope of spinal osteotomy are expanding. Treating deformity with osteotomy and instrumentation has got the recognition of most colleagues, especially for children who are still developing. My team and I were preparing to write *Spinal Osteotomy for Deformity Correction* to share our clinical experience with most of our colleagues and promote the development of spinal surgery 2 years ago.

This book is a reference for colleagues. It is a continuation based on the style of osteotomy and publication in the past 50 years while trying to illustrate with operation photos and typical cases. We did our best to produce the anatomical and radiographic pictures involved. At the same time, three-dimensional technology and digital medicine and simulation medicine are introduced to explain the operation process, so that readers can get familiarized with the relevant anatomy of the spine, and establish a good mindset to master the operation technique.

This book emphasizes the importance of traction, osteotomy, and instrumentation for spinal deformity in children who are growing and developing. After the golden age, it will bring difficulties to the correction of the spinal deformity. It puts forward the surgical strategies for congenital curvature of the spine, preventive early osteotomy, and correction of the deformity of the spine.

The contents of *Spinal Osteotomy for Deformity Correction* are divided into 4 parts and 53 chapters. The first part is a general introduction, which mainly describes the history of spinal osteotomy correction, spinal anatomy, biomechanics, clinical examination and diagnosis, simulation technology, postoperative external fixation, treatment of complications, and the application of the spine osteotome. The second part is the osteotomy correction for ASK. Various osteotomy techniques of ASK are described in detail with the combination of graphics and texts. The third part is about the osteotomy correction of spinal deformity for other etiologies, such as congenital, tuberculous, traumatic, degenerative, juvenile, and idiopathic tumors. The fourth part is about other conditions operated with osteotomes, such as discectomy, spinal canal decompression, anterior decompression of spinal cord grooving decompression with osteotome, and so on.

This book is practical, novel, and full of pictures and texts, containing more than 1700 high-definition pictures which shows techniques and steps of each osteotomy with graphics, so as to enable beginners to master surgical techniques quickly. References are attached at the end of each chapter for the reader's reference.

Thank you very much for the help and support of colleagues and experts in the process of compiling this book. Special thanks to Academician ShibiLu and John Chi-Yan Leong for their guidance and review despite their busy schedules, which makes this book perfect. Our thanks also go to the Sixth Affiliated Hospital of Xinjiang Medical University and the Second Affiliated Hospital of Kunming Medical University for the support and encouragement. We also thank Liang Zhou, Vice-President of Guangdong Science and Technology Publishing House, for his planning and guidance despite his busy schedule, so that the book can be brought to readers at an early date.

Due to the restriction of time and limitation of the author, this book might still contain unavoidable errors. We ask for criticism and correction by readers. The illustrations cited are listed in the references in the compilation of this book. As for any missing information please contact the authors of this book.

2016-3-27

Huizhong Tian
Yuan Ma
Jingming Xie

Introduction

Spinal Osteotomy for Deformity Correction is a monograph of introducing osteotomy for spinal deformity correction surgery. Its content is prominent and comprehensive. The unique arrangement with the combination of pictures and text is concise, intuitive, and vivid. It is a monograph for the needs of current clinical practice with reference value and teaching significance. The publication of *Spinal Osteotomy for Deformity Correction* expands the scope of application of osteotomy and the combined treatment with osteotomy and internal fixation. It solves the difficult problems treated only by simple instruments in the past and made spinal osteotomy further recognized by spinal surgeons in clinical application.

The Chinese version of *Spinal Osteotomy for Deformity Correction* was published by Guangdong Science and Technology Press in October 2018, including 4 articles and 53 chapters. The English version of *Spinal Osteotomy for Deformity Correction* was published by Springer, which is published in two volumes. The first volume is on spinal deformity osteotomy which consists of 13 chapters, including "History of the Development of Spinal Osteotomy," "Application of Tian's Spinal Osteotomes," "Transverse Laminectomy for Ankylosing Spondylitis Kyphosis," "V-Shape Laminectomy for Ankylosing Kyphosis," "Pedicle Subtraction Osteotomy for Ankylosing Kyphosis Deformity," "Vertebral Column Resection for Ankylosing Spondylitis Kyphosis," "Non-apex Osteotomy for ASK," "Apex Osteotomy for AS Kyphosis," "Spinal Osteotomy for Congenital Angular Kyphosis," "Hemivertebra Osteotomy," "Osteotomy for Tuberculosis Angular Kyphosis," "Posterior Vertebral Column Resection (PVCR) Correction for Severe Rigid Spinal Deformity," and "Osteotomy for Traumatic Spinal Deformity." They are various surgical methods of spinal osteotomy with Tian's osteotomes and also described in detail by pictures and text.

The feature of this book is to illustrate the method of surgical operation to achieve the purpose of enabling beginners to quickly grasp the surgical skills. A good book is a set of handy tools dedicated to the reader. We believe that readers will benefit from it and improve the ability and application level of spinal osteotomy and surgery.

We would like to express our deep appreciation to all the colleagues and experts for their great assistance and support in the translation and editing of this book! Thanks to the Sixth Affiliated Hospital of Xinjiang Medical University and the Second Affiliated Hospital of Kunming Medical University for their strong support and encouragement! Thanks to Zhou Liang, vice president, and Zeng Chong, editor of Guangdong Science and Technology Press, for your support! We would also like to thank Hu Bin, editor of Springer Press, and Jiao Guohui, editor of Springer, for taking time out of your busy schedules to plan and guide the book, so that it can be brought to the readers as soon as possible.

2020-11-25

Huizhong Tian
Yuan Ma
Jingming Xie
Yingsong Wang

Contents

1 **History of the Development of Spinal Osteotomy** 1
Huizhong Tian, Yuan Ma, Jingming Xie, Yingsong Wang, and Xia Lv

2 **Application of Tian's Spinal Osteotomes** 7
Huizhong Tian, Yuan Ma, and Xia Lv

3 **Transverse Laminectomy for Ankylosing Spondylitis Kyphosis** 21
Huizhong Tian, Jiangtao Sui, and Ying Zhang

4 **V-Shape Laminectomy for Ankylosing Kyphosis** 29
Huizhong Tian, Zhi Zhao, and Ni Bi

5 **Pedicle Subtraction Osteotomy for Ankylosing Kyphosis Deformity** 47
Huizhong Tian, Tao Li, and Zhibo Song

6 **Vertebral Column Resection for Ankylosing Spondylitis Kyphosis** 57
Huizhong Tian, Yuan Ma, and Jingming Xie

7 **Non-apex Osteotomy for ASK** 83
Yingsong Wang, Ying Zhang, and Huizhong Tian

8 **Apex Osteotomy for AS Kyphosis** 95
Yijian Liang, Shaoyu Liu, Huizhong Tian, and Junyi Ma

9 **Spinal Osteotomy for Congenital Angular Kyphosis** 107
Huizhong Tian, Weibin Sheng, Yilihamu Tuoheti, Li Li, and Junyi Ma

10 **Hemivertebra Osteotomy** 127
Huizhong Tian, Junjie Cheng, Tao Li, Zhibo Song, Zhiyue Shi, Zhi Zhao, Xu Zhu, Jie Dai, Junyi Ma, Jiangtao Sui, Weibin Sheng, Shaoyu Liu, and Quan Li

11 **Osteotomy for Tuberculosis Angular Kyphosis** 159
Huizhong Tian, Sikandaer Siyiti, Quan Li, Zhiyue Shi, Jie Dai, Xu Zhu, Yingsong Wang, Ni Bi, and Li Li

12 **Posterior Vertebral Column Resection (PVCR) Correction for Severe Rigid Spinal Deformity** 179
Jingming Xie

13 **Osteotomy for Traumatic Spinal Deformity** 187
Huizhong Tian, Yuan Ma, Yingsong Wang, and Li Li

Chief Editor Introduction

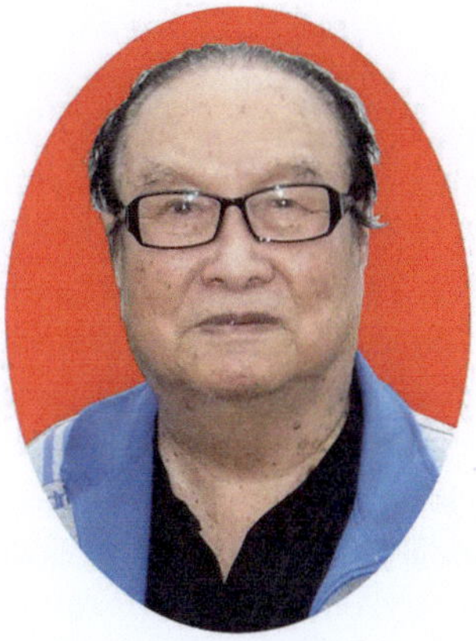

Huizhong Tian, male, born in 1925, graduated from the Medical College of National Henan University in 1949 and is professor, research fellow, PhD student supervisor, expert with State Department special allowance, honorary director of the Department of Spine Surgery of the Sixth Affiliated Hospital of Xinjiang Medical University, honorary director of the Research Institute of Spine Surgery in the Xinjiang Uygur Autonomous Region, and honorary president of Xinjiang Spinal Cord Injury Society. He has been engaged in orthopedics for 60 years and performed various surgical operations in more than 13,000 cases. He is one of the founders of Chinese spine surgery, and he has made outstanding contributions in the field of spinal surgery such as "Total Vertebral Column Osteotomy for Correction of Severe Scoliosis" which is the first international initiative. The inventions of Tian's spine osteotome and portable pediatric halo-pelvic ring traction device have obtained national patents, National Invention Award, and the International Gold Medal Award. He once had served as director of the Research Institute of Spine Surgery of Xinjiang Uygur Autonomous Region, president of Xinjiang Spine Surgery Hospital, visiting researcher of orthopedics of Tokyo University, visiting professor of orthopedics of Hirosaki University, vice-president of the American-Chinese Medical Association of orthopedics surgery society, chief editor of the *American Journal of Orthopaedics*, vice-president of Chinese Spinal Injury Research Society, deputy director of Research Institute of Spinal Cord Injury of Chinese Medical Sciences University, consultant of the Professional Committee of Spinal Cord Injury of Guangdong Province, etc. He has written and published 30 professional books such as *Spinal Deformity Surgery*, *Spinal Deformity & Osteotomy*, *Ankylosing Spondylitisacology*, *Practical Spinal Surgery*, *Practical Spine Surgery Atlas*, *Operative Orthopedics Gist & Atlas*, *Halo Pelvic Distraction Technique for Spinal Deformity*, *Cervical Spine Gist & Atlas*, *Pediatric Operative Orthopedics*, *Spinal Deformity Surgery*, *Surgical Techniques for the Cervical Spine*, and *Spinal Osteotomy Orthopedics*. Moreover, he has published more than 100 representative articles in national and international journals.

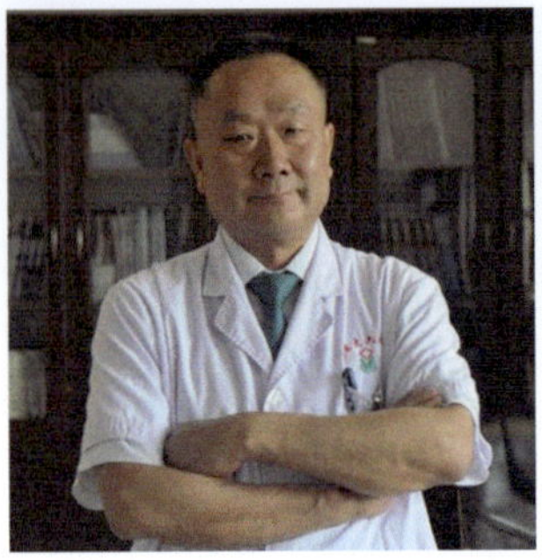

Yuan Ma is professor, PhD student supervisor, and director of the Department of Spine Surgery, Sixth Affiliated Hospital of Xinjiang Medical University. He has been engaged in orthopedics for 26 years and currently serves as vice-director of the Research Institute of Spine Surgery of the Xinjiang Uygur Autonomous Region, president of Xinjiang Spinal Cord Injury Society, national member of Spinal Surgery Group of the Chinese Medical Association, deputy director of Chinese Spinal Cord Injury Rehabilitation Society, council member of the Chinese Speaking Orthopedics Society, and committee member of Xinjiang Physical Disability Rehabilitation Society. He is in the editorial board of *Journal of Integrated Traditional Chinese and Modern Medicine* and *Orthopedics Journal of China*. Moreover, he has published dozens of articles in Chinese journals such as "Correction of Severe Kyphosis and Kyphoscoliosis by Total Spinal Osteotomy," "Total Enbloc Spondylectomy—A New Surgical Technique for Primary Malignant Vertebral Tumors," "Clinical Effect Analysis of Continuous Pedicle Screw for Scoliosis Correction," and "Clinic Effect Analysis of Translamina "V"-Shaped Osteotomy Internal Fixation to Correct Ankylosing Spondylitis." He has written and published ten professional books such as *Practical Spinal Surgery*, *Practical Spine Surgery Atlas*, *Internal Fixation Technique for the Spine*, and *Surgical Techniques for Spinal Tuberculosis*. He has won the Second Prize of Xinjiang Medical Science and Technology, a natural science grant by the Autonomous Region, and a national natural science grant by China.

As a visiting scholar, he studied spine surgery in Japan, Hokkaido University, especially in the field of cervical spondylosis and scoliosis correction surgery. He was instructed by famous professors of orthopedics of Hokkaido University in Japan including Professor Tamita and Professor Abumi. He has worked under the guidance of Professor Huizhong Tian for more than 20 years and accumulated abundant clinical experience and skills in the field of correcting spinal deformity, especially in the treatment of severe scoliosis and kyphosis deformity under the halo-pelvic ring traction, multilevel cervical spondylosis, and kyphosis deformity caused by old fracture. In 2010, he was selected as the leader of spine surgery discipline among the six affiliated hospitals of Xinjiang Medical University.

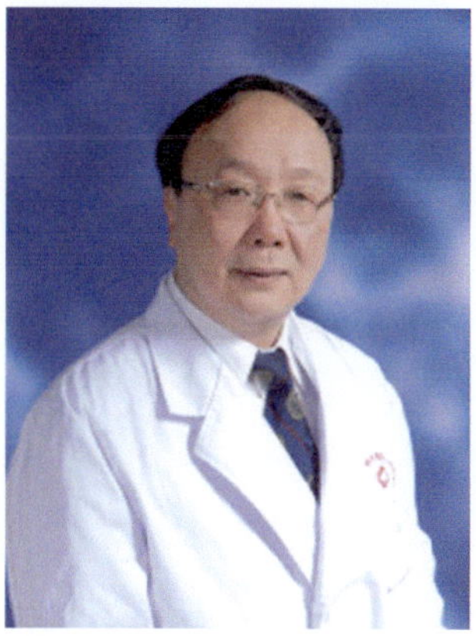

Jingming Xie is professor, PhD student supervisor, chief physician of the Department of Orthopaedics of the Second Affiliated Hospital of Kunming Medical University, and director of the Research Institute of Scoliosis and Spinal Deformity. He is an active member of Scoliosis Research Society, member of North American Spine Society, and member of AO Spine. He is in the editorial board of *International Journal of Orthopedics* and *BMC Musculoskeletal Disorders*. He enjoyed high reputation in the field of spine surgery home and abroad.

He has been devoting himself to the field of treatment of spinal deformities and related research. He is one of the first surgeons in the world applying "posterior vertebral column resection (PVCR)" to treat severe rigid spinal deformities. Over the past 10 years, he has been invited to give more than 60 presentations and academic exchange at international conferences, such as the Annual Meeting of Scoliosis Research Society, the Annual Meeting of the North American Spinal Society, and the Annual Meeting of the European Spinal Society, and his academic research results of treatment of severe rigid spinal deformity by PVCR got high recognition and praise from worldwide spine surgery peers. He was selected as tutor for the Scoliosis Research Society 2013 tutorial for global SRS members in 2013. In 2015, "Second PVCR Global Training Course" for international spine surgeons was successfully held, which improved and enhanced the treatment of severe rigid spinal deformity for the whole world. Over the past 30 years, he has always been adhering to the path of combining clinical and scientific research. Twenty-nine papers have been published in *Spine*, *European Spine Journal*, *Journal of Neurosurgery: Spine*, and other top international journals of spinal surgery, with a cumulative impact factor of 73.4. He invented 16 devices to treat early-onset scoliosis with national patent granted. He undertakes more than ten scientific research projects including with grant at national and provincial level.

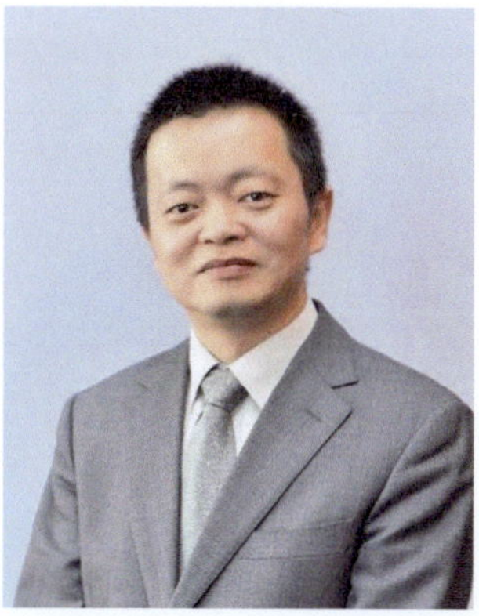

Yingsong Wang, MD, is professor, PhD student supervisor, Director of Orthopedics Department of the Second Affiliated Hospital of Kunming Medical University, with honored title of "Ten Thousand Famous Doctors" of Yunnan Province, Leading Youth Scholar of Yunnan Province, and Discipline Leader of Yunnan Health Commission. He is an elected member of Scoliosis Research Society (SRS) and member of the Education Committee; Deputy Director of Yunnan Orthopedics Association and Yunnan Pediatric Surgery Association; and Director of Bone, Joint and Rheumatic Disease Group of Yunnan Rehabilitation Medicine Association. He enjoys the First Prize and Second Prize of Yunnan Science and Technology Advancement Award. He has led or is leading six projects with grants from the National Natural Science Foundation. His research and clinical work focuses on spinal surgery.

Deputy Editor Chief

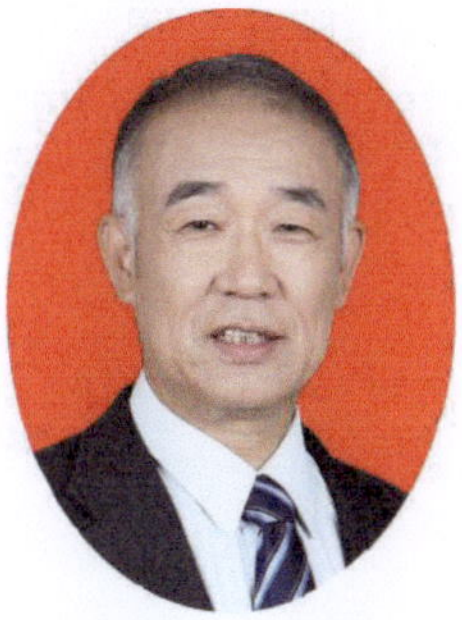

Shaoyu Liu
Chief Physician, Professor, Director, Department of Orthopedics.

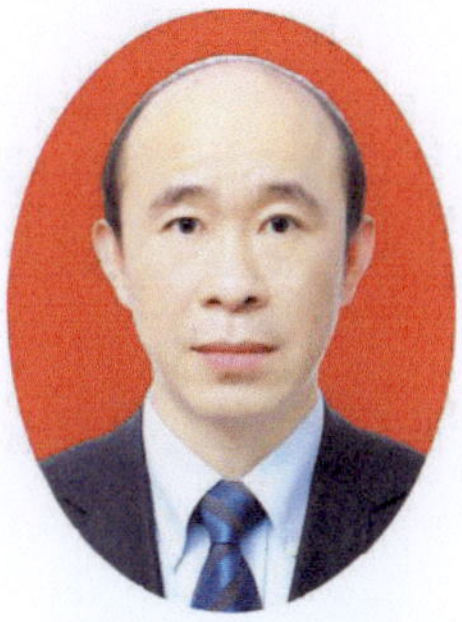

Weibin Sheng
Chief Physician, Professor, Director of Spine Surgery.

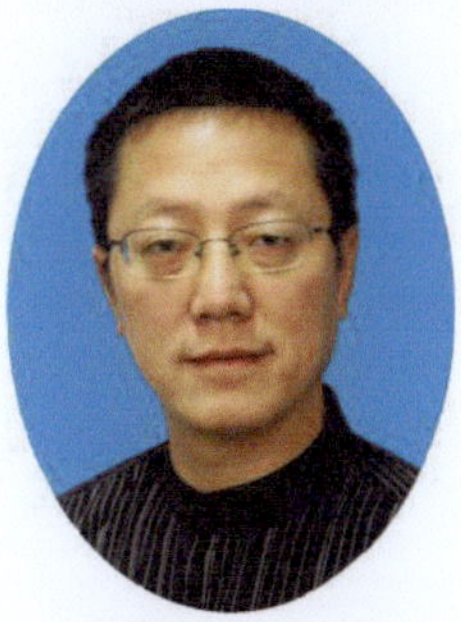

Yijian Liang
Chief Physician, Professor, Director of Spine Surgery.

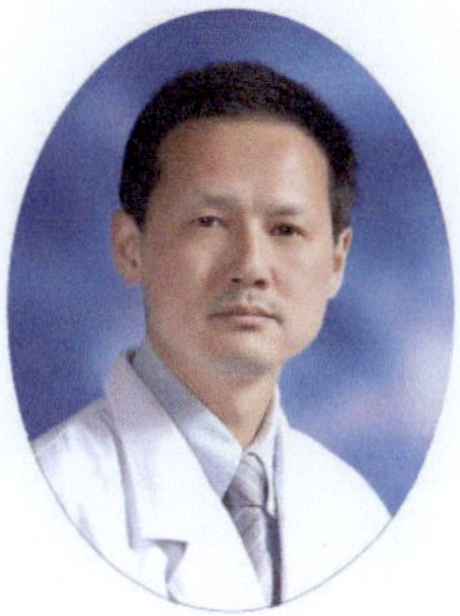

Ying Zhang
Chief Physician.

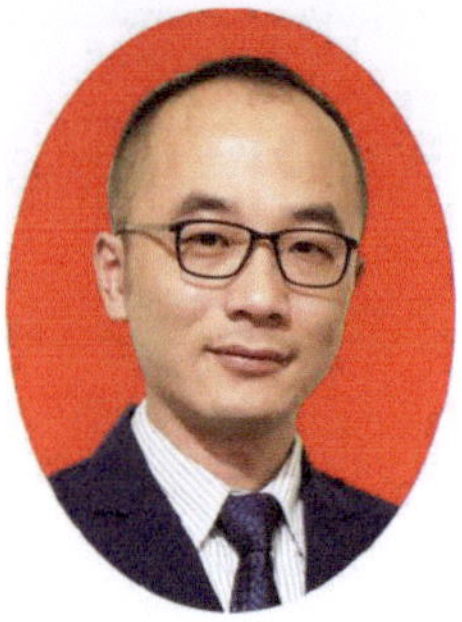

Zhi Zhao
Attending Doctor of Orthopedics.

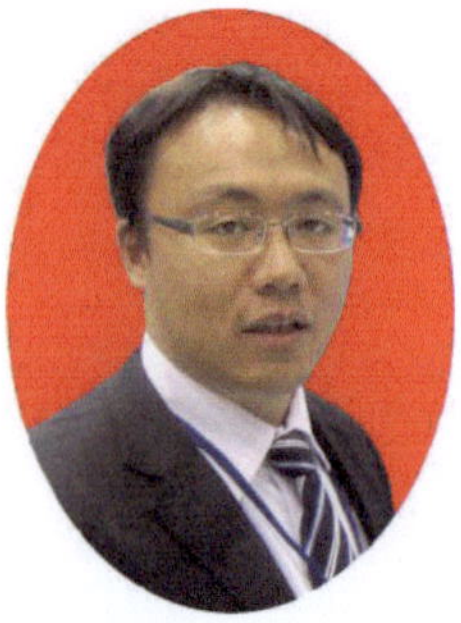

Tao Li
Attending Doctor of Orthopedics.

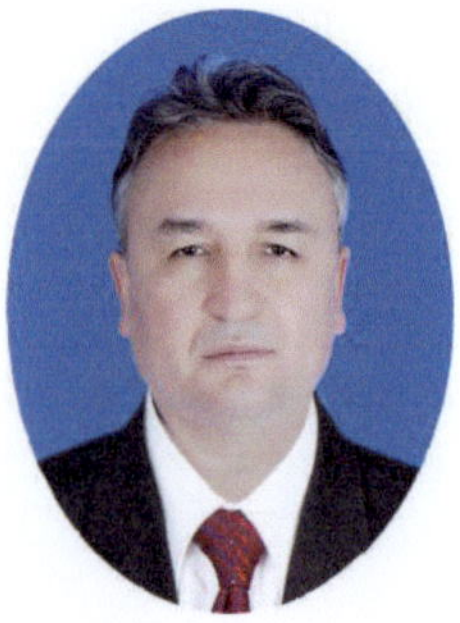

Yilihamu Tuoheti
Chief Physician.

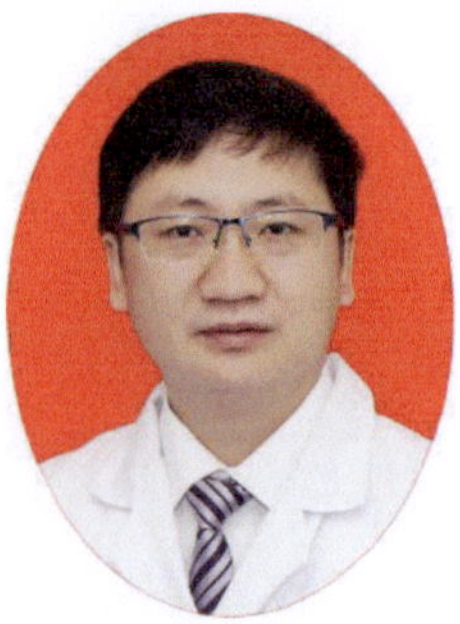

Jiangtao Sui
Deputy Chief Physician.

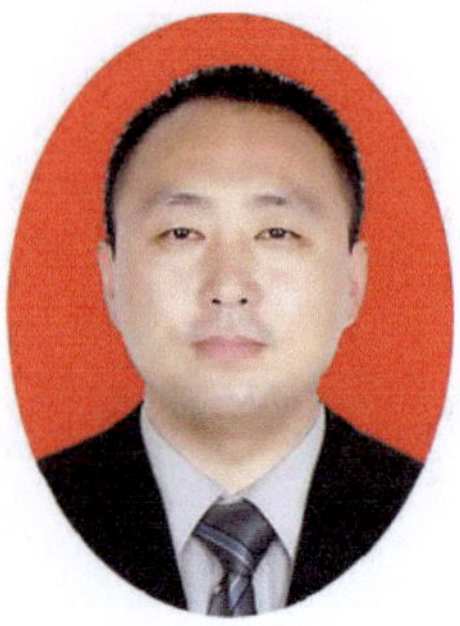

Junjie Cheng
Deputy Chief Physician.

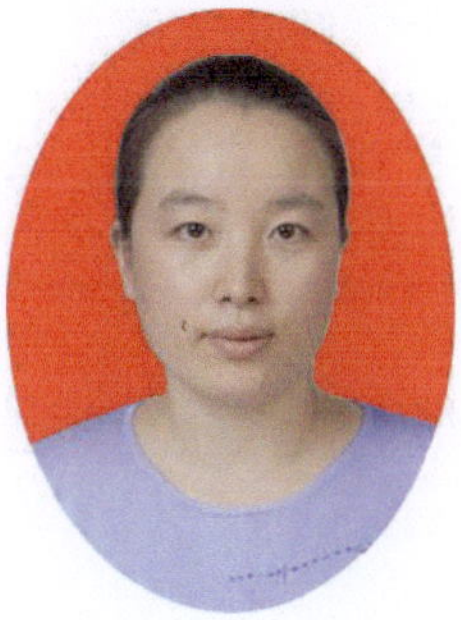

Xia Lv
Physician of Orthopedics.

List of Contributors

Ni Bi Department of Orthopedics, The 2nd Affiliated Hospital of Kunming Medical University, Kunming, China

Junjie Cheng Department of Orthopedics, Nanlang Branch, Zhongshan People's Hospital, Zhongshan, Guangdong, China

Jie Dai Spinal Surgery, The Sixth Affiliated Hospital of Xinjiang Medical University, Urumqi, China

Li Li Spinal Surgery, The Sixth Affiliated Hospital of Xinjiang Medical University, Urumqi, China

Quan Li Department of Orthopedics, The 2nd Affiliated Hospital of Kunming Medical University, Kunming, China

Tao Li Department of Orthopedics, The 2nd Affiliated Hospital of Kunming Medical University, Kunming, China

Yijian Liang Spinal Surgery, Affiliated Hospital of Southwest Jiaotong University, Chengdu, China

Shaoyu Liu Spinal Surgery, The Seventh Affiliated Hospital, Sun Yat-sen University, Shenzhen, China

Xia Lv Spinal Surgery, The Sixth Affiliated Hospital of Xinjiang Medical University, Urumqi, China

Junyi Ma Spinal Surgery, The Sixth Affiliated Hospital of Xinjiang Medical University, Urumqi, China

Yuan Ma Spinal Surgery, The Sixth Affiliated Hospital of Xinjiang Medical University, Urumqi, China

Weibin Sheng Spinal Surgery, The First Affiliated Hospital of Xinjiang Medical University, Urumqi, China

Zhiyue Shi Department of Orthopedics, The 2nd Affiliated Hospital of Kunming Medical University, Kunming, China

Sikandaer Siyiti Spinal Surgery, The Sixth Affiliated Hospital of Xinjiang Medical University, Urumqi, China

Zhibo Song Department of Orthopedics, The 2nd Affiliated Hospital of Kunming Medical University, Kunming, China

Jiangtao Sui Spinal Surgery, The Sixth Affiliated Hospital of Xinjiang Medical University, Urumqi, China

Huizhong Tian Spinal Surgery, The Sixth Affiliated Hospital of Xinjiang Medical University, Urumqi, China

Yilihamu Tuoheti Department of Orthopedics, The Seventh Affiliated Hospital of Xinjiang Medical University, Urumqi, China

Yingsong Wang Department of Orthopedics, The 2nd Affiliated Hospital of Kunming Medical University, Kunming, China

Jingming Xie Department of Orthopedics, The 2nd Affiliated Hospital of Kunming Medical University, Kunming, China

Ying Zhang Department of Orthopedics, The 2nd Affiliated Hospital of Kunming Medical University, Kunming, China

Zhi Zhao Department of Orthopedics, The 2nd Affiliated Hospital of Kunming Medical University, Kunming, China

Xu Zhu Spinal Surgery, The Sixth Affiliated Hospital of Xinjiang Medical University, Urumqi, China

History of the Development of Spinal Osteotomy

1

Huizhong Tian, Yuan Ma, Jingming Xie, Yingsong Wang, and Xia Lv

1.1 Ankylosing Spondylitis Osteotomy

The earliest spinal osteotomy for deformity correction was used in patients with ankylosing spondylitis and later developed to other spinal deformities including kyphosis and scoliosis which are caused by different etiological factors. However, different from ankylosing spondylitis, the anterior longitudinal ligament and intervertebral space structure in patients with other etiology deformities are not easy to rupture and open. Thus, the technique of simple posterior translaminar osteotomy is difficult to succeed.

In 1945, Smith Petersen, Larsont, and Aufranc performed lumbar osteotomy for ankylosing spondylitis kyphosis. According to the report, they treated six patients. The surgical procedures were to remove the spinous processes of L1, 2, and 3, and then to remove the lamina and the superior and inferior articular processes as a wedge shape, and to correct the deformity with over-extension position. The osteotomy site needed a bone graft. Postoperatively, patients care included casting for 2 months, and then Taylor brace for 1 year.

Lachapelle advocated the strategy of two-stage operation to correct the deformity. The first stage osteotomy was performed through a posterior approach under local anesthesia. After 2 weeks, the second stage of the anterior approach was performed to distract the anterior portion of the lumbar disc, and the bone plug was implanted in the open gap.

Briggs, Keats, and Schlesinger reported five patients treated with posterior lumbar translaminar wedge osteotomy to correct the deformity. The target for correction was located on the active axis of deformity (posterior edge of the L3-4 disc). Two patients were fixed with a metal plate following osteotomy and deformity correction.

Herbert advocated the strategy of one- or two-stage osteotomy. Firstly, the patient was taken to the prone position. If the spinal deformity could be corrected by posterior osteotomy, there is no need for a second-stage anterior approach.

Law reported a larger number of patients. He treated 120 patients, and among them, 10 died, and 6 patients encountered postoperative neurological complications.

In order to avoid excessive extension of the anterior column, many authors advocated the use of spinal shortening to correct deformities. Scudese and Calabro reported that they performed laminar osteotomy firstly in L2 and 3, and then removed a part of the upper vertebral body along the L2–3 disc. Thomasen has made further improvements to the surgical technique by removing the cancellous bone from the vertebral body. In the L2 osteotomy, the lamina was removed till extending to the pedicle, and the vertebral cancellous bone was removed as a wedge shape through the base of bilateral pedicles. Then L2 vertebral body was artificially fractured and the wedge-shaped gap was closed, so the posterior approach led to increased lumbar lordosis. Smith Petersen improved the procedure and corrected the deformity with a transpedicular internal fixation after osteotomy. McMaster has advocated the use of a strong internal fixation to maintain the corrected spinal column stabilization and prevent complications.

The pioneer of performing osteotomy for ankylosing kyphosis correction was Smith Petersen (1945). Just at the time, Smith Petersen named his laminectomy as "Spinal Osteotomy." Professor Tian Huizhong from the Xinjiang Institute of Spinal Surgery in China began to perform spinal osteotomy in patients with ankylosing spondylitis and kyphosis after 1961–1980 with reference to Smith Petersen's surgical approach. Tian's cases were chosen to be around 30 years old, and the curvature of the kyphosis was less than 80°. Under the general anesthesia of tracheal intubation, the translaminar osteotomy as transverse or V-shaped osteotomy was performed. During the operation, the osteotomy gap was

H. Tian · Y. Ma (✉) · X. Lv
The Sixth Affiliated Hospital of Xinjiang Medical University, Urumqi, China

J. Xie · Y. Wang
Department of Orthopedics, The 2nd Affiliated Hospital of Kunming Medical University, Kunming, China
e-mail: xiejingming@vip.163.com

H. Tian et al. (eds.), *Spinal Osteotomy Orthopaedics*, https://doi.org/10.1007/978-981-16-1387-6_1

closed by traction and manipulation press, and the harvested bone was implanted around the lamina. Postoperatively, trunk casting has been used, and then the casting vest was replaced after returning to the ward for 2 ~ 3 weeks. Tian treated 85 cases with ankylosing spondylitis in his method and get good treatment outcomes. From 1981 to 2011, patients with ankylosing kyphosis were divided into two types: mild (Cobb angle <80°) and severe (Cobb angle >80°). For the mild cases, the V-shaped osteotomy without internal fixation, and postoperative casting were used. Internal fixation was performed simultaneously with osteotomy and correction in severe cases. Subtotal vertebral body osteotomy or spinal column osteotomy was used in cases in which the intervertebral space could not be opened after osteotomy due to interbody rigid fusion.

In China, Tian Huizhong started spinal osteotomy earlier in 1961. The technique of treating ankylosing kyphosis was followed by Liu Runtian of Tianjin, Ma Jingkun of Shanxi, Wu Zhikang of Beijing, and Wan Nianyu of Qingdao. After 1980, the number of hospitals carrying out this technique in China has gradually increased, such as the major hospitals in Northeast China, Guangdong, Shandong, Fujian, Shanghai, Tianjin, and so on.

"Tian's Spine Osteotome" is a set of 20 thin-bladed osteotomes with different shapes and curvatures developed by Professor Tian Huizhong in combination with more than 50 years of orthopedic clinical experience. In 1979, the Chinese National Trauma Orthopaedic Conference was held in Datong, Shanxi. He met with orthopedic colleagues throughout China and was highly praised by the ancestors of the orthopedic community. Professors such as Ye Yanqing, Shang Tianyu, and Wu Zhikang gave the series instrumentation high marks. In particular, Professor Wu Zhikang, after the meeting, invited Tian to go to the Beijing People's Liberation Army 301 Hospital to perform the application of "Tian's Spine Osteotome" and proposed improvement suggestions. Later, it developed into "Type II Tian's Spine Osteotome." In the early 1990s, the "Type III Tian's Spine Osteotome" was officially put into production at Tokyo Mizuho Co., Ltd in Japan, and its products were sold to China, Japan, the United States, and European countries. Subsequently, the series osteotome has been continuously improved in application, and has been transformed into a "Type VI Tian's Spine Osteotome." This type is divided into two subtypes: simple subtype and spinal column osteotomy subtype, which has 10 and 20 different osteotomes, respectively. The appearance of the Tian's Spine Osteotomes has promoted the development of spinal column osteotomy. In addition to the application in ankylosing kyphosis, it was turned to considered to be a higher value in deformity correction in patients with angular kyphosis, such as tuberculosis or congenital. However, using osteotome for spinal surgery is technically demanding, the surgeon needs to have a sophisticated anatomical concept and a well-trained special skill and basic skills for surgery using a thin-edged osteotome.

Since the appearance of the Tian's Spine Osteotome in 1979, a "milestone" has been established in the history of spinal osteotomy in China. The progression involved the path from applying simple instruments to correct the curvature of the spine, to combined traction and instrument to correct the curvature of the spine, and finally to achieve traction and osteotomy and instrument correction. Especially, facing the cases of ankylosing kyphosis, if lacking "spine osteotomy," correction of kyphosis should be an impossible mission. Thus, in patients with ankylosing kyphosis, simple lamina osteotomy with external casting, lamina osteotomy with internal fixation, transpedicular vertebral body subtotal osteotomy with internal fixation, and spinal column osteotomy with internal fixation are the main techniques for the treatment of ankylosing kyphosis.

1.2 History of Spinal Osteotomy in China

In the previous textbooks, it was stipulated that the operation on the spine with the osteotome was not allowed, because the vibration of the osteotome was great, and it was difficult to grasp its depth. Once surgeons' hand was lost, it would cause serious spinal cord injury. But the author Tian Huizhong began to study the application of thin-edged sharp bone knife in wedge-shaped osteotomy, grooving, and clearing, etc. on the spine in the late 1950s, which can be easily solved and used more quickly than any electric drill or saw and can be more comfortable and able to handle and master the scale. If the surgeon is proficient in his/her skills, there is no risk of damage to the spinal cord or nerve tissue. Our spinal surgeons should also learn the fine traditions of the old artists and can engrave the basic skills of caving the Eight Immortals Crossing the Sea on a peach core. In the late 1950s, the author devoted himself to the use of thin-blade osteotomes with various curvatures and shapes to perform experimental osteotomy on the spine of fresh corpses. It is believed that both the vertebral body and the pedicle are made of cancellous bone. The combination of strong bones is very suitable for slicing with a thin-blade osteotome. Because the thin-blade osteotome is hit into the pedicle or vertebral body, the resistance is small and the vibration is light, which will not cause shock damage to the spinal cord and nerve tissue. Also, since the bone tissue is removed by the osteotome from the outside to the inside until the inner cortical layer close to the dural tube is touched, the hand feeling is relatively obvious, so there is no consideration of damage to the nerve tissue. On the contrary, if the rongeur is used to bite the bone tissue close to the dural tube, the jaw must be inserted between the medial cortex and the dura sac to bite off part of the bone tissue, so there is a high risk of crushing and injuring nerve root or nerve. If someone can really master the basic skills of using a thin-blade osteotome, you can completely eliminate the concerns of nerve tissue damage.

In order to promote the application of spinal deformity osteotomy procedures, in 1997, the authors began to cooperate with the Institute of Spinal Cord Injury of China Medical University and established four spinal centers in various parts of the country where there is a high incidence of ankylosing spondylitis, such as Liaodong Peninsula, Shandong Peninsula, and Eastern Guangdong. The center of the spine, namely the Dalian Spine Center, the Gaozhou Spine Center, the Yangjiang Spine Center, and the Foshan Spine Center. Thirty surgical sites have been established in grassroots hospitals (surgery hospitals) across the country, and surgeons from the spine center have been assigned to assist in surgery and training surgeons for the profession.

From 1997 to 2011, a total of 825 cases of spinal osteotomy and correction surgery were performed at the peripheral spine center and 30 surgical sites. A large number of young doctors who can use the thin-edged osteotome for spinal surgery have promoted the clinical application of osteotomy.

1.2.1 A Brief History of Spinal Osteotomy with Thin-Edged Osteotome

At the time of the first author, Tian, started the surgical clinical practice in 1950, patients with ankylosing spondylitis kyphosis or tuberculous kyphosis were always refused—because there was no good treatment method for their disease—as "Incurable disease," just launched outside the door. But deep in my heart I always feel unspeakable, can it be said that such obvious spinal deformity is not the object of treatment by our surgeons? Seeing the "incurable disease" as a shame of our surgeons, lurking in my heart until the late 1950s, prompted me to work on osteotomy to correct spinal deformities. First, I used pig bones or dog bones to experiment and found that the pig and dog bones were too hard and strong. Later, the experimental study of the thin scalpel on the fresh corpse confirmed that the osteotomy with the thin-edged osteotome can achieve free slicing, no vibration, and no resistance. At the same time, it can produce a neat cut surface, which is convenient for bone wax to control bleeding. In the late 1950s, many experimental studies and animal experiments were performed for the application of thin-edged osteotomes for spinal osteotomy, which laid a solid foundation for future clinical applications. In 1961, patients with ankylosing spondylitis kyphosis were treated with simple laminar osteotomy, which achieved remarkable results. Since then, the use of thin-edged bone cutters for lamina osteotomy begun. The technique at that time was similar to that of Smith Petersen's lamina osteotomy, but the surgical procedure was completely different from that of Smith Petersen. We used a sharp thin-edged osteotome to cut the lamina and without internal fixation. Postoperatively, the patient was placed on a flatbed until the kyphosis deformity is gradually corrected by body position, then an extension casting vest was given for 6–8 months until posterior bone graft and anterior interbody gap were proved as rigid fusion. Operation was performed on a total of 85 patients between 1961 and 1981. During the 30 years from 1981 to 2011, the curved kyphosis (ankylosing spondylitis, Scheuermann's disease), angular kyphosis (congenital kyphosis, tuberculous spine, Post-traumatic kyphosis), scoliosis, and kyphoscoliosis were successfully treated by various spinal osteotomies, including laminar osteotomy, laminar V-shaped osteotomy, transpedicular osteotomy, and spinal column osteotomy. In the 30 years, a total of 1820 cases of spinal osteotomy were performed in Tian's major spinal center, and 825 cases in the peripheral spine center, so a total of 2645 cases of spinal deformity underwent osteotomy and correction surgery. The number of spinal deformity cases treated by Tian was one of the worldwide largest data group.

During this period, the invention of the design of the Tian's Spine Osteotome was developed from Type I to Type VII. Type III Tian's Spine Osteotome (20 sets each) are produced by Tokyo Mizuho Co., Ltd. and are sold to countries all over the world. Type VI Tian's Spine Osteotome (10 sets each) has a simple subtype, low in price, and is sold well in China, all of which have obtained national patents.

During this period, as the editor-in-chief, Tian has published Monographs on spinal deformity and spinal osteotomy in Chinese People's Health Publishing House, People's Military Medical Publishing House, and several local Publishing House, respectively, such as: Spinal deformity Surgery, Spinal Deformity and Osteotomy, Therapeutics of Ankylosing Spondylitis, Practical Spinal Surgery, Practical Spinal operation Illustration, Key Points and Illustrations of Orthopedic Surgery, Cranio-Pelvic Traction Technique in Treatment of Spinal Deformity, Key Points and Illustrations of Cervical Spine Surgery, Cervical Spine Surgery Technology, Spine Deformity: Osteotomy and Correction, Spine Deformity Operation, Thoracic and Lumbar Spine Surgery Points and Illustrations, a total of 12 monographs. In addition, more than 30 papers on the treatment of spinal deformity by osteotomy and correction have been published in domestic and foreign, Chinese, English, and Japanese magazines. These achievements fill the gaps in spinal osteotomy at home and abroad.

Type VII Tian's Spine Osteotome has been redesigned on the basis of the former VI type and was released in 2013. Type VII Tian's Spine Osteotome has been carefully studied to make it more suitable for a posterior approach to bypass the dural sac and spinal nerve root for the need of anterior vertebral osteotomy. Further modifications have been made to the curvature and shape of the instrument. The number of osteotomes has increased to 23, making this device meet the needs of various surgical procedures in spinal surgery (Fig. 1.1).

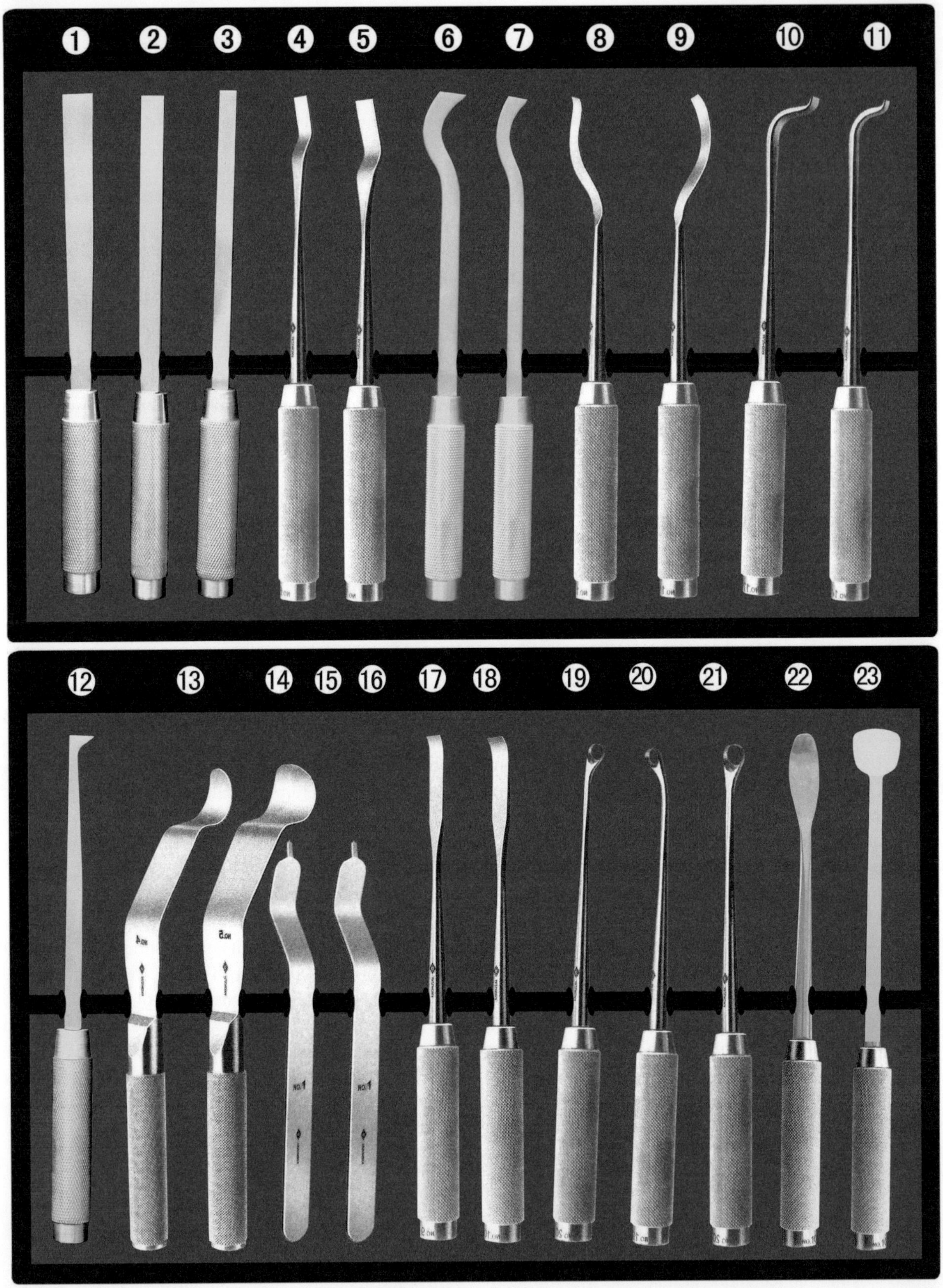

Fig. 1.1 Type VII Tian's spine osteotome set of 23: 1–3 straight osteotome (large, medium, and small); 4–5 blade osteotome (large and small); 6–7 crescent osteotome (large and small); 8–9 left/right curved osteotome; 10–11 push down osteotome (large, small); 12 oblique sharp osteotome; 13–14 seesaw osteotome (wide, narrow); 15–16 nerve root pull hook; 17–18 anonymous peeler (large, small); 19–21 hollow spatula (left, right, straight); 22 Tian's small stripper; 23 Tian's large stripper

1.2.2 The Support and Praise from Chinese Spinal Experts

The national spine surgery colleagues have a consensus on the work of Tian Huizhong to perform spinal osteotomy for spinal deformity correction in China. Tian Huizhong, a researcher at the Institute of Spinal Surgery in Xinjiang Uygur Autonomous Region, began the osteotomy surgery for ankylosing spondylitis kyphosis in 1961, which was the first case in China. During the 20 years from 1961 to 1981, 85 patients had achieved good results, and no one died. The osteotomy procedure was performed according to Smith Petersen's opening osteotomy method. However, the operation of Tian was completely different from that of Smith Petersen, on the tools used and detailed steps of osteotomy. Tian Huizhong used a thin-edged spine osteotome developed by himself to make a transverse or V-shaped regular osteotomy on the lamina, built the 8–12 mm osteotomy gap, and then compression force led the osteotomy gap closing, with the intervertebral space of the anterior border of the vertebral body opening. However, this method can only be used for ankylosing spondylitis kyphosis correction initially. Because the anterior longitudinal ligament and intervertebral disc of ankylosing spondylitis are weak due to the change of inflammation, and correction step can result in the opening of the anterior intervertebral space and the tearing of the anterior longitudinal ligament. As long as the case is properly selected, the operation is not difficult.

When the National Orthopaedic Conference was held in Datong, Shanxi Province in 1979, Professor Wu Zhikang was very interested in the surgical method of using the "Tian's spine osteotome" to bypass the dural tube and remove the vertebral body. After the meeting, Tian Huizhong was invited to perform surgery at the Beijing People's Liberation Army (301) Hospital. Professor Wu put forward many valuable opinions on the design of Tian's osteotomes, and then it changed from Type I "Tian's spine osteotome" to Type II. Under the guidance of Professor Wu, the treatment range of spinal osteotomy is from simple ankylosing spondylitis to spinal deformity caused by other reasons, such as congenital scoliosis and kyphoscoliosis, traumatic scoliosis, or kyphoscoliosis. In the development of spinal osteotomy, Professor Wu Zhikang has given a lot of help and inspiration (Fig. 1.2). Gradually, with improvement of the surgical tools and surgical methods, with expanding of the indication, "Tian's spine osteotome" has transitioned from type I to type VII. Thanks to Professor Wu for his unforgettable and helpful spirit. Professor Wu held Tian's hand before he died: "You must carry forward the work of spinal osteotomy for the treatment of spinal deformity!" Professor Wu has done his utmost to promote the development of spinal surgery in China. He dedicated to raising the popularity of hospitals that can perform spinal surgery in the whole country to the international level. This was his lifelong wish and our goals that have been pursued.

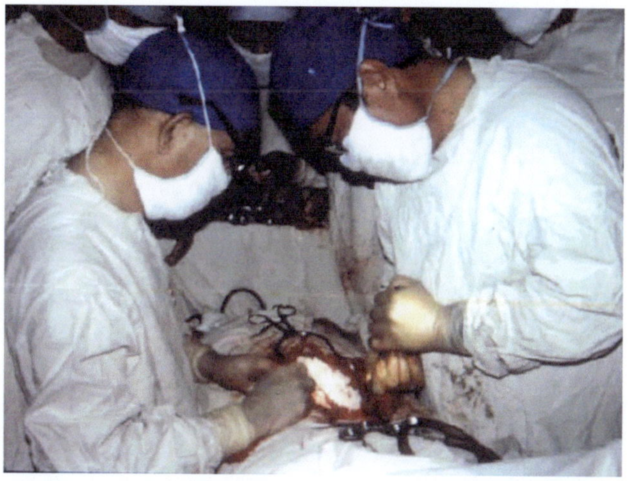

Fig. 1.2 Professor Wu Zhikang (left) and Professor Tian Huizhong (right) on the operation for scoliosis correction

1.3 Surgical Skills and Qualities of Spine Surgeons

Spinal surgery is full of difficulty and risk, especially for spinal osteotomy procedures. It can cause hemorrhagic shock due to large blood loss during surgery, or it can cause lifelong paralysis or nerve damage due to damage to the spinal cord and nerve roots. The incidence of early or late postoperative complications is high, making it difficult for doctors to completely eliminate them. Experienced doctors can only prevent the occurrence of serious complications, detect complications early, and make response early. The common reasons for the mistakes are: (1) improper clinical thinking methods; (2) lack of professional knowledge; and (3) improper surgical methods and poor surgical skills. Firstly, surgeons who only understand the surgical methods and procedures do not have the qualifications to perform the operation independently. They must have a pure anatomical concept and biomechanical point of view. It is also necessary to have all aspects of the whole process of surgical treatment and prevent accidents and rescue measures in order to complete the task of spinal osteotomy independently. Doctors doing spinal osteotomy should deal with the anatomical knowledge of the spine and spinal cord and form a clear concept in the brain. In any anatomical abnormality or deformity, the position can be correctly judged and recognized without losing direction. Secondly, the selection and use of the osteotomy tools should be applied clinically after training on the corpse or in the animal laboratory to achieve mastery. Both rongeur and grinding are not a substitute for Osteotomes. Osteotomy with an osteotome is the basic skill of an orthopedic surgeon. The spine surgeon should learn to use the thin-edged spine osteotome to perform osteotomy on the spine while keeping the spinal cord and nerve roots intact. This is the real basic surgery skill. Spine surgeons should study the fine craftsmanship of the old artists and sculptors, who familied in China. They can engrave the spirit of "Eight Immortals Crossing the Sea" on a peach core, using different curvatures and different shapes of bone knives. Performing spinal osteotomy by osteotomes, developing China's traditional advantages, can be regarded as Chinese's own distinctive features. On the other hand, there were many surgical techniques and various kinds of spinal internal fixation devices imported from abroad. If they have not been absorbed or deeply understood by spine surgeons on their own, they may not be necessarily safe and reliable for use on the patients.

Professor Rao Shucheng pointed out: We must recognize the advantages and disadvantages of various methods, we must not emphasize that a certain method is absolutely good. In addition to constantly reading books and magazines, we must be good at summing up experience, including our own and others' experiences and lessons, especially from failure cases. The knowledge that benefits our life is summed up. Even if you have a very successful operation, you should be good at summing up the shortcomings, and try to find a place that should be improved, and strive for excellence. For new operations, the initial surgery can be successful after sufficient preparation; most of the problems occur when two or three similar operations are performed. Therefore, facing some difficult and dangerous operations, the surgeon should not simply rely on self-courage or a rough understanding to perform operation, but should reach the depth of grasping various surgical rules. An increasingly mature doctor will inevitably correct some of his views and understandings in his lifetime of medical practice, thus enriching himself and constantly improving.

Basic knowledge that spine surgeons must have: (1) comprehensive knowledge of orthopedics; (2) comprehensive knowledge of the general theory of surgery; (3) all subdisciplines of surgery, especially the knowledge of craniocerebral, chest and abdomen, urinary damage; (4) detailed anatomical knowledge of spinal surgery, and related biomechanical knowledge and clinical pathology knowledge; (5) spine surgery, clinical examination and diagnostic knowledge; and (6) the proposed treatment, the evolution of the procedure and the instruments used, the design and biomechanical principles, the application methods, and possible complications.

Suggested Reading

1. Tian H. Application of "Tian's spinal bone knife" in orthopaedic surgery. Chinese Journal of Orthopaedics. 2003;11(15):1073–5.
2. Tian H. Spinal surgeons should be good at using rongeurs and osteotome. Chinese Journal of Modern Operative Surgery. 2002;6(1):67–8.
3. Tian H. Surgical treatment of kyphosis kyphosis. Chinese Journal of Orthopaedics. 1992;12(3):162–5.
4. Tian H, Tian Y, Xiang Z, Tian S. Posterior invasion and vertebral osteotomy. Spinal Deformation. 1992;7(1):4–11.
5. Tian H, Li F. Spinal deformity and osteotomy. Xi'an: World Book Publishing Company; 2001. p. 662–734.
6. Tian H, Lin Q, Tan Y. Therapeutics of ankylosing spondylitis. Guangzhou: World Book Publishing Company; 2005. p. 1–415.
7. Tian H, Li M, Ma Y. Spinal deformity osteotomy orthopedics, vol. 5. Beijing: People's Medical Publishing House; 2011. p. 3–339.
8. Tian H. A brief history and popularization of spinal osteotomy with thin blade bone knife. Chinese Journal of Orthopaedics. 2012;20(23):2207–8.
9. Tian H. History of treatment of spinal deformity in China. Chinese Journal of Orthopaedics. 2009;17(9):706–7.
10. Tian H, Zhang H, Liang Y. Surgical treatment of spinal deformity. Guangzhou: Guangdong Science and Technology Press; 2012. p. 1–19.
11. Tian H, Wang B, Lv X, et al. Correction and fixation of ankylosing kyphosis and osteotomy. Chinese Journal of Orthopaedics. 2005;13(7):509–12.
12. Tian H, Liu S, Ma Y. Practical spine surgery illustration. Beijing: People's Military Medical Press; 2008. p. 1–450.
13. Tian H, Lv X, Tian B. Correction of osteotomy of cervical and thoracic kyphosis with ankylosing spondylitis. Chinese Journal of Orthopaedics. 2006;14(7):522–3.
14. Tian H, Ma Y, Lv X. Minimally invasive V-shaped osteotomy for correction of ankylosing kyphosis. Chinese Journal of Orthopaedics. 2008;16(5):349–52.
15. Tian H, Liu S, Ma Y. Practical Spine Surgery. Guangzhou: Guangdong Science and Technology Press; 2008. p. 1–459.
16. Tian H, Li M, Wang Z. Key points and diagrams of thoracolumbar surgery. Beijing: People's Medical Publishing House; 2012. p. 3–374.
17. Tian H, Li M. Ankylosing spondylitis spinal deformity osteotomy and orthopedic surgery skills. Beijing: People's Medical Publishing House; 2014. p. 1–28.
18. Tian H, Lv X, Ma Y. Treatment of severe spinal curvature with total spine osteotomy and internal fixation with head-sleeve ring. Chinese Journal of Orthopaedics. 2007;15(3):167–72.
19. Tian H. Tuberculous kyphosis osteotomy orthopedic surgery. Chinese Journal of Orthopaedics. 2011;19(23):1937–40.
20. Tian H, Alken AD, Du P, et al. Posterior hemiverteectomy for congenital horny kyphosis. Chinese Journal of Orthopaedics. 2010;18(15):1250–1253.
21. Tian H, Alken AD, Ma Y. Prophylactic osteotomy for the treatment of congenital lateral paravertebral vertebral body. Chinese Journal of Orthopaedics. 2011;19(07):541–544.
22. Tian H, Liang Y, Ma Y, et al. Treatment of ossification of thoracic ligamentum flavum with total osteotomy and decompression with Tian's bone knife. Chinese Journal of Orthopaedics. 2010;18(20):1693–6.
23. Tian H. Report of 25 cases of traumatic paraplegia treated with posterior spinal decompression by posterior approach. Chinese Journal of Orthopaedics. 2006;07:549–50.
24. Tian H, Ma Y, Jie J. Spinal osteotomy orthopedics. Guangzhou: Guangdong Science and Technology Press; 2018. p. 2–8.

2 Application of Tian's Spinal Osteotomes

Huizhong Tian, Yuan Ma, and Xia Lv

2.1 Overview

Spinal osteotomy is also the same as limb osteotomy. It is necessary to use an osteotome to make a wedge osteotomy, and then close the wedge gap to correct the deformity, so that the spine can achieve normal alignment. But the difference is that the spinal canal contains the spinal cord, and on both sides, there are spinal nerve roots from the intervertebral foramen. This makes it extremely difficult for 3-column osteotomy, so it is not like a limb with straight osteotomes. However, the status of spinal osteotomy in the correction of spinal deformity is increasingly valued by surgeons, especially in the whole spinal osteotomy correction of angular kyphosis such as congenital or tuberculous, it is difficult to achieve correction without special equipment.

"Tian's Spinal Osteotomes" was invented in orthopedics and spine surgery for more than 60 years. It was invented according to the need for osteotomy to bypass the spinal canal and gradually reform the shape and curvature of the osteotomes. From type I, type II, type III (Fig. 2.1) to Type VII, a set of spinal surgery tools has been developed.

The author has gained more than 50 years of experience in spinal surgery with spinal osteotomies and believes that the vertebral arch and vertebral body composed of cancellous bone and cortical bone can be removed with sharp thin blade spinal osteotomes, and the resistance is very small, which is not likely to cause spinal cord injury due to concussion. But the conditions of using spinal osteotomes are: (1) must be sharp thin spinal osteotomes; (2) must be stable spine or the spine under cranial pelvic traction; (3) the surgeon has a clear concept of the anatomy of the spine; and (4) the surgeon has excellent surgical skills. The first two are essential, while the second two are based on an in-depth understanding of spinal anatomy and animal model training, combined with clinical experience and surgical skills to achieve mastery. It is more convenient and faster to perform osteotomy or decompression surgery on the spine with spinal osteotomes, and it is less likely to damage the spinal cord and nerve roots than simply using bone rongeur or electric and pneumatic drills. Due to the tight contact between the compressed spinal cord and bone protrusions, when forced insertion with bone rongeur, due to the thickness of bone rongeur mouth occupied, there is the possibility of spinal cord injury. The bone was laminated from the outside to the inside with a bone knife until the thin layer of bone near the dural canal was removed. Then the bone was pushed out with a pushing knife and a removal forceps, so as to avoid the risk of squeezing the spinal cord with the mouth of the rongeur. Drilling is a method like ants gnawing at a bone, and it is a waste of time and is not as fast and reliable as spinal osteotomies. If it is used for thoracolumbar deformities, the removal of a large amount of bone tissue is required.

"Tian's spine osteotomes" has opened a new page in the development of spine osteotomy: since 1945 when Smith-Peterson adopted the treatment method of spinal osteotomy for kyphosis caused by ankylosing spondylitis, for a long period of time, full laminectomy was referred to as spinal osteotomy, which was only limited to the correction of ankylosing kyphosis. Later, staging anterior and posterior osteotomy was used to correct spinal deformity, but posterior approach total spinal osteotomy, which involves spinal arch and vertebral body, has not been reported. The main reason is that the center of the spine contains the spinal cord and nerve. Therefore, the circular osteotomy of the whole spine is regarded as the biggest problem. Since 1945, nearly half a century, spinal osteotomy is only within the scope of simple laminectomy, vertebral arch vertebral body subtotal osteotomy, and staging anterior and posterior osteotomy, and its treatment is mostly limited to the kyphosis caused by ankylosing spondylitis. In contrast, angular kyphosis, such as congenital and tuberculous angular kyphosis, requires full spinal circular osteotomy and wedge resection to resolve the

H. Tian · Y. Ma · X. Lv (✉)
The Sixth Affiliated Hospital of Xinjiang Medical University, Urumqi, China

H. Tian et al. (eds.), *Spinal Osteotomy Orthopaedics*, https://doi.org/10.1007/978-981-16-1387-6_2

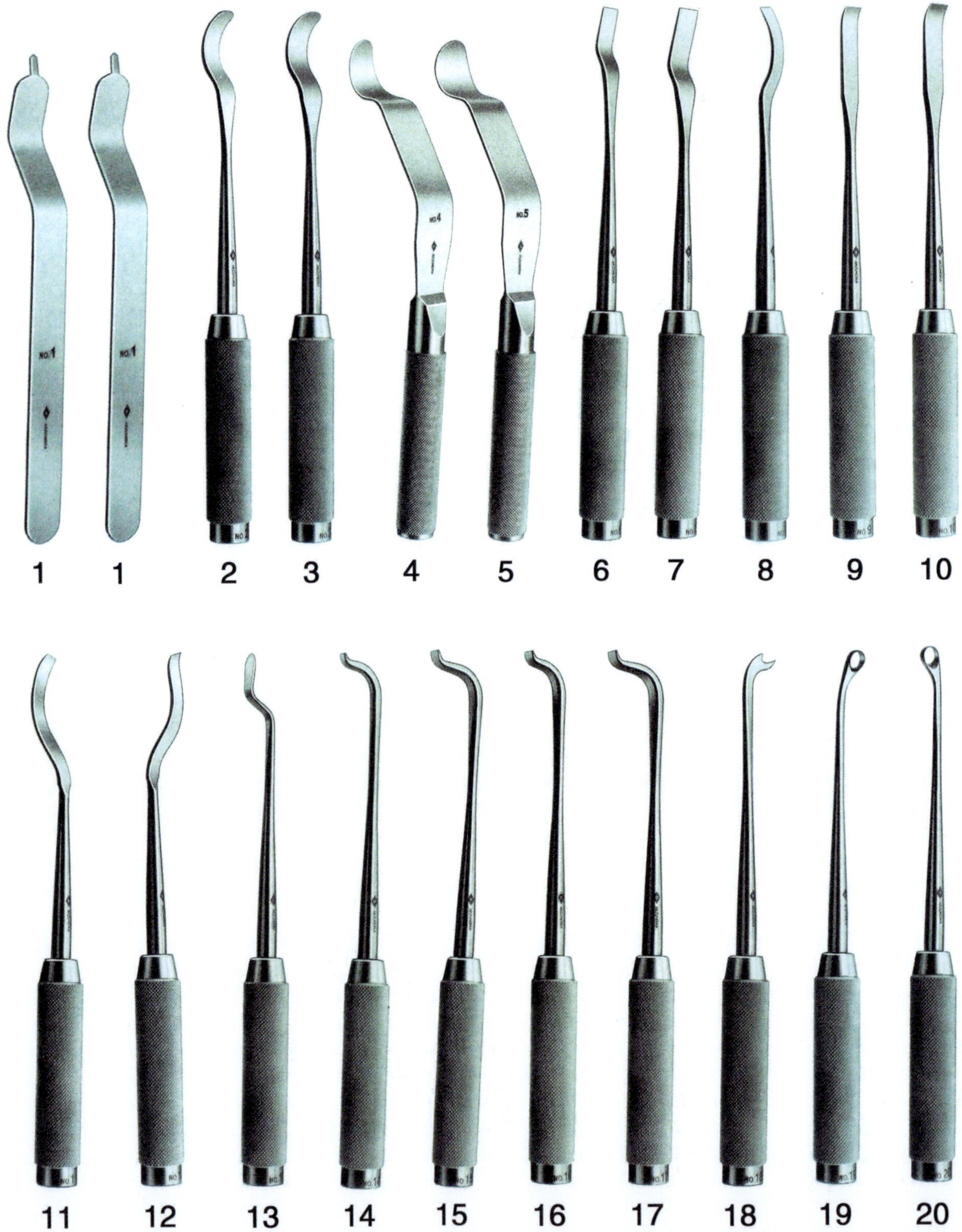

Fig. 2.1 Type III Tian's spinal osteotomes: 1. Nerve root retractors; 2–3. Vertebral dissectors; 4–5. Lever plates; 6–7. Shovel osteotomes; 8. Crescent osteotome; 9–10. Anonymous strippers; 11–12. Left and right osteotomes; 13. Posterior longitudinal ligament stripper; 14–17. Push osteotomes; 18. Posterior edge of vertebral body osteotome; 19–20. Hollow scraper spoons

problem. This is the biggest problem in osteotomy today, and the Tian's spine osteotomes were designed to solve this problem. The various shapes of the osteotomes (Fig. 2.2) were used to achieve circular osteotomy and wedge resection around the dural tube to correct spinal deformity. The author has used this set of osteotomes to perform a total spinal

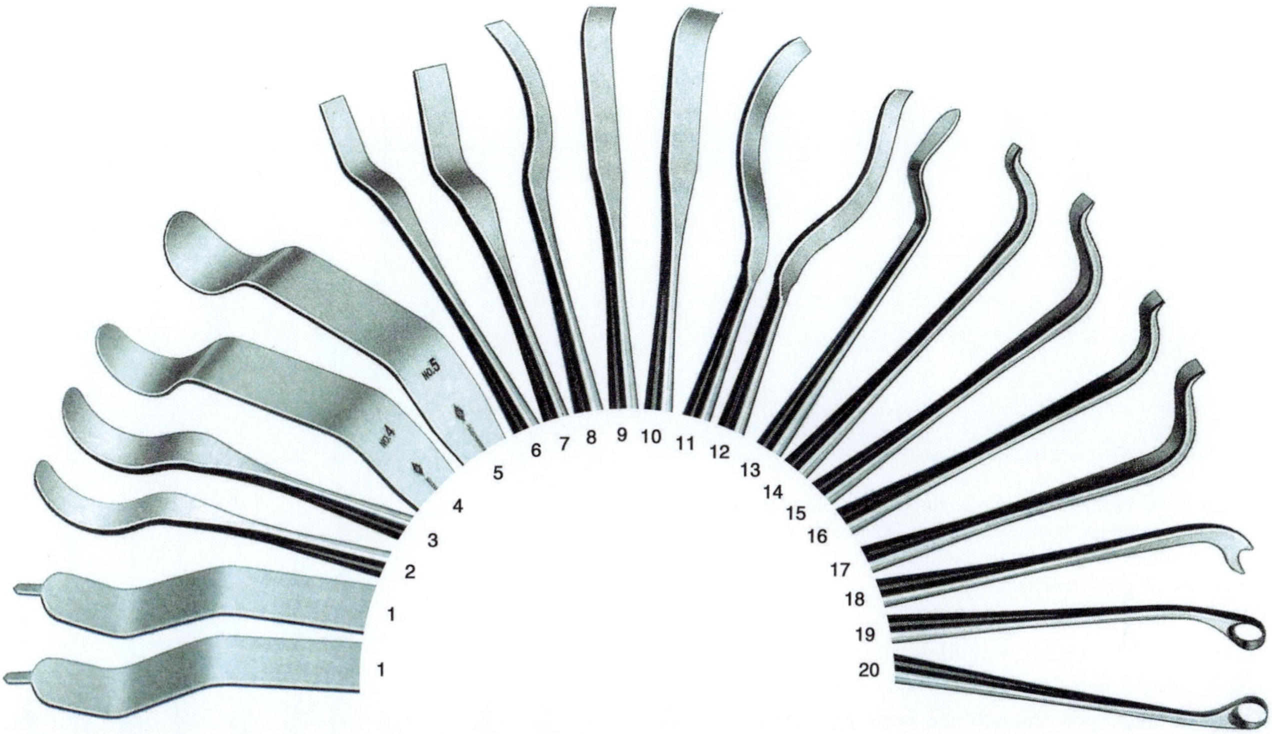

Fig. 2.2 Type III Tian's spinal osteotomes: The vertebral body was resected bypass the Spinal dural, and combined vertebral arch osteotomy was performed by using its different degrees of curvature, so as to avoid the phenomenon of extruding, touching, or abrasion of the spinal cord by surgical instruments. This is the greatest advantage of Tian's spinal osteotomes for the total vertebral column resection

circular osteotomy and wedge resection (cutting the width of the wedge base 3 ~ 6 cm) plus instrument correction for 255 patients. The correction rate of spinal curvature deformity reached 70.32%, and none of the 255 cases suffered paraplegia or incomplete paraplegia due to surgery. Takahiro Kurokawa, Masahiro Harada, Masahiro Takenaka, Bingzhong Liang, and Roy Camille all appreciated this approach. Mizuho Corporation of Japan purchased the type III spine osteotomes for preparing for the operation. It is agreed that by means of "Tian's spine osteotomes" to treat spinal deformity has opened a new page for spinal osteotomy.

Tian's spine osteotomes were designed and invented by Professor Tian Huizhong. The Tian's spine osteotomes were presented to the national orthopedic fellows at the first National Orthopaedic Trauma Conference held in Datong, Shanxi Province in 1979. During the meeting, Tian's spine osteotomes were praised by well-known experts such as Ye Yanqing, Feng Chuanhan, Shang Tianyu, and Wu Zhikang. After the meeting, Professor Wu Zhikang invited Professor Tian Huizhong to the Beijing 301 Hospital to perform the application of Tian's spine osteotomes. Under the guidance of Professor Wu Zhikang, Tian's spine osteotomes were developed from type I to type II. After long-term clinical application of osteotomes domestically till 1990, it was finally accepted by the world's orthopedic colleagues at the Hong Kong International Orthopaedic Conference. In particular, Professor Takasu Kurokawa from the medical department of the University of Tokyo, Japan, personally led a surgical team with five members to the sixth affiliated hospital of Xinjiang Medical University, on December 28, 1990, to visit and learn the clinical application of Tian's spine osteotomy. From then on, Tian Huizhong was invited as a visiting research fellow to the University of Tokyo, Japan. From 1991 to 1995, he went to the Tokyo University twice a year to perform operations for doctors and postdocs (specially approved by the Ministry of Foreign Affairs of Japan). Tokyo Mizuho Co, Ltd manufactured Type III Tian's spine osteotomes in Japan and the osteotomes are not only sold in Japan but also available throughout Asia, in the USA, and European markets. Type VI Tian's spine osteotomes sold well in China because they are simple, with 10 sets of each, and the price is low.

"Type VI Tian's spine osteotomes" (Fig. 2.3) is further modified on the basis of the original one, which is the original 20 sets of instrument decreased to the 10 sets; thus, it is easy to carry. In addition to the full spine osteotomy, it needs to be compatible with the type III osteotome, which is suitable for various common operations in spinal surgery, such as: interlaminar fenestration in lumbar disc surgery; total laminectomy for semi-laminectomy; enlargement of the spinal canal and root canal stenosis; fenestration exposure from posterior interbody fusion or Cage surgery; V-shaped osteotomy for kyphosis; apical resection of scoliosis; congenital

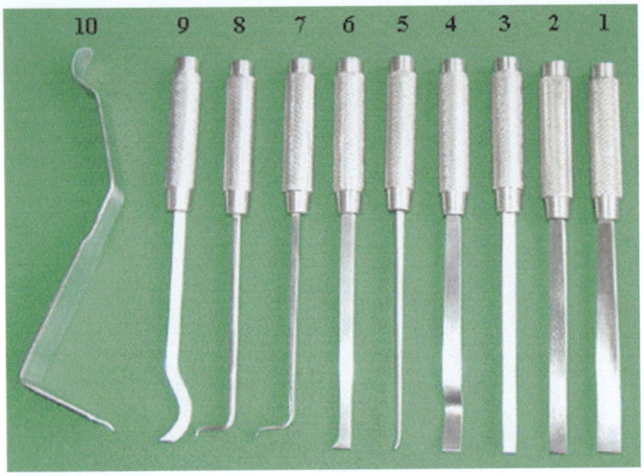

Fig. 2.3 Type VI Tian's spinal osteotomes: 1–3. Straight osteotomes; 4. Shovel osteotomes; 5. Anonymous; 6. Oblique tip osteotome; 7–8. Push osteotomes; 9. Crescent osteotomes; 10. Lever plates and single side exposed dual-purpose retractor

hemivertebra resection in children; total spinal osteotomy with kyphosis; anterior vertebral body margin resection for thoracolumbar burst fracture and bone grafting or Kaneda surgery; cervical anterior bone grafting, etc. This set of instruments can be used successfully to complete the whole process of surgery, in order to save the operation time and avoid the occurrence of squeezing nerve roots or wire drawing when the vertebral plate is removed with a rongeur.

With more than 50 years of clinical application, the Tian's spine osteotomes have been evolved from type I to type VI and have been gradually improved and perfected. Due to the increased number of users, we have further updated and improved the design of the new type VII Tian's spine osteotomes on the basis of the former VI type to meet the demands of the spine surgery colleagues.

There are 23 osteotomes in type VII Tian's spine osteotomes. They are three straight osteotomes (large, medium, and small); two shovel osteotomes (large and small); two crescent osteotomes (large and small); left and right osteotomes; two push osteotomes (large and small); one oblique tip osteotome; two Lever plates (wide and narrow); two nerve root retractors; two anonymous strippers; tree hollow scraper spoons (left, right and straight); and two Tian's stripper (small and big) (Fig. 2.4).

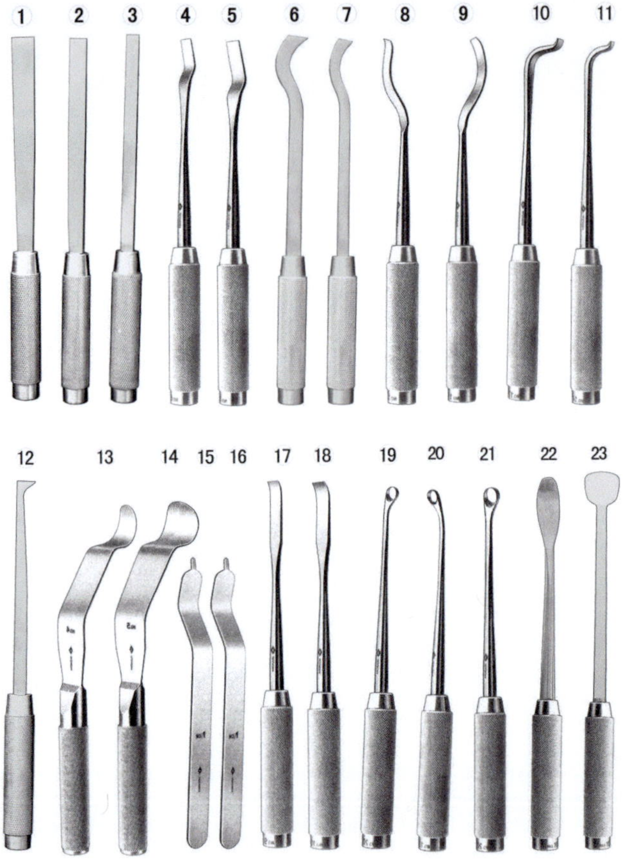

Fig. 2.4 Type VII Tian's spinal osteotomes: A set of Type VII Tian's spinal osteotomes

2.2 Surgical Indications for Type VII Tian's Spine Osteotomes

1. Ankylosing spondylitis kyphosis osteotomy
2. Tuberculous angular kyphosis osteotomy
3. Traumatic kyphosis osteotomy
4. Idiopathic scoliosis osteotomy
5. Congenital scoliosis osteotomy
6. Adolescent kyphosis and multiple intersegmental osteotomy
7. Thoracic spine, ossification of flavum ligament
8. Semi-laminectomy for decompression and lumbar spinal canal enlargement
9. Thoracic discectomy
10. Lumbar discectomy
11. Artificial lumbar disc replacement
12. Internal fixation of spondylolysis of vertebral arch without spondylolisthesis
13. Thoracic posterior longitudinal ligament ossification
14. Thoracolumbar burst fracture, anterior surgery
15. Congenital hemivertebra resection
16. Spinal tuberculosis or spinal tumor decompression and bone graft
17. Tuberculous kyphosis osteotomy
18. All kinds of thoracolumbar anterior and posterior approaches are adapted to use the Tian's spine osteotomes.
19. Various cervical vertebrae surgery can occasionally be done with the Tian's spine osteotomes, but the Tian's spine osteotomes are mainly applied to the thoracolumbar spine.

2.3 Usage of Type VII Tian's Spine Osteotomes

The "Type VII Tian's spine osteotomes" (Fig. 2.5) has been further improved in curvature and shape, and the number of pieces has changed from 20 to 23. With such a set of instruments, various osteotomy procedures can be performed without the need for other instruments. In addition to the anterior and posterior operations of the thoracolumbar spine and lumbosacral spine, the bone grafting of the cervical vertebrae can also be used in conjunction with other instruments. Therefore, type VII Tian's spine osteotomes are widely used in spinal surgery. Examples are given to illustrate the application of each device as follows:

NO. 1–3 Straight osteotomes (large, medium, and small): They are mainly used for osteotomy and grooving on the lamina or vertebral body, resection of the lamina or vertebral body exposure, decompression of dural canal and spinal nerve root, especially in the removal of the pedicle and the lateral part of the vertebral body, it is an indispensable and advantageous tool. The straight osteotomes are divided into three: large, medium, and small ones, and large straight osteotomes are used to perform V-shaped or transverse osteotomy on the lamina, or complete laminectomy of thoracic and lumbar vertebrae. The middle straight osteotomes are used for hemilaminectomy and transversectomy. Small straight osteotomes are used in minimally invasive discectomy, vertebral posterior margin osteophyte resection, cervical posterior nerve root decompression, etc. (Fig. 2.6a–d).

NO. 4–5 Shovel osteotomes (large and small): They are used for lamina and vertebral body resection and clear the bottom and planning the groove, especially suitable for cervical vertebral body or thoracolumbar vertebral body central part resection, combined with crescent osteotomes to complete the central part of the vertebral body resection (Fig. 2.7a–d).

NO. 6–7 Crescent osteotomes (large and small): They are divided into two sizes, mainly used for the resection of the central part of the vertebral body, and the combination of shovel osteotomes as a favorable tool for the resection of the vertebral body. It can be used for ASK anteriorly vertebral ossification resection (Fig. 2.8a–c).

NO. 8–9 Left and right osteotomes (left and right): They are used for intervertebral bone grafting via posterior approach, planing grooves on the vertebral body, spinal tuberculosis or tumor to remove vertebral lesions and using its curvature to bypass the dural canal for vertebral body resection (Fig. 2.9a, b).

NO. 10–11 Push osteotomes (large and small): They are used to push the thin layer of bone slices close to the dural canal from the inside without damaging the spinal cord, such as pushing temporarily retained posterior vertebral margin to avoid bleeding from the pre-dural venous plexus. For a burst fracture of the thoracolumbar segment, push down the broken bone fragments at the posterior margin of the vertebral body which protruding into the vertebral canal (Fig. 2.10a–e).

NO. 12 Oblique tip osteotome: Tt is used for discectomy, incision of the annulus fibrosus on the intervertebral space to remove the intervertebral disc, and osteophytes in the posterior margin of the vertebral body can also be removed. It is used for removing the posterior margin of the vertebral body in total spine osteotomy. Its special role is to bypass the dural tube to remove the pre-dural bone tissue or intervertebral disc (Fig. 2.11a, b).

NO. 13–14 Lever plates (wide and narrow): They are used to pry open the anterior longitudinal ligament and the paravertebral soft tissue, and to block the segmental arteries and veins across the lumbar vertebra, so as to avoid the complicated work of ligating the segmental vessels. When the whole vertebral body resection is performed, the entire vertebral body can be fully exposed (Fig. 2.12a–c).

NO. 15–16 Nerve root retractor: When vertebral body osteotomy is performed, the nerve roots through the upper and lower intervertebral foramen are pulled away, and the tip of the retractor is inserted into the vertebral body bone to prevent sliding, so as to block the spinal nerve roots and fully expose the vertebral body (Fig. 2.13a, b).

NO. 17–18 Anonymous strippers (large and small): It is very advantageous for the subperiosteal peeling exposure; especially when the rib head is removed, it is very advantageous to peel off the rib joint. It is also a useful tool to expose the pedicle and lumbar vertebra by anterior pedicle dissection along the lateral side of the pedicle (Fig. 2.14a–d).

NO. 19–21 Hollow scraper spoons (left, right and straight): It is a favorable tool for interbody fusion. It is very convenient and quick to scrape the intervertebral disc and nucleus pulposus. The left and right are used to scrape the nucleus pulposus on both sides. The straight scraper spoons are used to scrape most of the nucleus pulposus in the center of the vertebral body (Fig. 2.15a–c).

NO. 22–23 Anonymous strippers (large and small): It is specially used to peel off the segmental blood vessels of the vertebral body to ensure that the segment is strictly removed from the subperiosteum without damaging the segmental vessels. The segmental vessels are completely blocked outside the surgical field and then blocked by the action of the lever plates to achieve the purpose of not ligating the segmental blood vessels (Fig. 2.16a–g).

2.4 Essentials and Notes

1. Type VII Tian's spine osteotomes have been clinically applied for more than 50 years. Based on the former type VI, it has been further improved and upgraded. It is the most suitable instrument for 3-column osteotomy by

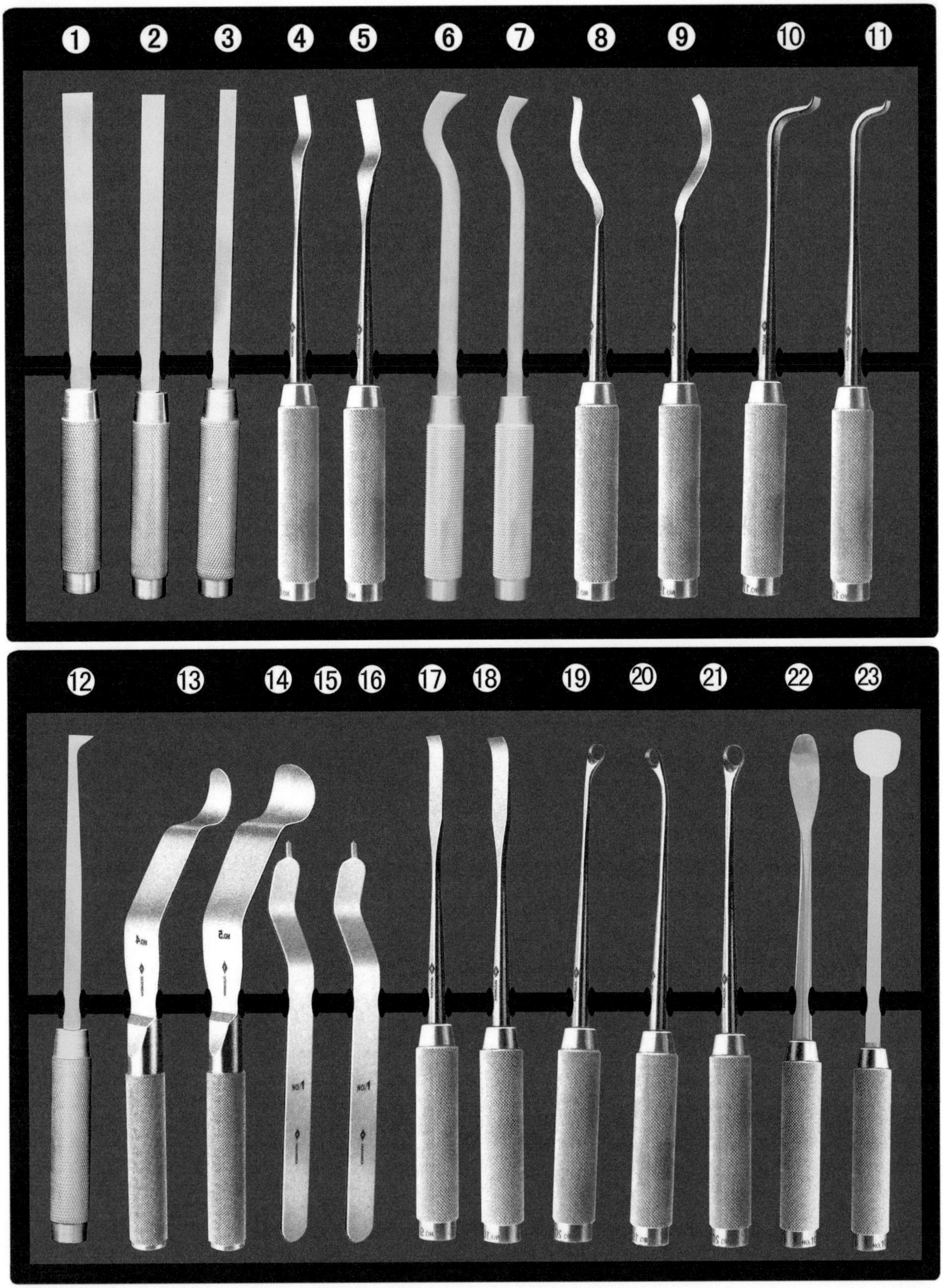

Fig. 2.5 Type VII Tian's spinal osteotomes 1–3. Straight osteotomes; 4–5. shovel osteotomes; 6–7. Crescent osteotomes; 8–9. Left and right osteotomes; 10–11. Push osteotomes; 12. Oblique tip osteotome; 13–14. Lever plates; 15–16. Nerve root retractors; 17–18. Anonymous strippers; 19–21. Hollow scraper spoons; 22. Tian's small stripper; 23. Tian's big stripper

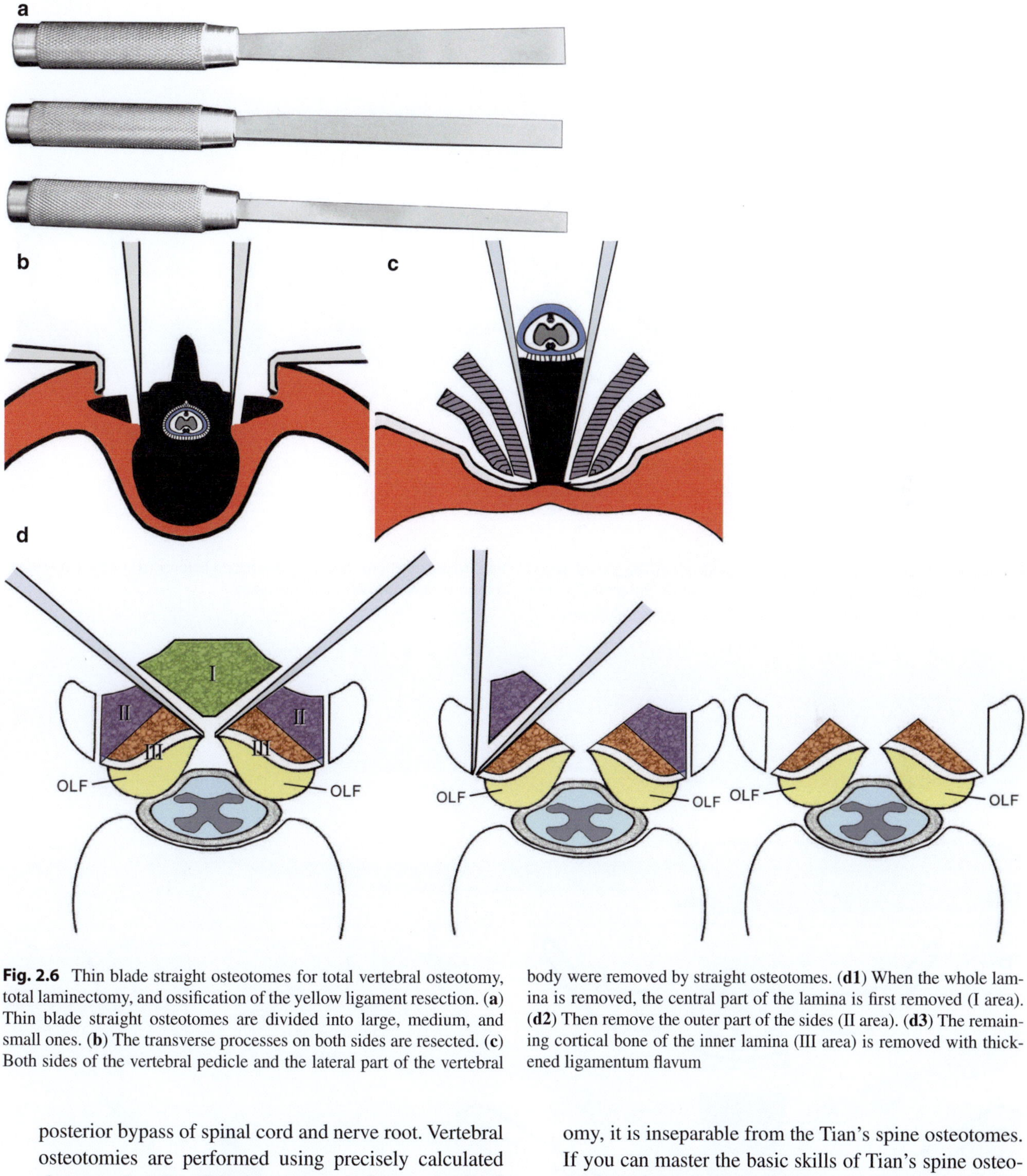

Fig. 2.6 Thin blade straight osteotomes for total vertebral osteotomy, total laminectomy, and ossification of the yellow ligament resection. (**a**) Thin blade straight osteotomes are divided into large, medium, and small ones. (**b**) The transverse processes on both sides are resected. (**c**) Both sides of the vertebral pedicle and the lateral part of the vertebral body were removed by straight osteotomes. (**d1**) When the whole lamina is removed, the central part of the lamina is first removed (I area). (**d2**) Then remove the outer part of the sides (II area). (**d3**) The remaining cortical bone of the inner lamina (III area) is removed with thickened ligamentum flavum

posterior bypass of spinal cord and nerve root. Vertebral osteotomies are performed using precisely calculated shapes and angles of the instruments to bypass the dural canal and spinal nerve roots, replacing the anterior and posterior approaches. It is truly minimally invasive and innovative to change two-stage operation into a one-stage operation.

2. There are a total of 23 Tian's spine osteotomes, which can be used for various surgeries in the field of spinal surgery. From lumbar discectomy to total spinal osteotomy, it is inseparable from the Tian's spine osteotomes. If you can master the basic skills of Tian's spine osteotomes and the surgical techniques of osteotomy, you can greatly expand your treatment range in spinal surgery and turn what you once considered a difficult case into a treatable one.
3. The application of the spine osteotome is a kind of craftwork. It is similar to the old artist who can engrave the "Eight Immortals" on the peach core. It belongs to the same nature. This is the specialty of our Chinese people.

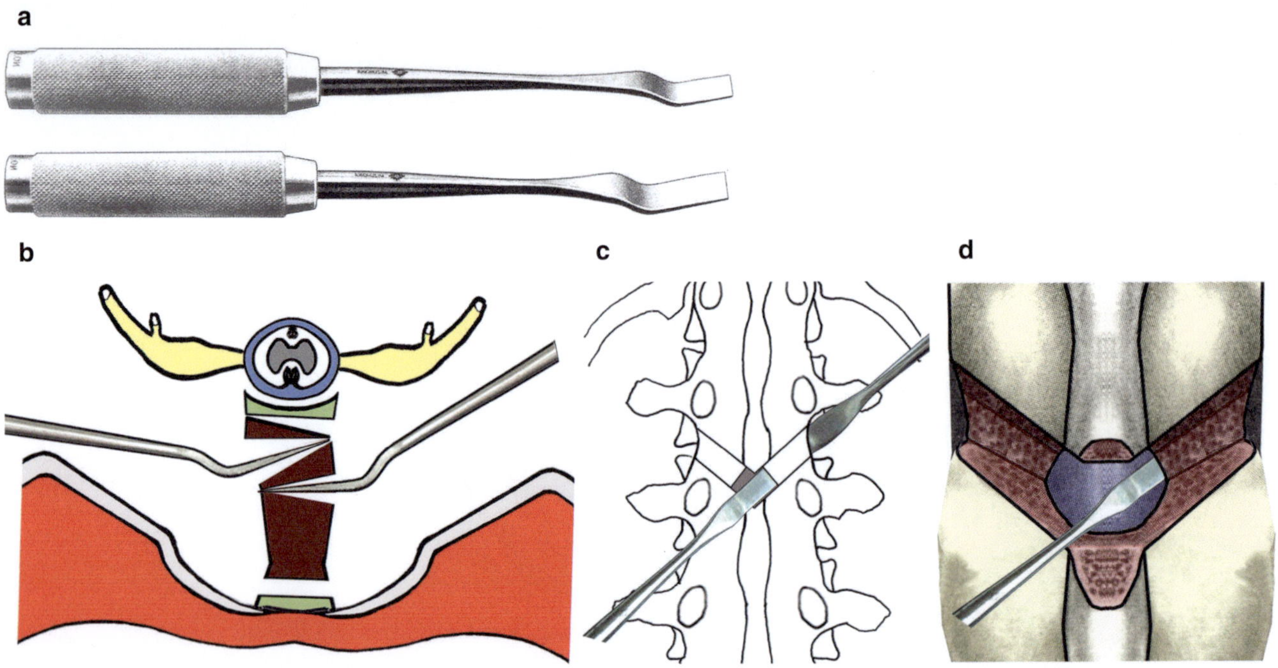

Fig. 2.7 Different uses of the shovel osteotomes. (**a**) The shovel osteotomes are divided into two sizes. (**b**) Used to remove the central part of the vertebra. (**c**) In a V-shaped lamina osteotomy, shovel osteotomes are used to remove both ends of the V-shaped lamina. (**d**) Use shovel osteotomes to clean the bottom of the plane

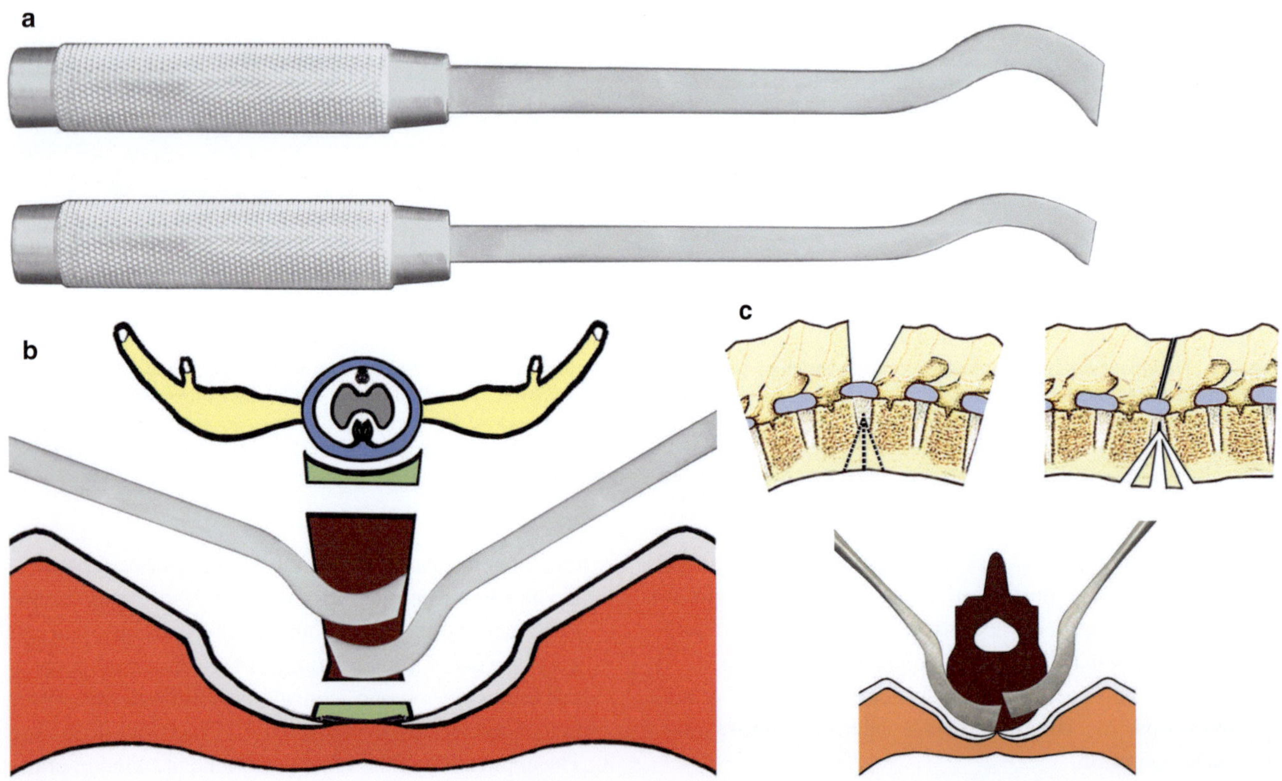

Fig. 2.8 Crescent osteotomes are used to remove the central portion of the vertebra, often in conjunction with shovel osteotomes. (**a**) Crescent osteotomes are divided into two sizes, (**b**) Used to remove the central part of the vertebra, (**c**) When the reduction is difficult after ASK laminectomy, the crescent osteotomes can be used to bypass the vertebral arch through the posterior approach and resect the anterior 1/3 of the vertebral body

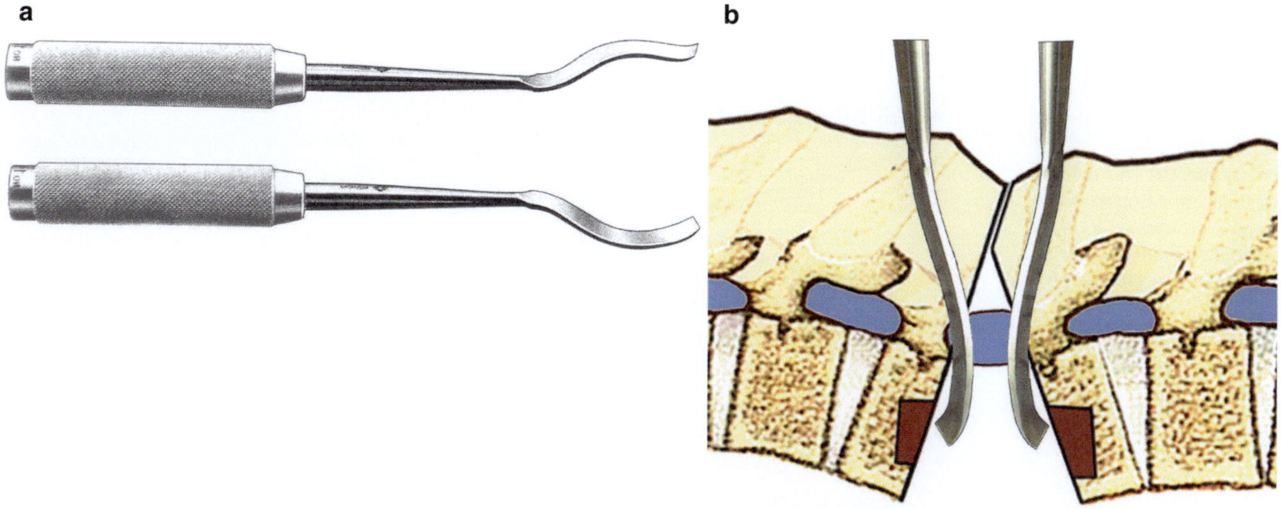

Fig. 2.9 By using its curved shape to bypass the vertebral canal, it is convenient and quick to gouge bone grafting on the vertebral body at the cranial end and the caudal end. (**a**) Left and right osteotomes, (**b**) Application of left and right osteotomes

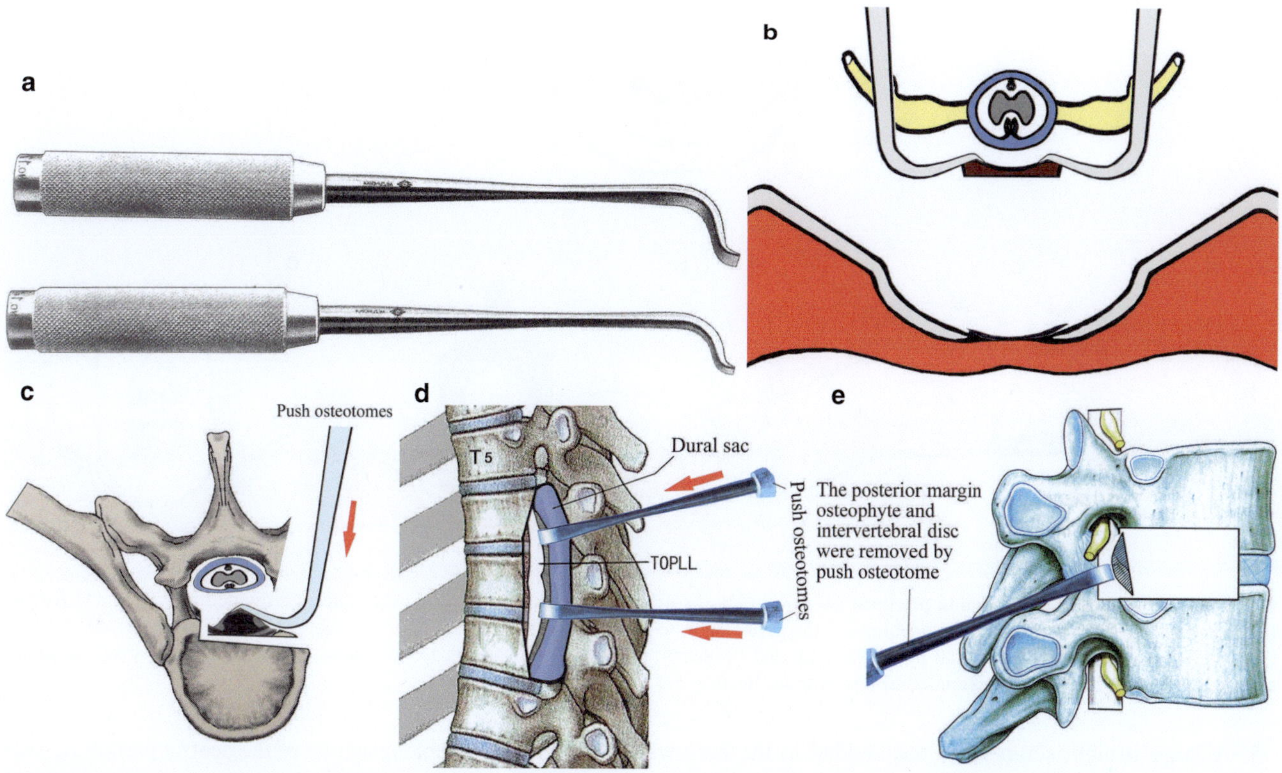

Fig. 2.10 Different applications of Push osteotomes. (**a**) Push osteotomes are divided into two sizes. (**b**) The push osteotomes toppled the temporarily retained thin layer of the posterior margin of the vertebral body. (**c**) The posterior longitudinal ligament was torn down and excised by using Push osteotomes in ossification of the posterior longitudinal ligament of the thoracic spine. (**d**) The posterior longitudinal ligament was torn down and excised on the lateral view. (**e**) The posterior margin osteophyte and intervertebral disc were removed

Only those who have the heart can learn and understand the real basic skills through hard training and real comprehension. Anatomical concepts and operational skills must form indelible concepts in your mind.

4. According to the width of osteotomy required for vertebral ossification in ankylosing spondylitis, the crescent osteotomes were widened the width and the arc again, making it more in line with the width and shape required for cutting the anterior margin of the vertebral body through the posterior approach. It makes the effect of anterior opening and posterior closure more reliable after anterior margin cutting.

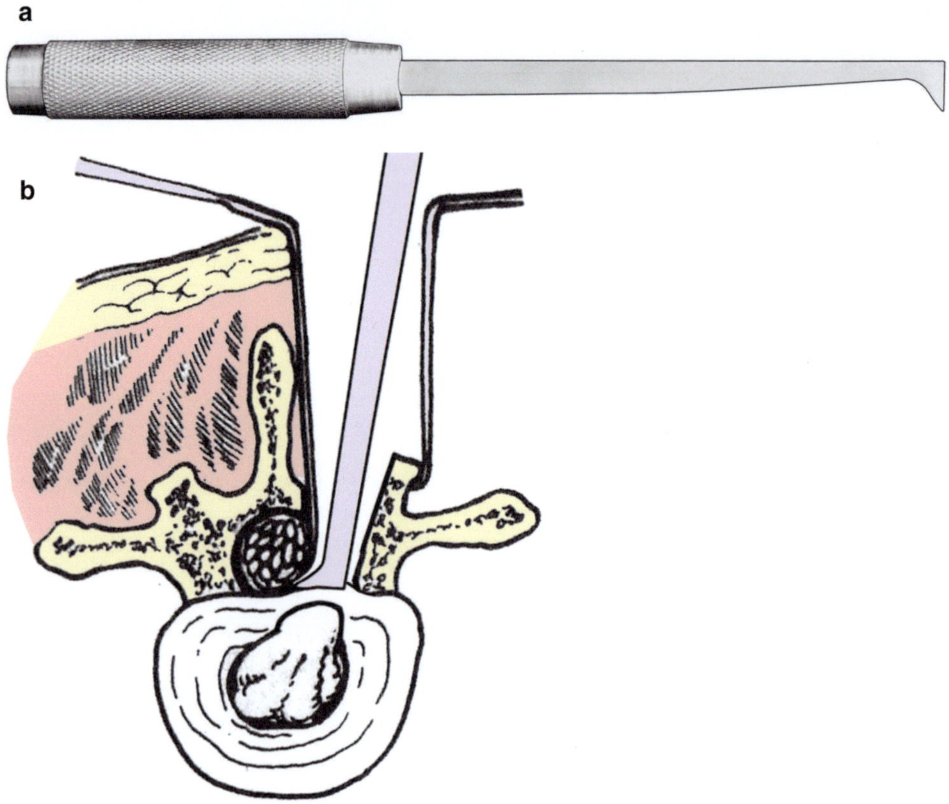

Fig. 2.11 This oblique tip osteotome is used to remove protruding discs and osteophytes at the posterior margin of the vertebral body. (**a**) One oblique tip osteotome. (**b**) This oblique tip osteotome is used to remove protruding discs and osteophytes at the posterior margin of the vertebral body

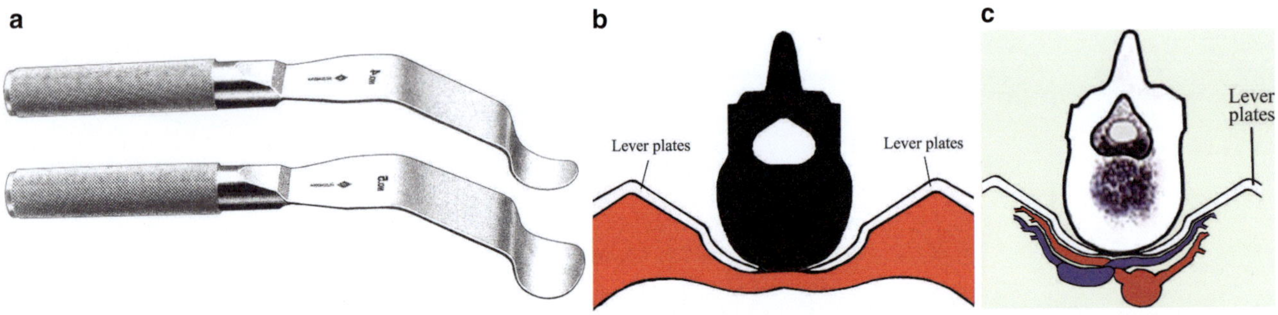

Fig. 2.12 The lever plates are used to pry open the paravertebral soft tissue and the anterior longitudinal ligament under the periosteum, to keep the segmental vessels out of the operative field, and to clearly expose the vertebral body and intervertebral disc without ligating the segmental vessels. (**a**) Lever plates are divided into wide and narrow sizes. (**b**) Expose the entire vertebra. (**c**) The segmental arteries and veins are blocked by Lever plates, and the segmental vessels need not be ligated

5. A large straight scraper has been added to the hollow scraper spoons, which can be used to completely remove the intervertebral disc and the central part of the upper and lower cartilaginous plates in lumbar fusion surgery more quickly and conveniently. Left and right scraping spoons are used to scrape the intervertebral space on both sides. The combined application of these three instruments saves a lot of time in clearing the intervertebral space and facilitates the intervertebral bone graft fusion or installing a fusion cage.
6. According to the need for resection of the central part of the vertebral body, the angle of the shovel osteotomes was changed again, which is conducive to more convenient and reliable resection of the central part of the vertebral body.
7. The addition of two sizes of the Tian's stripper not only ensured the greater safety of subperiosteal dissection but also protected the segmental blood vessels.
8. The trailing edge osteotome was replaced with an oblique tip osteotome. The oblique tip osteotome is used for the removal of central disc herniation or posterior margin of the vertebral body during lumbar discectomy.
9. The lever plates are slightly wider than the original lever plates, which are used for long segment vertebral body resection. After the entire vertebral body resection, the

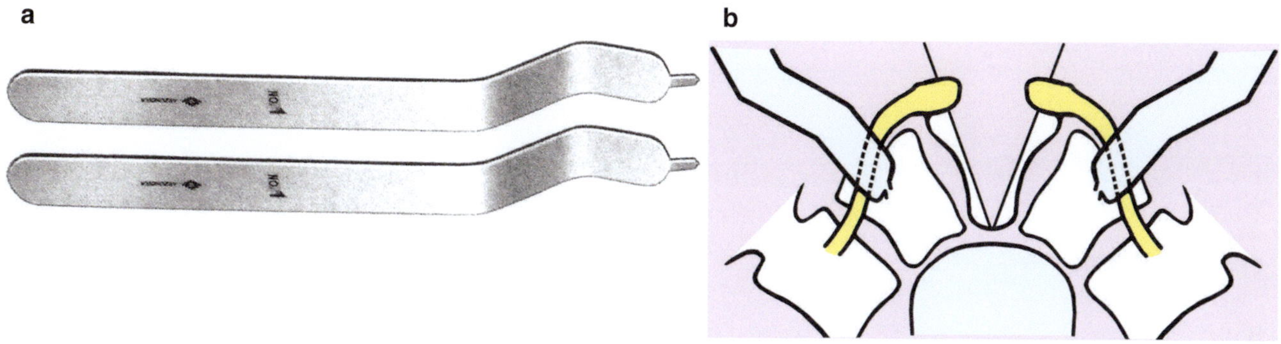

Fig. 2.13 Application of nerve root retractor. (**a**) Two nerve root retractors. (**b**) The nerve roots from the upper and lower intervertebral foramen are kept out of the operative field in vertebral body resection

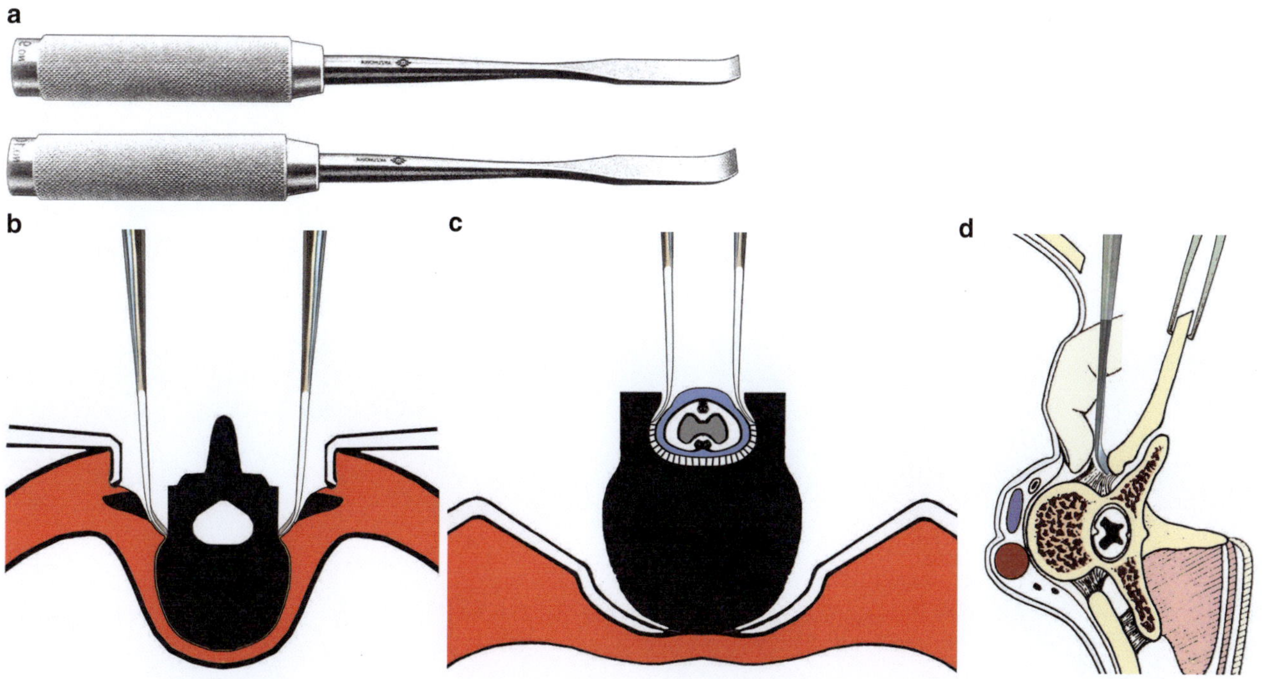

Fig. 2.14 Different applications of anonymous strippers. (**a**) Two size anonymous strippers. (**b**) Stripping both sides pedicle and vertebral body. (**c**) Stripping epidural adhesion in spinal tuberculosis. (**d**) When a lateral approach is required to expose the vertebra, an anonymous stripper is convenient to remove the costal capitulum

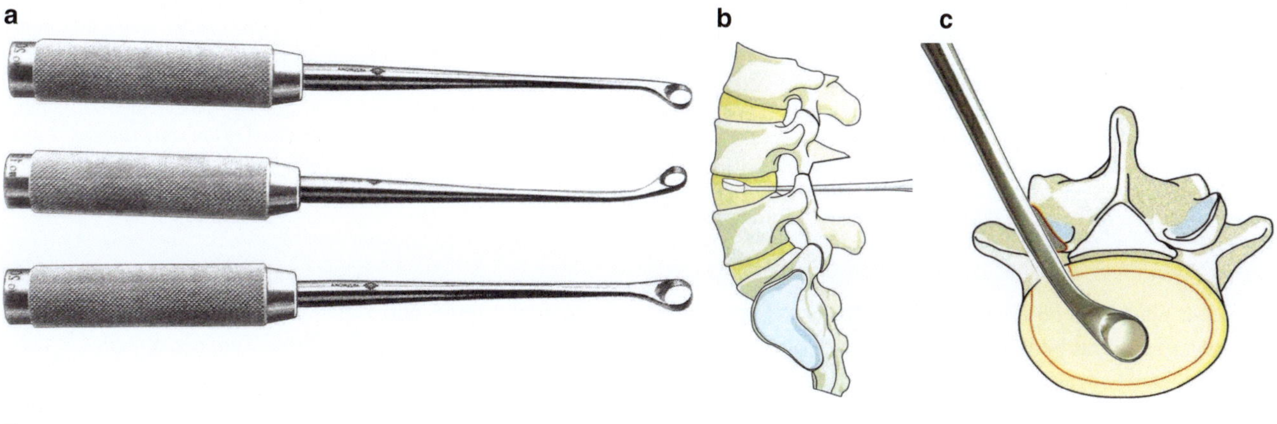

Fig. 2.15 Applications of hollow scraper spoons. (**a**) Three hollow scraper spoons (left, right, and straight). (**b**) A straight scraper scoop is used to scrape the central portion of the intervertebral disc, nucleus pulposus, and cartilage plate during lumbar interbody fusion. (**c**) A bent scraper scoop is used to scrape the edges of the intervertebral disc, nucleus pulposus, and cartilage plate during lumbar interbody fusion

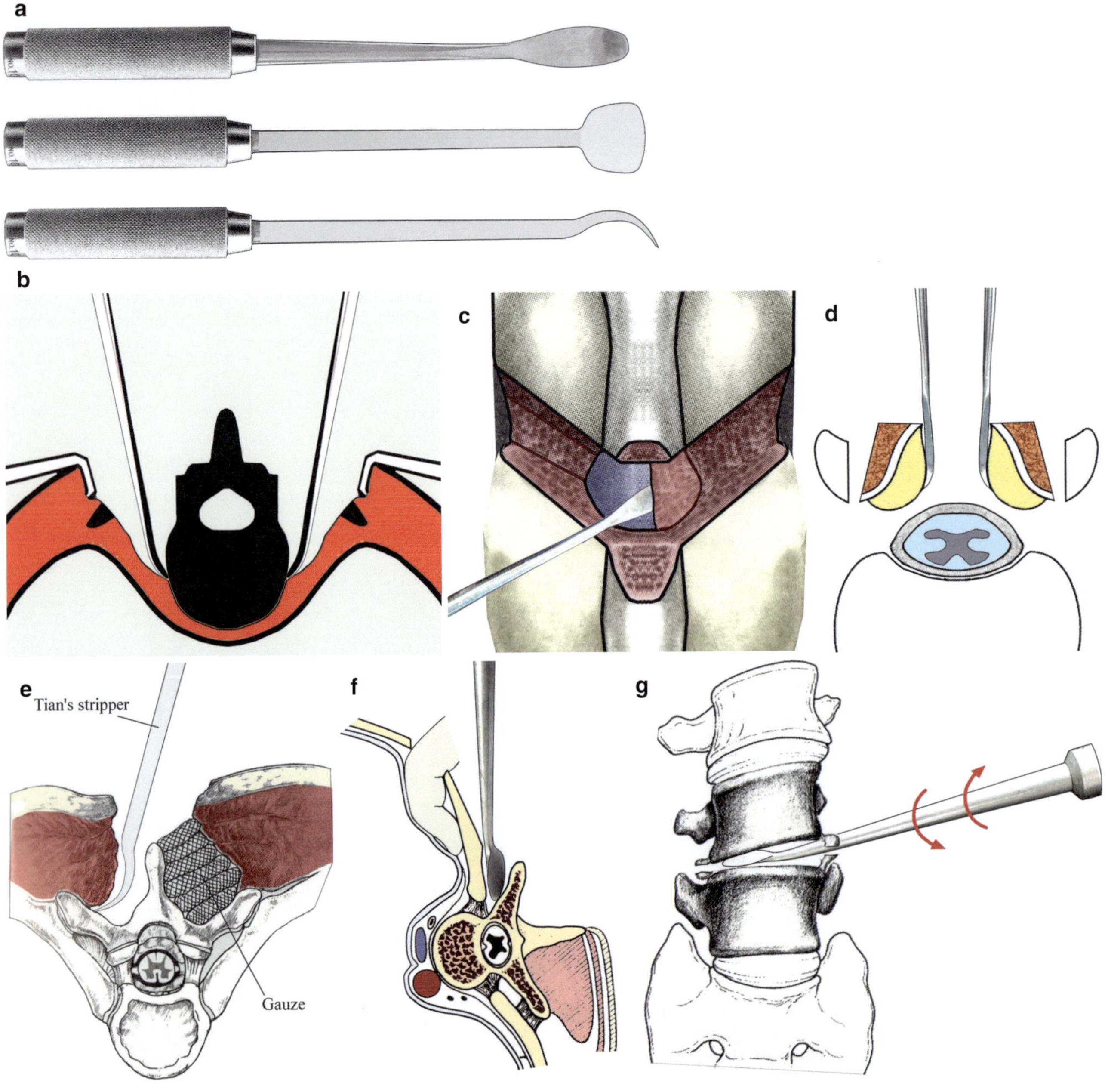

Fig. 2.16 (**a–d**) Applications of Tian's small stripper. (**a**) Tian's strippers are divided into two sizes. (**b**) The vertebral body was dissected along with Tian's small stripper to the anterior longitudinal ligament, and then the lever plates were replaced. (**c**) When the ASK lamina V-shaped osteotomy, the Tian's small stripper was inserted into the central space of the ligamentum flavum and inserted between the cortical layer of the lamina and the ligamentum flavum, and peeled forward along the osteotomy space to separate the gap between the ligamentum flavum and the medial cortex. Then, the osteotomy removes the full lamina. (**d**) In the case of ossification of the thoracic ligamentum flavum, the ossified ligamentum flavum and the medial bony cortex of the lamina were dissected from the inside out with Tian's small stripper to decompress the spinal cord. (**e–g**) Applications of Tian's big stripper. (**e**) Tian's big stripper is used to expose the spinous process, lamina, articular process, and transverse process. (**f**) Tian's big stripper is used for the separation and exposure of the costal vertebral joints. (**g**) Tian's big stripper is used in the vertebral body space pry reduction

lever plates can block the leading edge of the upper and lower vertebral bodies.

10. The Tian's stripper is divided into two sizes, and it can be used for the peeling of the vertebral body. These two Tian's strippers can be used in a variety of operations. The small Tian's stripper is designed to peel off the segmental arteries and veins of the vertebral body and protect it from damage. The large Tian's strippers are used to expose the outer edge of the vertebra and annulus of fiber. When the degenerative lumbar interspace is not equally widened or being dislocated, the reduction is achieved by leverage using the large strippers.

Suggested Reading

1. Tian H. Surgical treatment of kyphosis kyphosis. Chinese Journal of Orthopaedics. 1992;12(3):162–5.
2. Tian H, Tian Y, Zheng X, Tian S. Posterior invasion and vertebral osteotomy. Spinal Deformation. 1992;7(1):4–11.
3. Tian H, Xiang Z. Spinal deformity surgery. Xinjiang: Science and Technology Medical Press; 1994. p. 271–324.
4. Tian H. Hemilaminectomy and total spinal canal decompression in the treatment of spinal canal stenosis: a report of 50 cases. U.S. Chinese Journal of Orthopaedics. 1996;2(2):144.
5. Tian H. Resection of vertebral posterior border bone mass with column fender bone grafting. U.S. Chinese Journal of Orthopaedics. 1996;2:243.
6. Tian H, Zhao J, Huang W, et al. Lumbar disc extraction by using UL model osteotomy and fenestration of lateral fossa: a report of 500 cases. U.S. Chinese Journal of Orthopaedics. 1996;2(3):172.
7. Li J, Ge B, Lu S, et al. Complete works of surgery: volume of Orthopaedic surgery. Beijing: People's military Medical Publishing House; 1996. p. 45–1613.
8. Tian H, Li F. Spinal deformity and osteotomy. Xi'an: World Book Publishing Company; 2001. p. 377–735.
9. Chen A, Xu W. Spinal surgery atlas. Beijing: People's Medical Publishing House; 2001. p. 77–233.
10. Tian H. Spinal surgeons should be good at using rongeurs and osteotome. Chinese Journal of Modern Operative Surgery. 2002;6(1):67–8.
11. Tian H. Reconstruction surgery of thoracic kyphosis for scoliosis combined with thoracic lordosis. Chinese Journal of Modern Operative Surgery. 2002;6(1):52–3.
12. Tian H. Application of "Tian's spinal bone knife" in orthopaedic surgery. Chinese Journal of Orthopaedics. 2003;11(15):1073–5.
13. Xu S, Ge B, Xu Y. Practice of orthopaedics. 2nd ed. Beijing: People's Military Medical Publishing House; 2003. p. 598–636.
14. Bradford DS, Zhang Y, Wang Y. The spine. Shenyang: Liaoning Science and Technology Press; 2003. p. 279–92.
15. Lei W, Li Q. Application guides for spinal implant system. Xi'an: The Fourth Military Medical University Press; 2004. p. 1–423.
16. Tian H, Lin Q, Tan Y. Therapeutics of ankylosing spondylitis. Guangzhou: World Book Publishing Company; 2005. p. 127–261.
17. Tian H, Wang B, Lv X, et al. Correction and fixation of ankylosing kyphosis and osteotomy. Chinese Journal of Orthopaedics. 2005;13(7):509–12.
18. Hou S. Spinal surgery. Beijing: People's Military Medical Publishing House; 2005. p. 444–610.
19. Tian H, Lv X, Tian B. Correction of osteotomy of cervical and thoracic kyphosis with ankylosing spondylitis. Chinese Journal of Orthopaedics. 2006;14(7):522–3.
20. Tian H. Report of 25 cases of traumatic paraplegia treated with posterior spinal decompression by posterior approach. Chinese Journal of Orthopaedics. 2006;07:549–50.
21. Tian H, Lv X, Ma Y. Treatment of severe spinal curvature with total spine osteotomy and internal fixation with head-sleeve ring. Chinese Journal of Orthopaedics. 2007;15(3):167–72.
22. Tian H, Liu S, Ma Y. Practical spine surgery. Guangzhou: Guangdong Science and Technology Press; 2008. p. 87–409.
23. Tian H, Liu S, Ma Y. Practical spine surgery illustration. Beijing: People's Military Medical Press; 2008. p. 152–675.
24. Tian H, Ma Y, Lv X. Minimally invasive V-shaped osteotomy for correction of ankylosing kyphosis. Chinese Journal of Orthopaedics. 2008;16(5):349–52.
25. Tian H, Ma Y, Lv X. Halo pelvic distraction and elastic growing rods fixation for treatment of scoliosis during growing period. Orthopedic Journal of China. 2008;16(21):1660–3.
26. Tian H, Bai J, Liu S. Operative orthopaedics Gist & Atlas. Beijing: People's Medical Publishing House; 2009. p. 46–165.
27. Tian H, Ma Y, Lv X. Rib plasty with halo pelvic wearing for treatment of collapsed chest. Orthopedic Journal of China. 2009;17(11):836–8.
28. Tian H. History of treatment of spinal deformity in China. Chinese Journal of Orthopaedics. 2009;17(9): 706–7.
29. Ma Y, Liu S, Zeng Z. Internal fixation techniques for the spine. Beijing: People's Military Medical Publishing House; 2010. p. 189–304.
30. Tian H, Liang Y, Ma Y, et al. Treatment of ossification of thoracic ligamentum flavum with total osteotomy and decompression with Tian's bone knife. Chinese Journal of Orthopaedics. 2010;18(20):1693–6.
31. Tian H, Alken AD, Du P, et al. Posterior hemiverteectomy for congenital horny kyphosis. Chinese Journal of Orthopaedics, 2010, 18 (15): 1250-1253.
32. Tian H, Wan Y, Li M. Halo-Pelvic distraction techniques for the spinal deformity. Guangzhou: Guangdong Science and Technology Press; 2010. p. 1–305.
33. Tian H. Principles of diagnosis and treatment for scoliosis with diastematomyelia. Orthopedic Journal of China. 2010;18(20):1753–5.
34. Tian H, Alken AD, Ma Y. Prophylactic osteotomy for the treatment of congenital lateral paravertebral vertebral body. Chinese Journal of Orthopaedics, 2011, 19 (07): 541-544.
35. Tian H. Selection of internal fixation after osteotomy and correction of ankylosing kyphosis. Orthopedic Journal of China. 2011;19(9):784–6.
36. Tian H, Li M, Ma Y. Spinal deformity osteotomy orthopedics, vol. 5. Beijing: People's Medical Publishing House; 2011. p. 3–339.
37. Tian H. Tuberculous kyphosis osteotomy orthopedic surgery. Chinese Journal of Orthopaedics. 2011;19(23):1937–40.
38. Tian H. Pedicle lateral screw-rod system for the treatment of scoliosis. Orthopedic Journal of China. 2011;19(13): 1149–51.
39. Tian H, Elken A, Ma Y, et al. Lateral anterior approach osteotomy for thoracic disc herniation. Orthopedic Journal of China. 2012;20(5):459–62.
40. Tian H, Elken A, Ma Y, et al. Minimally invasive thoracolumbar anterior decompression and bone grafting with L-shaped plate internal fixation for the treatment of burst fractures or severe compression fractures with spinal cord injury. Orthopedic Journal of China. 2012;20(14):1330–2.
41. Tian H, Ma Y, Lv X. Osteotomy through anterolateral approach for ossification of the posterior longitudinal ligament of the thoracic spine. Orthopedic Journal of China. 2012;20(21): 1995–6.
42. Tian H. A brief history and popularization of spinal osteotomy with thin blade bone knife. Chinese Journal of Orthopaedics. 2012;20(23):2207–8.
43. Tian H, Zhang H, Liang Y. Surgical treatment of spinal deformity. Guangzhou: Guangdong Science and Technology Press; 2012. p. 1–483.
44. Tian H, Li M, Wang Z. Key points and diagrams of thoracolumbar surgery. Beijing: People's Medical Publishing House; 2012. p. 1–470.
45. Huang W, Tian H, Lv X, et al. Lateral anterior decompression for late paralysis of thoracic tuberculosis. Orthopedic Journal of China. 2012;20(7):647–9.

46. Dove J, Hsu LC, Yau AC. The cervical spine after halo-pelvic traction. An analysis of the complications of 83 patients. J Bone Joint Surg Br. 1980;62-B(2):158–61.
47. Susan S. GRAY'S anatomy. Beijing: Peking University Medical Press; 2006. p. 14–98.
48. Tian H. Total spinal osteotomy for the treatment of kyphosis and kyphoscoliosis. Japanese Scoliosis Society program of the 25th Annual Meeting, l991;25:23.
49. Tian H, Li F, Tan J. Children's spinal operative orthopaedics. Guangzhou: Guangdong Science and Technology Press; 2016. p. 1–443.
50. Tian H, Li M. Ankylosing spondylitis spinal deformity osteotomy and orthopedic surgery skills. Beijing: People's Medical Publishing House; 2014. p. 1–28.
51. Tian H, Ma Y, Xie J. Spinal osteotomy orthopedics. Guangzhou: Guangdong Science and Technology Press; 2018. p. 2–541.

3 Transverse Laminectomy for Ankylosing Spondylitis Kyphosis

Huizhong Tian, Jiangtao Sui, and Ying Zhang

3.1 Overview

The surgical technique of transverse laminectomy for ankylosing kyphosis is performed in accordance with the original design of Smith Petersen in 1945. The spinous process and the inferior articular process of the osteotomy level are first removed to expose the upper edge of the lower lamina and superior articular process and then a transverse osteotomy and wedge resection is performed on the lamina, posterior to the intervertebral foramen on both sides. The width of wedge resection is generally about 8 mm (Fig. 3.1). The gap of wedge osteotomy should not be too wide, so as to avoid the narrowing of the intervertebral foramen and compression of spinal nerve roots due to the closure of the osteotomy gap after the corrective procedure. This method, or Smith Petersen's original technique, is simple and easy to implement. Professor Tian Huizhong introduced this technique in 1961 to treat ankylosing kyphosis with a kyphotic Cobb angle <80°. It is often performed only under local infiltration anesthesia. Since the width of the wedge resection of the transverse osteotomy is not big, it is generally not a problem to correct the deformity and spontaneously close the osteotomy gap. Sometimes after the transverse laminectomy and wedge resection, the osteotomy gap can be closed without any traction or manipulation for correction. To remove the bone fragments in the intervertebral foramen on both sides, the osteotomy gap needs to be opened with a spreader first. After the osteotomy gap is closed, place the long bone block resected on the osteotomy gap for posterior grafting. Place a negative pressure drainage tube behind the lamina, close the incision in layers to finish the operation. Treat cases with a small kyphosis angle by the above simple method is safe, reliable, simple, and convenient. Kyphotic deformity correction is achievable. After the operation, the spine is just stabilized by the external plaster vest in overextension to achieve good outcomes.

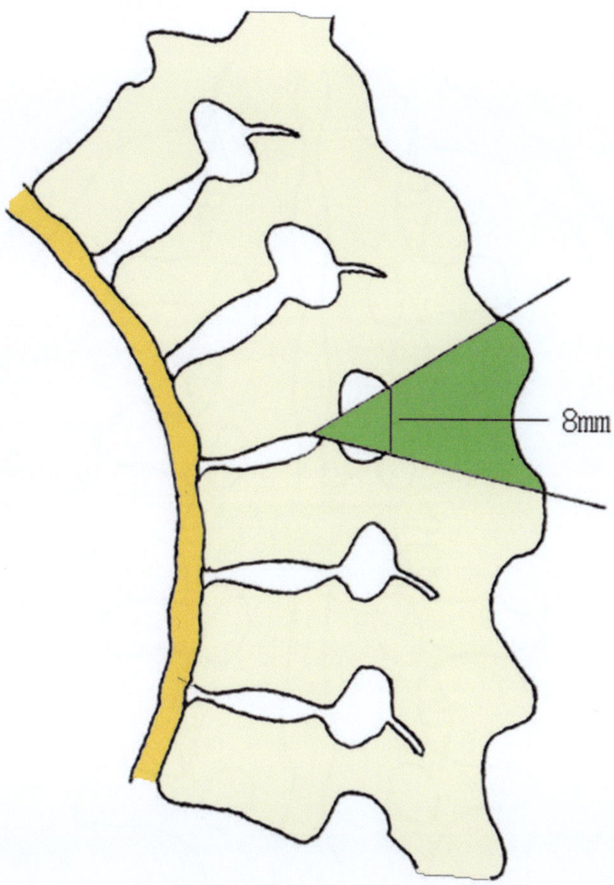

Fig. 3.1 The angle of lamina osteotomy, from the spinous process to the posterior edge of the vertebral body, is generally about 40–45°. The angle and width of the osteotomy are determined according to the severity of the kyphosis. The width of the osteotomy is 8 mm at the bone cortex on the inner side of the lamina

H. Tian (✉) · J. Sui
The Sixth Affiliated Hospital of Xinjiang Medical University, Urumqi, China

Y. Zhang
Department of Orthopedics, The 2nd Affiliated Hospital of Kunming Medical University, Kunming, China

H. Tian et al. (eds.), *Spinal Osteotomy Orthopaedics*, https://doi.org/10.1007/978-981-16-1387-6_3

3.1.1 Modified Methods of Transverse Laminectomy

Try to keep the spinous processes at both ends of the osteotomy gap from being removed (Fig. 3.2). At the level of disc space, use a sharp thin-blade osteotome to perform a transverse wedge resection, so that the lamina and spinous process will have a bone-on-bone approximation. Compared with resecting the spinous processes above and below the osteotomy gap, this method is more stable by not only relying on the stability of the lamina, it facilitates internal fixation on the retained spinous processes. As the ossified spinous process and the interspinous space form a longitudinal thick bone wall, it is very advantageous to use it for internal fixation to hold the spinous process. It is more advantageous compared with the technique of removing the adjacent spinous process and only rely on the lamina. The alignment will be more stable and reliable. A bony contact surface between the lamina and the spinous process is produced, which is favorable for bony fusion. It is especially suitable for the dynamic double Luque rod fixation technique.

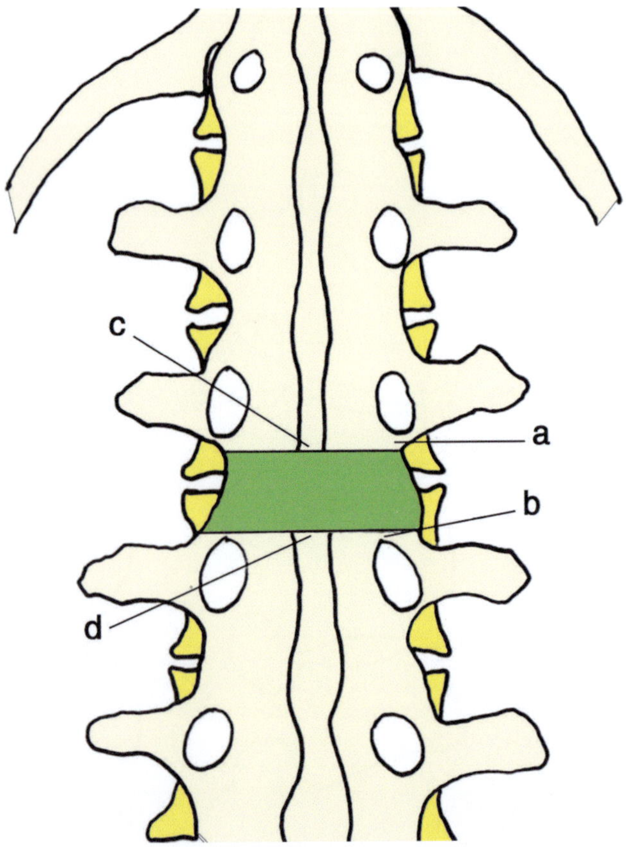

Fig. 3.2 Transverse laminectomy, anatomical landmarks. (**a**) 1 ~ 2 mm below the lower edge of the pedicle. (**b**) 1 ~ 2 mm above the upper edge of the pedicle. (**c**) Upper edge of the spinous process. (**d**) Lower edge of spinous process. Osteotomy width: 8 mm. Osteotomy gap: single gap

3.1.2 Location of Transverse Laminectomy

According to AP X-ray, to observe the opening of the interspinous space of the apical vertebrae, and then according to the lateral X-ray, evaluate the degree of extension of the upper and lower diameters of the intervertebral foramen of the apical level, to determine the apical vertebrae. If the apical vertebrae is T12 ~ L1, the osteotomy is performed between T12 ~ L1, so apical vertebra osteotomy may not always be between L2 ~ L3, but on the true apical level. This is the so-called apical osteotomy. However, osteotomy is limited to T10 ~ L4, because the spinal canal diameter of T10 ~ L4 is relatively wide and it is not prone to produce spinal stenosis after osteotomy and correction. In addition, this segment is not limited to the chest cage and ribs. The width of lamina osteotomy is commonly 8–12 mm. After the operation, head and foot traction and manual correction are performed to achieve the closure of the osteotomy gap, which makes the anterior edge of the vertebral body open and extend the spine. A short segment of post lamina elastic compression fixation is applied. After the operation, the patient should return to the ward and lie in a flatbed to allow self-correction or manual reduction. Upon satisfactory correction, the patient should wear a plaster vest for external immobilization. Eight months after the operation, the plaster is removed after examination shows that bone healing occurs in the osteotomy space.

3.2 Surgical Procedure

Spinal osteotomy bears the same principle as long bone osteotomy. It requires a wedge-shaped osteotomy with osteotomes, and then closes the wedge-shaped gap to correct the deformity so that the spine restores its alignment. Transverse laminectomy is a traditional technique as used by Smith Petersen. This method has been applied by the author since 1961 for spinal osteotomy. The method is simple and suitable for beginners. It is also a good technique to treat ankylosing spondylitis with kyphosis.

1. Device preparation: A set of Tian's spinal osteotome (Fig. 3.3), pedicle finder, and implants and instruments as needed. Alternatively, the patient may go back to the ward without internal fixation and lie in a flatbed for self-correction after osteotomy. After satisfying correction is achieved, a plaster vest is applied for external immobilization.
2. Anesthesia: Local infiltration anesthesia or tracheal intubation anesthesia
3. Position: Prone or lateral position
4. Surgical procedure:

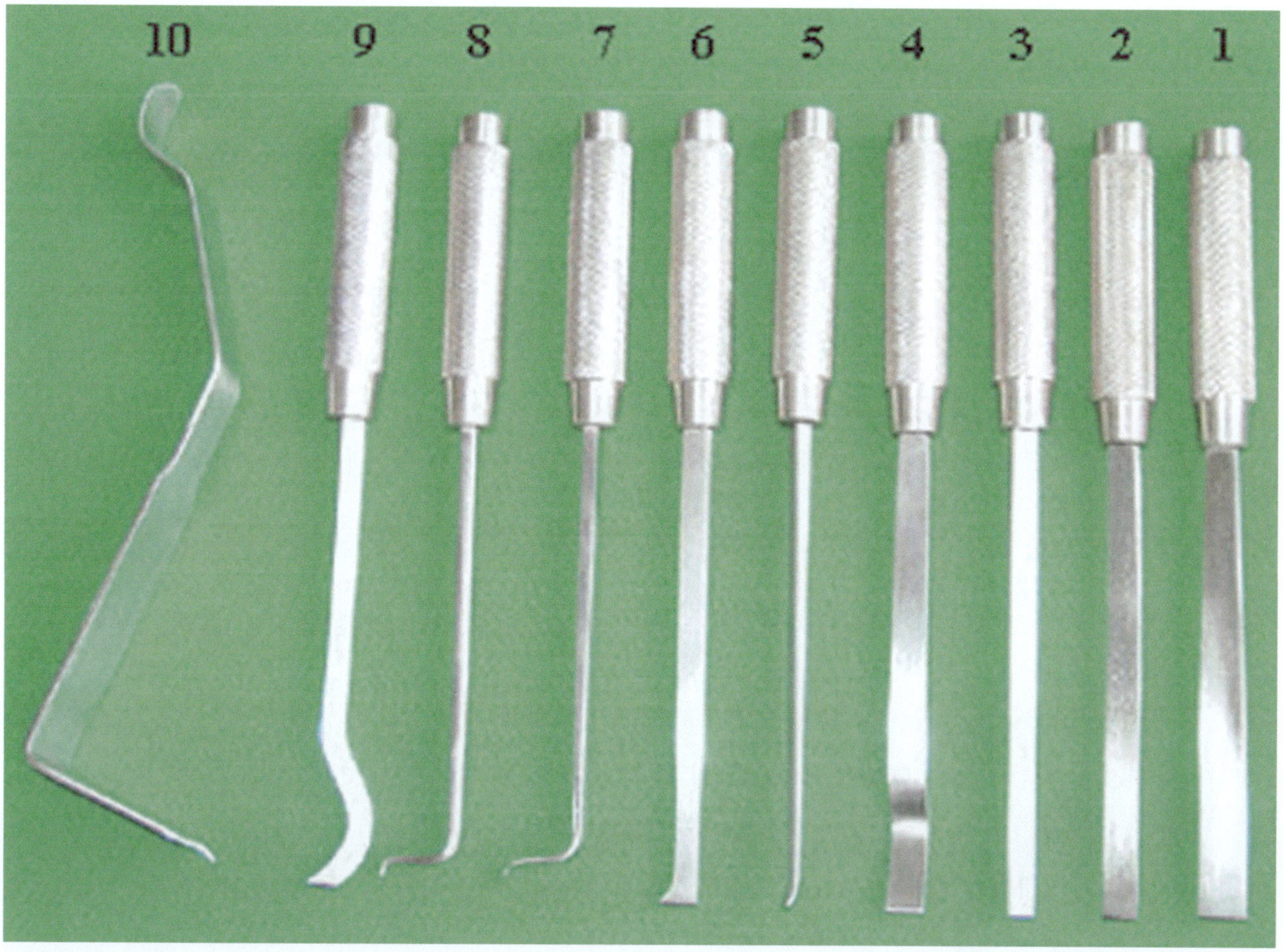

Fig. 3.3 A set of Type VI Tian's osteotome

Step 1: Place the patient prone on the operating table. Adjust the operating bed to a reverse V shape. Put 10 cm diameter cloth rolls under both sides of the trunk to free the abdomen. Mark the spinous process (Fig. 3.4), and disinfect and drape.

Step 2: Make a longitudinal incision along the spinous process, about 10 ~ 15 cm in length. Cut the skin and subcutaneous tissue, dissect and expose the spinous process, lamina and transverse process with a cautery. Retract the paraspinal muscles with an automatic retractor. Confirm the osteotomy space. Expose to the lateral till the transverse process (Fig. 3.5).

Step 3: Use the pedicle finder (Fig. 3.6a, b) to find out the distance between the intervertebral foramen and the upper and lower pedicles, and then determine the osteotomy site (Fig. 3.7a–c).

Step 4: Use a thin-blade straight osteotome to perform a transverse wedge resection from the spinous process to the posterior edge of the vertebral body. The width of the

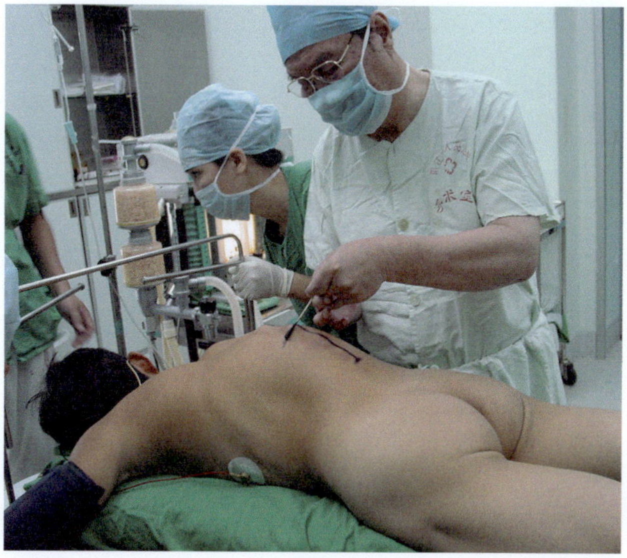

Fig. 3.4 Mark the incision along the spinous process on top of the apex of the kyphosis

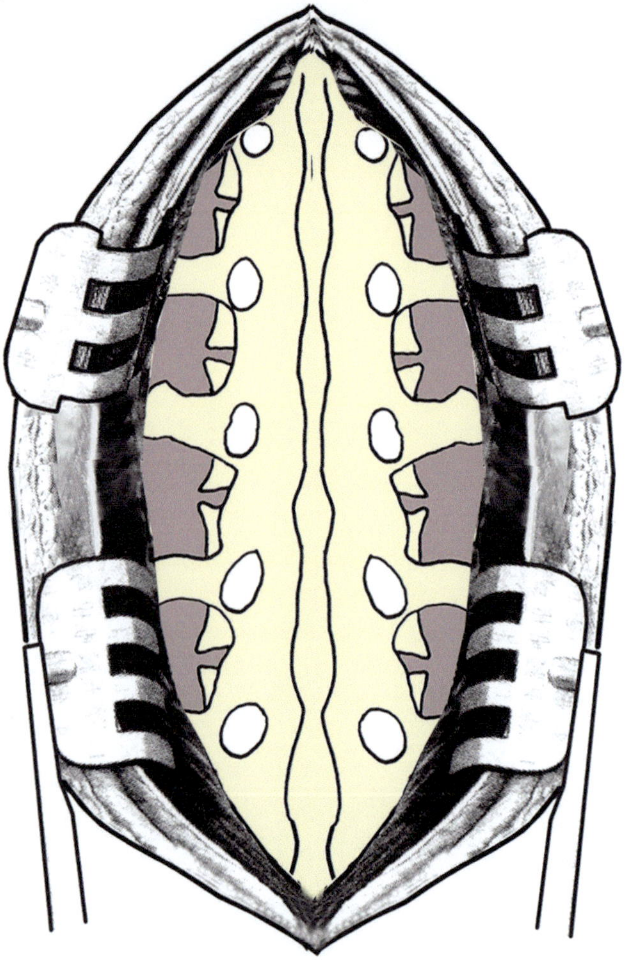

Fig. 3.5 According to the severity and needs of the kyphosis, the length of the internal fixation and incision is determined. The spinous process, lamina, and transverse process are exposed

wedge resection is 8–12 mm wide between the lamina (Fig. 3.8).

Step 5: Scope of transverse osteotomy: Draw a parallel line 1 ~ 2 mm below the lower edge of upper pedicles on both sides, and another parallel line 1 ~ 2 mm above the upper edge of the lower pedicles. Between the two parallel lines is the scope of transverse osteotomy (Figs. 3.9 and 3.10).

Step 6: After the transverse osteotomy is done, use a spreader to open the osteotomy gap to completely remove the epidural bone fragments and ligamentum flavum. Osteophytes protruding inward along the margin of the osteotomy should be removed (Fig. 3.11), so as to avoid spinal cord compression after hyperextension reduction.

Step 7: Remove the spreader, adjust the reverse V shape operating table to a V shape. Gently compress and perform head and foot traction outside the aseptic zone to put the spine into hyperextension, close the osteotomy gap, and open the anterior edge of the vertebral body. Fix with Luque rods and interspinous wiring (Fig. 3.12a, b). However, it is important to avoid excessive pressure during compression which may force the truncated spine to be displaced, resulting in paraplegia.

Step 8: Internal fixation includes interspinous wiring compression (Fig. 3.13), pedicle screw–rod compression and fixation, or hook–rod compression and fixation. However, pedicle screws or hooks should be placed before osteotomy. These steps should be done before the osteotomy is completed to avoid displacement of the osteotomy gap.

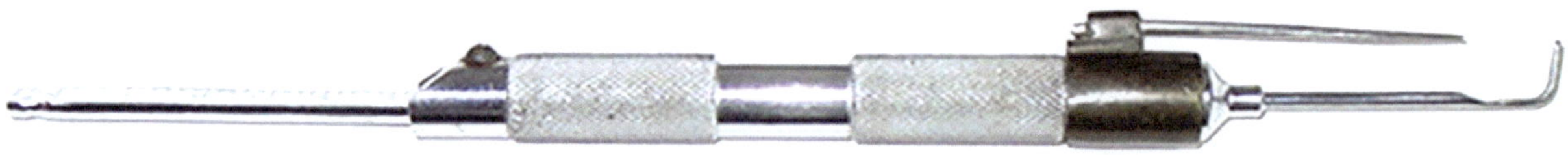

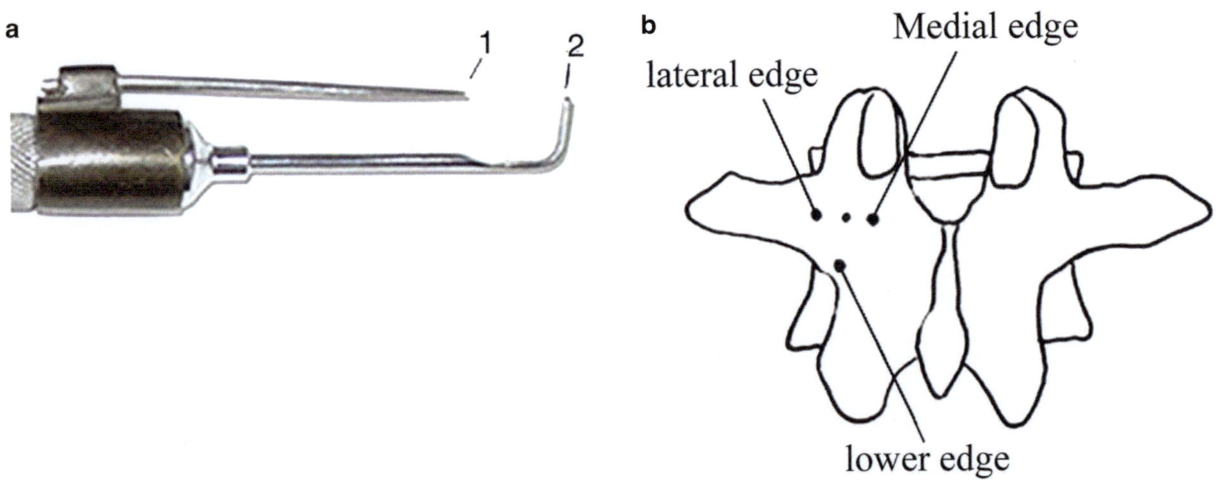

Fig. 3.6 (a) Pedicle finder, 1. probe; 2. stylus. (b) Position of pedicle back to the lamina: the entry point is between the medical edge and lateral edge; the lower edge point is the reference value

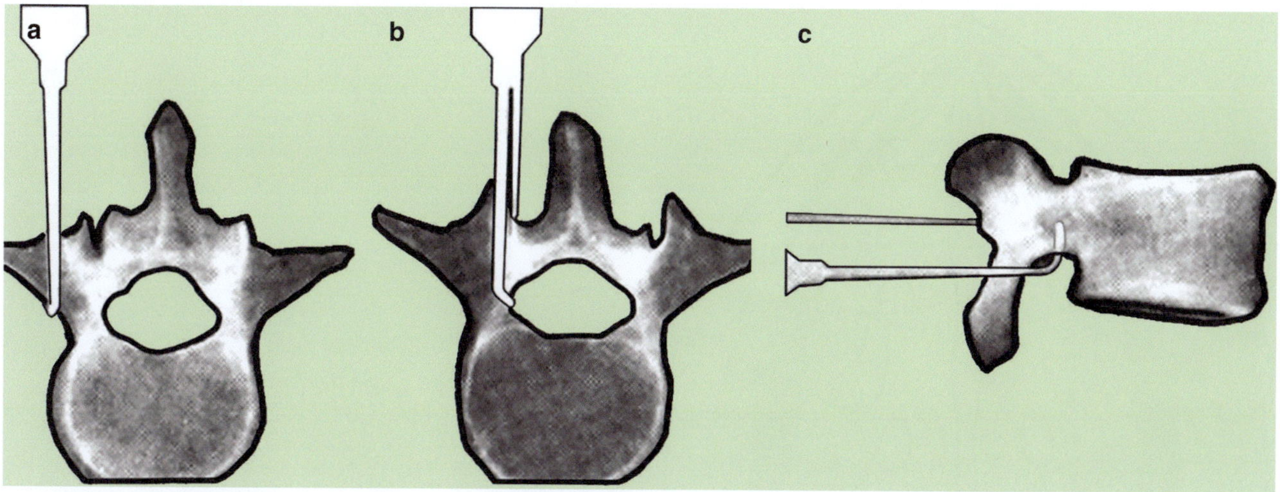

Fig. 3.7 The relationship between the finder and the pedicle. (**a**) Determination of the outer edge; (**b**) Determination of the inner edge; (**c**) The probe tip and pointer tip of the finder are located exactly at the central point of the upper and lower dimension of the pedicle

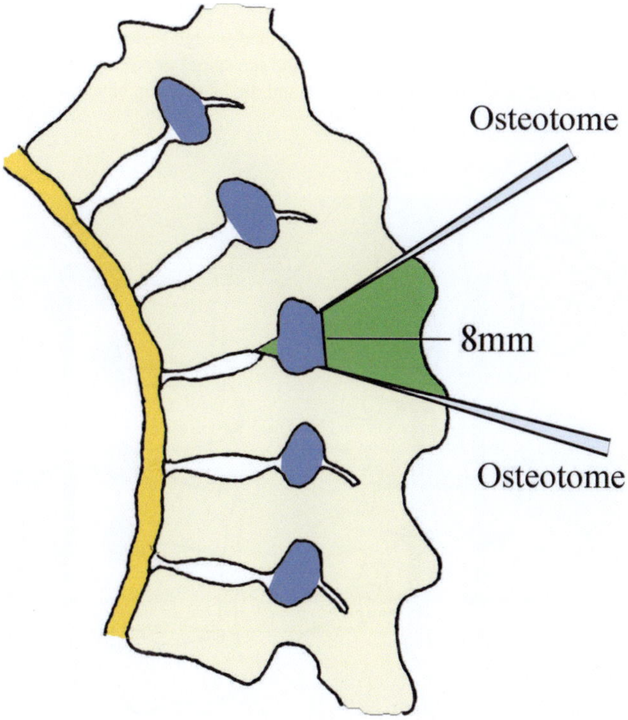

Fig. 3.8 According to the severity of the kyphosis, the width of the transverse laminectomy is determined. Generally, the width of the osteotomy between the lamina is 8–12 mm

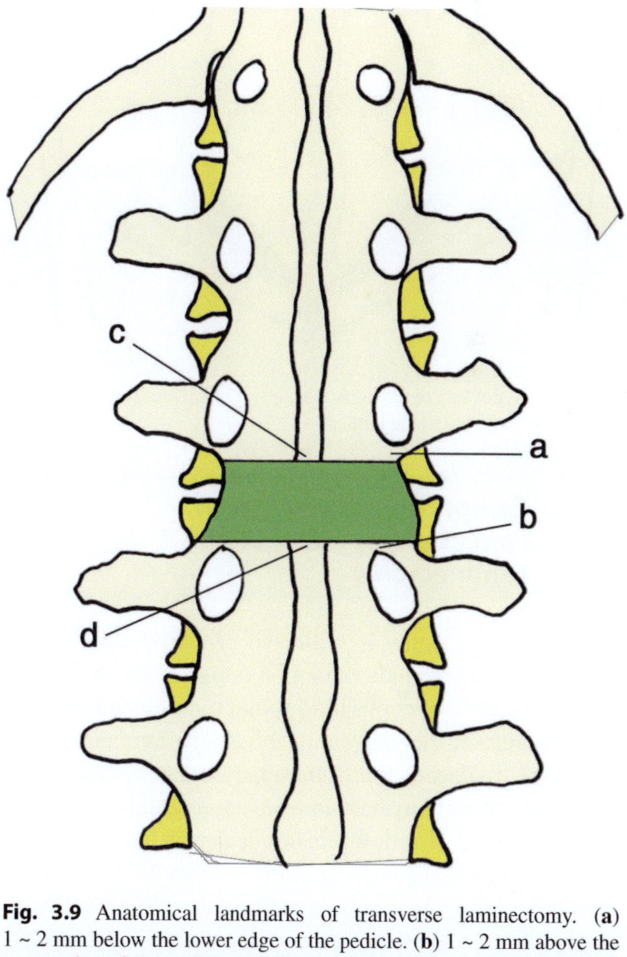

Fig. 3.9 Anatomical landmarks of transverse laminectomy. (**a**) 1 ~ 2 mm below the lower edge of the pedicle. (**b**) 1 ~ 2 mm above the upper edge of the pedicle. (**c**) Upper edge of the spinous process. (**d**) Lower edge of spinous process. Osteotomy width: 8 mm. Osteotomy level: single level

Step 9: Irrigate the wound followed by hemostasis. Place T tubes on both sides of the spinous process for negative pressure drainage.

5. Postoperative management:

The postoperative drainage volume is 100 ~ 300 ml is a sign that there is no blood collection in the wound. The drainage tube is removed 24 ~ 48 h after surgery. After the stitches are removed, the patient is externally immobilized with a plaster vest in a hyperextension position (Fig. 3.14a, b) for 8–12 months.

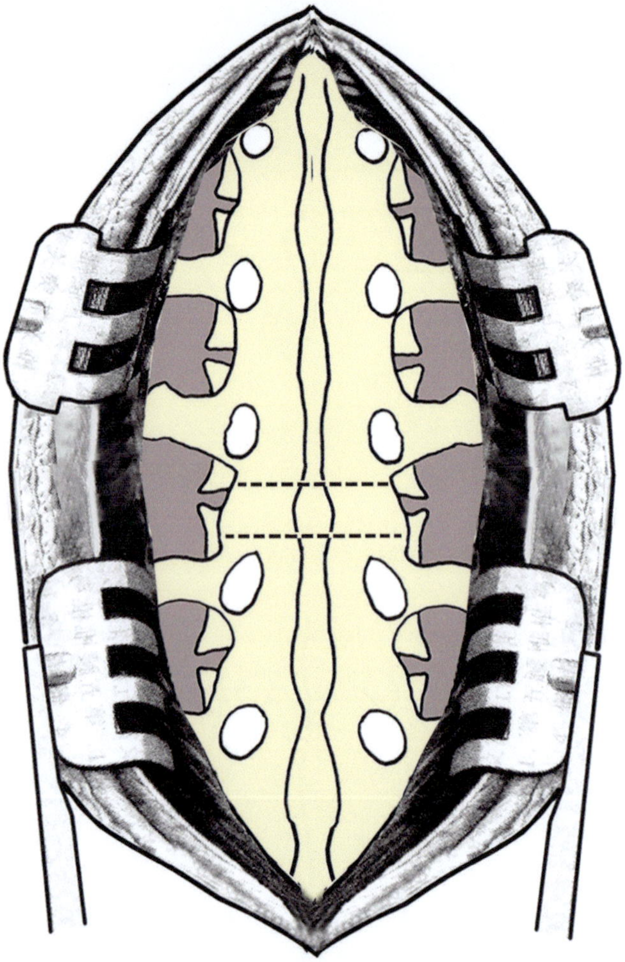

Fig. 3.10 According to the kyphosis angle, mark a predetermined osteotomy line posterior to the lamina

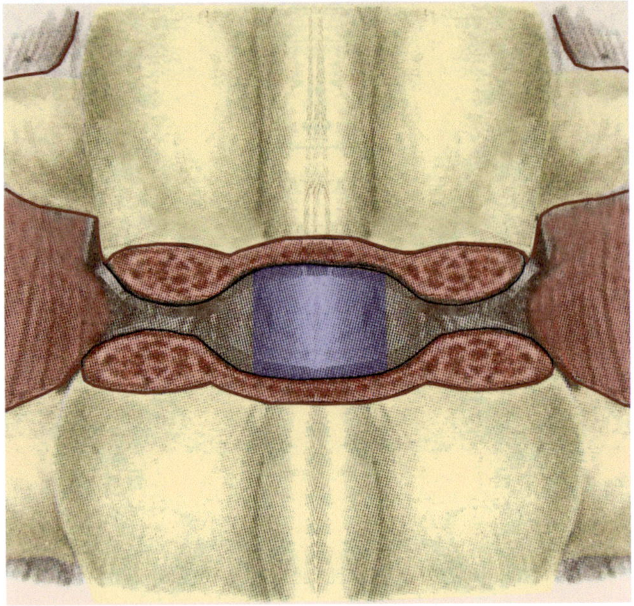

Fig. 3.11 The transverse laminectomy and wedge resection has been completed, exposing the dural canal and the spinal nerve roots on both sides. As shown, the spinous process and the lamina cap have formed a flat cut surface

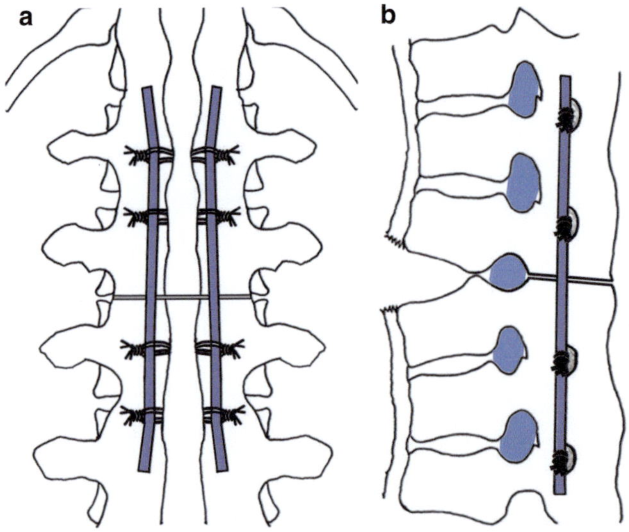

Fig. 3.12 Transverse laminectomy is an osteotomy that opens the anterior and closes the posterior. Luque rods and wires are used to fix the spinous processes firmly and reliably because the spinous processes of ankylosing spondylitis are fused with each other to form a thick wall which is very suitable for fixing between spinous processes

3.3 Comparison of Transverse Laminectomy and V-Shape Laminectomy

Transverse osteotomy is criticized primarily for the fact that the osteotomy ends cannot be impacted by each other and is incapable of controlling spinal rotation and dislocation. Therefore, the conventional V-shape laminar osteotomy has replaced the transverse laminar osteotomy. V-shape laminectomy has more advantages than transverse osteotomy, and it follows anatomical and biomechanical better. However, the latter is more technically demanding. Therefore, surgeons on the learning curve of spinal osteotomy should start with transverse laminectomy to understand the basics and move on to V-shape osteotomy to achieve better surgical results.

Ankylosing kyphosis and tuberculosis or congenital kyphosis require a completely different osteotomy correction technique. Ankylosing kyphosis is a round kyphosis, while tuberculosis or congenital kyphosis is an angular kyphosis. For the osteotomy of ankylosing kyphosis, the non-apical osteotomy is often applied to correct the deformity. In other words, to change the round curve kyphosis (C-shaped kyphosis) into a “figure of 3” kyphosis (Fig. 3.15). Thus, the patient’s lumbar

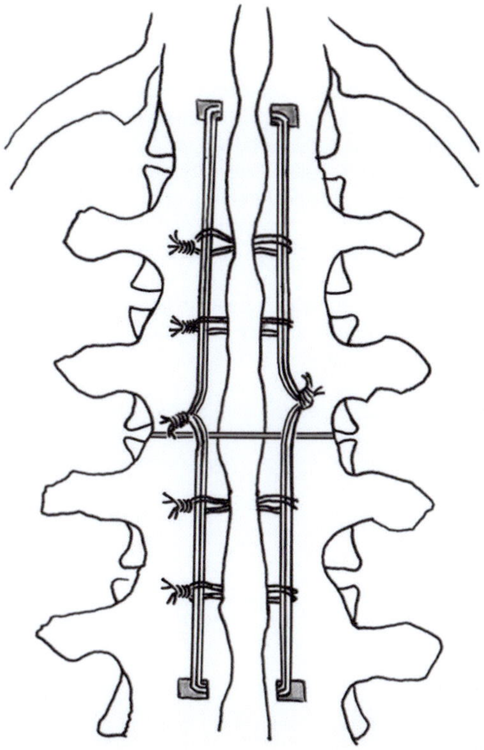

Fig. 3.13 In transverse laminectomy, the spinous process should not be removed. After reduction, good stability is achieved between the lamina and between the spinous process as well as additional interspinous process wiring compression fixation. It is a simple and reliable fixation technique

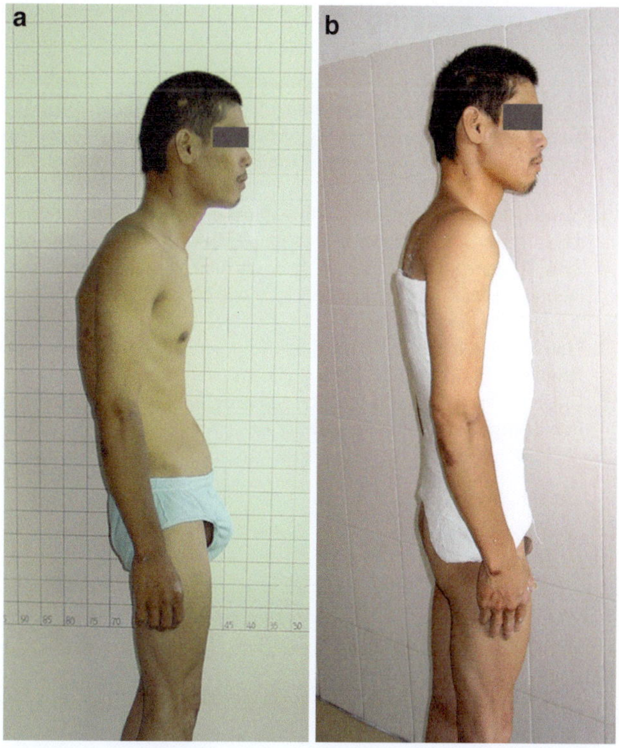

Fig. 3.14 Mild ankylosing kyphosis, transverse laminectomy, simple interspinous wiring. Reliable plaster vest external immobilization for 8–12 months after surgery to allow solid bony fusion. (**a**) Appearance before operation. (**b**) External immobilization of plaster vest after operation

lordosis is increased to compensate for the thoracic kyphosis, to achieve horizontal vision, to increase the distance between the xiphoid and the pubic symphysis, to solve the problem of abdominal compression, poor appetite, and digestive dysfunction. At the same time, the diaphragm is freed to have better contraction to improve abdominal respiration. Thus, the CO_2 and O_2 exchange as well the life quality and status of the patient are improved.

The pathological change of ankylosing spondylitis is a pathological change similar to rheumatoid arthritis. The surrounding joint capsules, ligaments, and intervertebral discs are replaced by fragile granulation tissues, especially the vertebral bodies, intervertebral discs, and anterior longitudinal ligaments. Become very fragile. Therefore, only the method of laminectomy can cause the closure of the laminectomy space, the tearing of the anterior longitudinal ligament, and the opening of the anterior vertebral body space under compression and traction. For cases of tuberculosis kyphosis, congenital kyphosis, and traumatic kyphosis, the purpose of correcting kyphotic deformity cannot be achieved with simple interlaminar osteotomy.

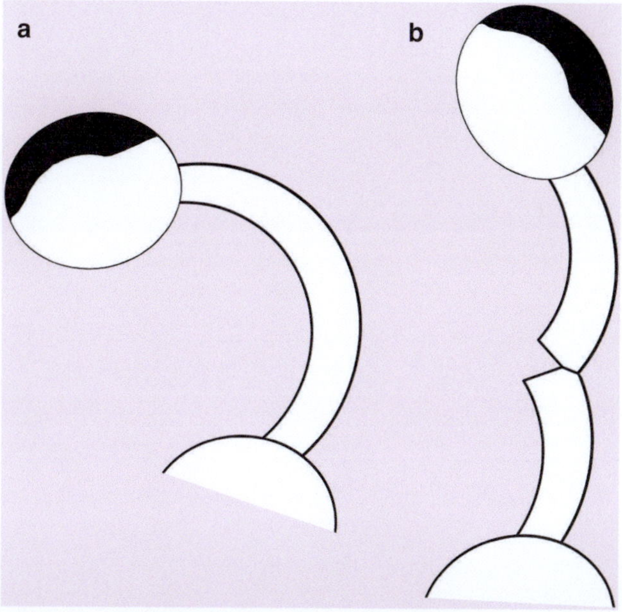

Fig. 3.15 Non-apical osteotomy. (**a**) Large C-shaped kyphosis before surgery. (**b**) The surgery converts it into a "figure of 3" double-curved kyphosis, which restores normal physiological functions

Suggested Reading

1. Tian H, Lin Q, Tan Y. Therapeutics of ankylosing spondylitis. Guangzhou: World Book Publishing Company; 2005. p. 165–95.
2. Tian H, Wang B, Lv X, et al. Correction and fixation of ankylosing kyphosis and osteotomy. Chinese Journal of Orthopaedics. 2005;13(7):509–12.
3. Tian H. Application of the "Tian's spinal osteotomes" in orthopaedic surgery. Chinese Journal of Orthopaedics. 1994;14(4):236–40.
4. Tian H. Selection of internal fixation after osteotomy and correction of ankylosing kyphosis. Orthopedic Journal of China. 2011;19(9):784–6.
5. Tian H, Liu S, Ma Y. Practical spine surgery illustration. Beijing: People's Military Medical Press; 2008. p. 316–21.
6. Chen A, Xu W. Spinal surgery atlas. Beijing: People's Medical Publishing House; 2001. p. 181–273.
7. Tian H, Ma Y, Lv X. Minimally invasive V-shaped osteotomy for correction of ankylosing kyphosis. Chinese Journal of Orthopaedics. 2008;16(5):349–52.
8. Liang Z. Transpedicular osteotomy for the treatment of kyphosis caused by ankylosing spondylitis. Chinese Journal of Orthopaedics. 1997;17(6):351–2.
9. Tian H, Li M, Ma Y. Spinal deformity osteotomy orthopedics, vol. 5. Beijing: People's Medical Publishing House; 2011. p. 101–279.
10. Tian H, Li M, Wang Z. Key points and diagrams of thoracolumbar surgery. Beijing: People's Medical Publishing House; 2012. p. 375–417.
11. Tian H, Liang Y. Ankylosing spondylitis spinal deformity osteotomy and orthopedic surgery skills. Beijing: People's Medical Publishing House; 2014. p. 1–328.

4 V-Shape Laminectomy for Ankylosing Kyphosis

Huizhong Tian, Zhi Zhao, and Ni Bi

4.1 Overview

Ankylosing spondylitis (AS) is a systemic disease, occurring mostly in young men. Its early symptoms mainly involve progressive pain of sacroiliac joints which may extend upward along the spine. Other common symptoms include nocturnal pain, morning stiffness, hyperhidrosis, and emaciation. As a response to the nocturnal pain and sleep deprivation, patients are often forced to keep the knee and hip in flexion and bend the back when sitting. The long-term impact leads to the development of ankylosing kyphotic deformity toward the late stage of the disease.

Early-stage ankylosing spondylitis is primarily managed with drugs. When proper drugs are used with sound compliance, ankylosing kyphosis deformity in the late stage could be delayed. Some AS patients are cured by drugs only, for example, drugs tend to work well for women. Appropriate medical therapy provides significant control over pain while additional sports therapy or swimming shows a positive effect on the disease.

Ankylosing spondylitis usually starts from the sacroiliac joint and may extend upward along the spine all the way up to C1 and C2. On X-ray, blurred ossification of the bilateral facet joint space is the first sign to see, followed by ossification of the interspinal ligament, and then ossification of the intervertebral joints which look like segments of bamboo. In the process of ossification, the nocturnal pain forces the patient to constantly bend the back when sitting. Kyphotic deformity of the spine is thus formed over time. Mild kyphosis is defined as kyphotic Cobb <80°. Severe kyphosis is defined as kyphotic Cobb >80°.

Most cases of mild ankylosing kyphosis are treated with V-shaped laminectomy, reduction, internal fixation, to close the osteotomy site. The long bone block cutoff is grafted between the lamina. A negative pressure drainage tube is placed. The incision is then closed by layers to finish the procedure. For severe kyphosis, vertebrae column resection (VCR) should be considered.

On the basis of Smith Petersen transverse laminar osteotomy, we further modified it to "laminar V osteotomy" (Fig. 4.1a, b) in which the V-shaped tips are inserted into each other to prevent lateral displacement and rotational deformity after osteotomy. The operation of V-shape osteotomy is more complex than transverse osteotomy, and requires certain surgical skills and special tools, i.e., "thin blade osteotomes with multiple angle options." Performing a V-shaped osteotomy with this osteotome is fast and convenient, and the cross-section of the osteotomy is smooth. After correction, the V-shaped edges are impacted with each other without a gap, which is conducive to bone fusion.

The advantages of V-shape osteotomy include: (1) V-shape osteotomy is a good option for kyphotic ankylosing spondylitis, as the procedure is less traumatic, with short operation time, and less bleeding. The average blood transfusion is 200 ~ 600 ml. (2) Spine Osteotomy for the spine with a thin blade osteotome is a special surgical technique. Once this skill is mastered skillfully, it is safe and reliable, with low potential of damaging the dura mater, spinal cord, and nerve root. It is just a kind of surgical craftsmanship. (3) The direction of V-shape osteotomy of vertebral lamina should be oriented slightly cranial. After closing the V-shape osteotomy, the osteotomy surface forms an overlapping sealing, which can prevent lateral and superior-inferior displacement.

4.2 Surgical Procedure

1. Instruments preparation: Tian's spine osteotome set × 1, pedicle screw and rod system × 1, pedicle finder, Luque wire 0.8–1.2 mm diameter, Luque rods; and general instruments.

H. Tian (✉)
The Sixth Affiliated Hospital of Xinjiang Medical University, Urumqi, China

Z. Zhao · N. Bi
Department of Orthopedics, The 2nd Affiliated Hospital of Kunming Medical University, Kunming, China

H. Tian et al. (eds.), *Spinal Osteotomy Orthopaedics*, https://doi.org/10.1007/978-981-16-1387-6_4

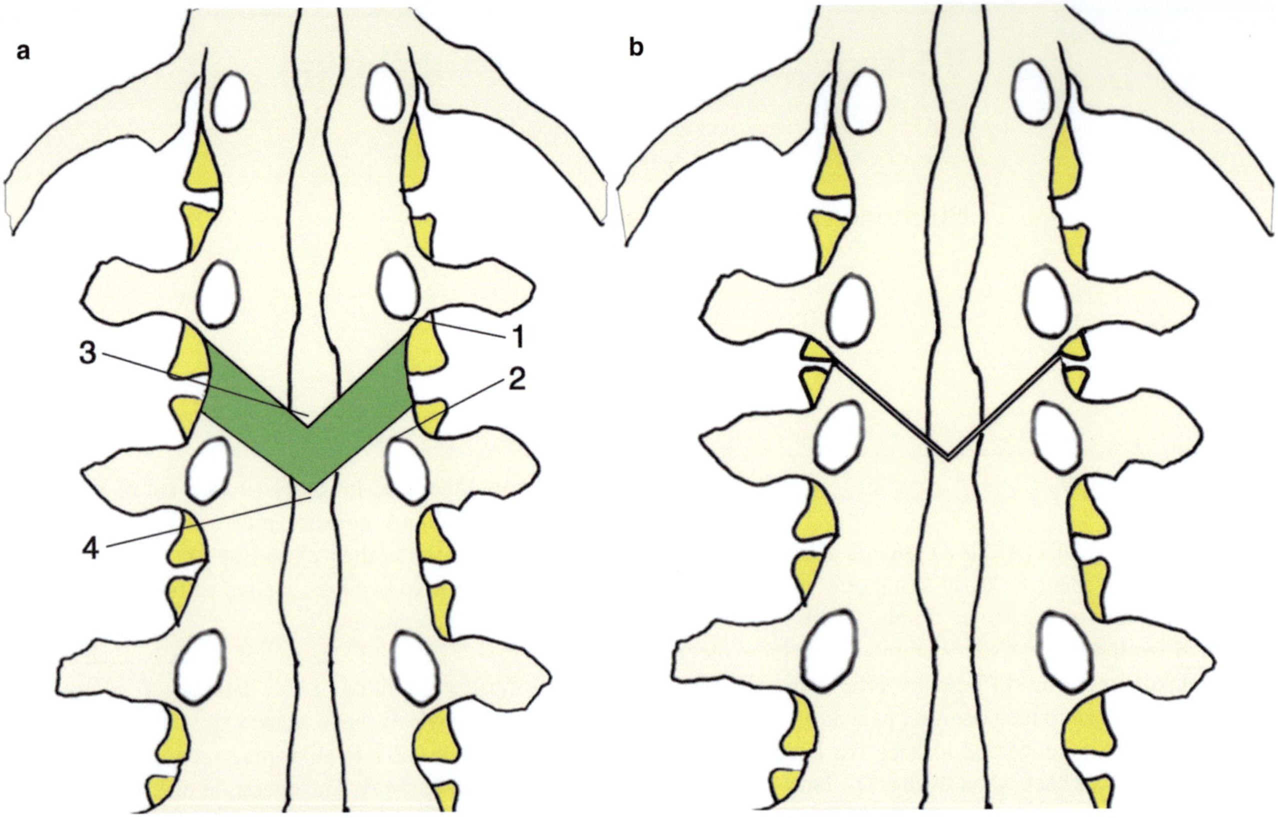

Fig. 4.1 (**a**) Schematic diagram of lamina V osteotomy. 1. Lower edge of pedicle; 2. Upper edge of pedicle; 3. Lower edge of spinous process; 4. Upper edge of the spinous process; Osteotomy width is 8–12 mm. (**b**) After the reduction and closure of the V-shaped lamina osteotomy, the cutter faces the cutter to form a V-shaped osteotomy line, which is tightly and neatly combined, stable and reliable, and creates good conditions for future bone fusion

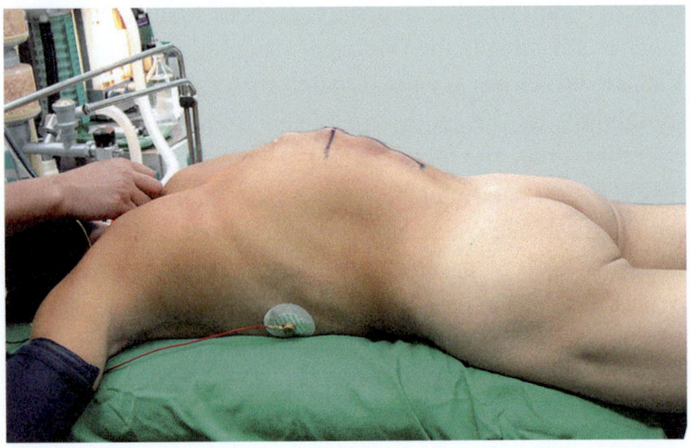

Fig. 4.2 Prone position for small kyphosis angle

2. Anesthesia: local infiltration anesthesia or general anesthesia with tracheal intubation.
3. Patients position: generally in prone position (Fig. 4.2). According to the degree of kyphosis of the patient, the operating table should be set into an inverted V shape. The waist bridge should be raised, and the shoulders should be raised with a special shoulder support cushion for severe kyphosis (Figs. 4.3 and 4.4). The head of the patient should be placed on the head frame that can be adjusted automatically, and the feet should be fixed on the end of the table. Pads should be used to fill the space under the ventral side thus after osteotomy the pads are to be removed or the table to be set flat to close the osteotomy site and straighten the trunk. Place the 10 cm wide traction bands made from sheets under the axilla. When the osteotomy is done, with the bands unscrubbed personnel will apply traction on the head and foot to straighten the trunk of the patient and close the osteotomy gap before applying internal fixation (Fig. 4.5).
4. Surgical procedure
   Step 1: Make a skin incision along the spinous process or midline of the back and dissect subcutaneous tissue. Dissect Supraspinal Ligament along the spinous process which are interconnected and ossified between adjacent levels. Elevate subperiosteumly along the spinous process and lamina bilaterally to the transverse process. The site and level of osteotomy are determined (Figs. 4.6 and 4.7) to get ready for lamina V-shape osteotomy (Figs. 4.8 and 4.9).

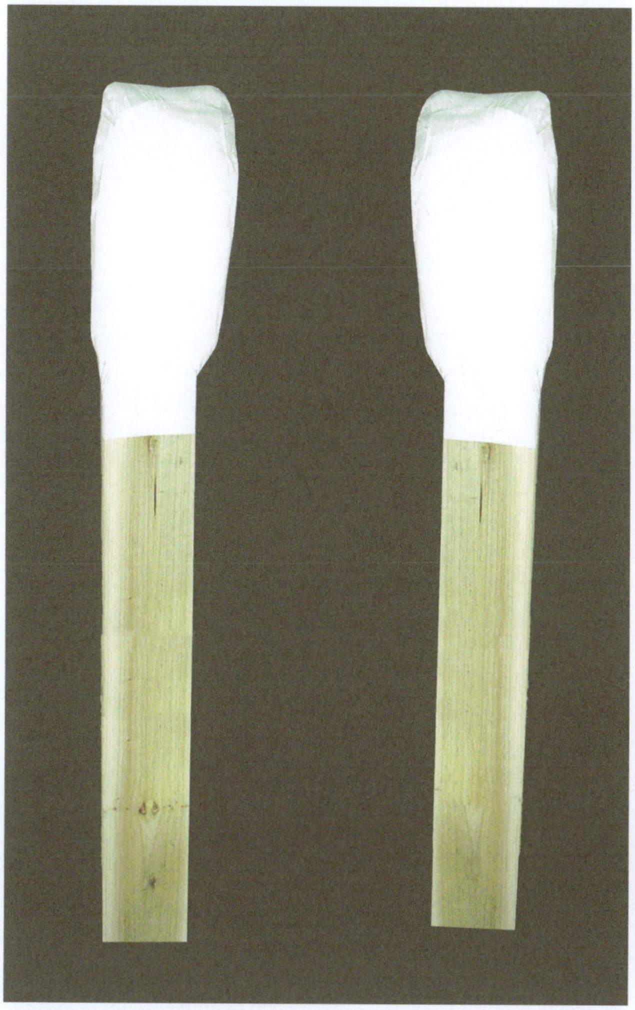

Fig. 4.3 Special shoulder cushion

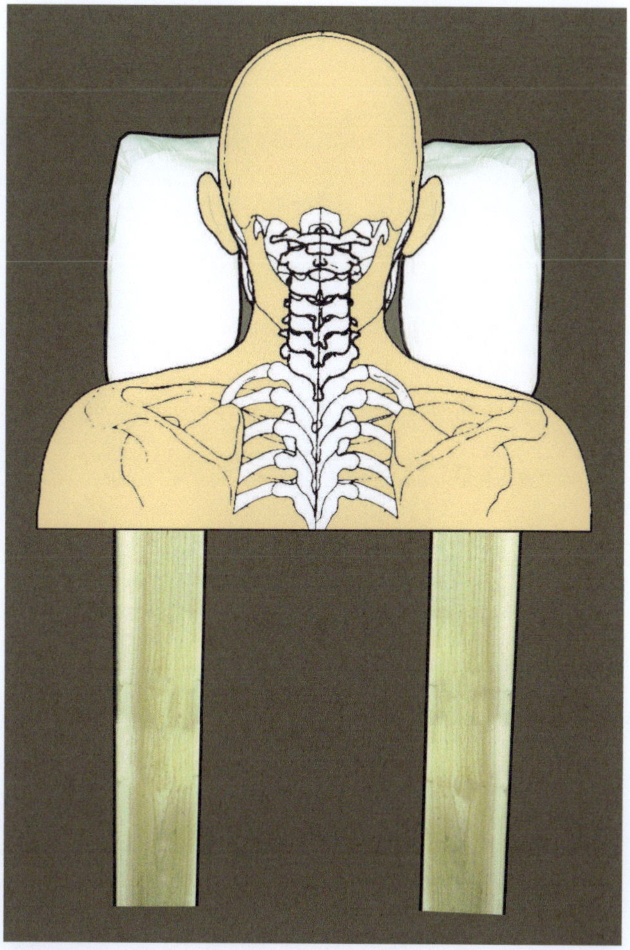

Fig. 4.4 Schematic diagram of raising two shoulders with special shoulder cushion

Step 2: The landmarks of the V osteotomy of the vertebral lamina include the superior and inferior margins of the intervertebral foramen for the lateral side, and between the two spinous processes next to the osteotomy site (see Fig. 4.1a). First, an osteotome is used to create an indentation marking V shape osteotomy on the lamina. According to the degree of kyphosis, the width of the osteotomy gap is determined. The width of the laminectomy is usually 8 ~ 12 mm, as 8 mm is the width of a small straight osteotome while 12 mm is the width of a large straight osteotome. If the osteotomy space is too narrow, carrying out the technique inside will be difficult. The direction of osteotomy is slightly toward the cranial, so that the lamina, once closed, may naturally form an overlapping structure (Figs. 4.10a, b and 4.11a, b).

Step 3: The whole process of osteotomy should be done with a thin blade osteotome. It is required to make a smooth cutting surface so that the osteotomy gap is to be closed seamlessly. Blunt osteotome or rongeur, which makes the cutting surface rough and irregular and difficult to approximate, should be avoided, otherwise there is a higher risk of non-union. The ossified interspinal ligament is transected with a wide straight osteotome to access the plane of the lamina (Fig. 4.12). The two lateral ends of "V" are created upward and outward (Fig. 4.13). The direction is from the interspinous process to the neural foramen, and the width is 8–12 mm (Fig. 4.14). The superior edge of the osteotomy line is the inferior edge of the pedicle of the upper level, while the inferior edge is the superior edge of the pedicle of the lower level (see Fig. 4.1a).

Step 4: The osteotomy is performed with a wide thin-bladed straight osteotome. The V-shape gap on the right side is made first, followed by the left side. The width is set to 8 mm (Fig. 4.15). The depth is from the posterior cortex of the lamina to the medial cortex (Fig. 4.16). The site is cleaned with a shovel cutter until the inner cortex of the lamina is exposed (Figs. 4.17 and 4.18). From the interspinous part, the inner cortex is excised to expose the

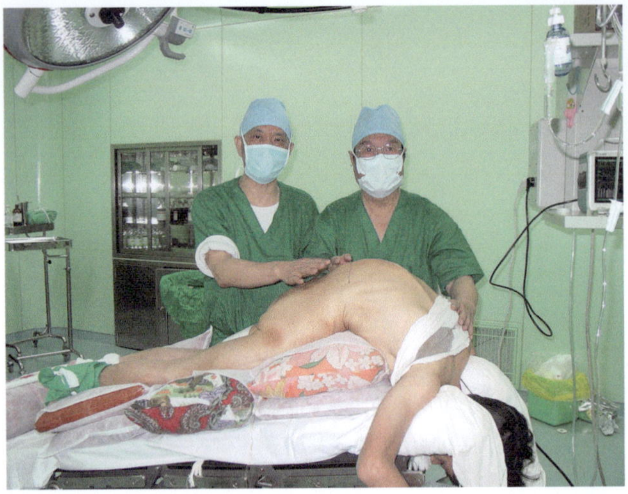

Fig. 4.5 A patient with severe kyphosis was put into a prone position. Shoulder cushions were padded well to hold the shoulders so that the head of the patient was out of the table and stayed below, and the forehead on the orange which can be adjusted automatically. The table was set to an inverted V shape. The abdomen and the anterior superior iliac spine were cushioned firmly, and fix the feet at the end of the table with bandages to prevent the patient from sliding forward. The traction band is placed under the axilla for traction after the osteotomy was completed

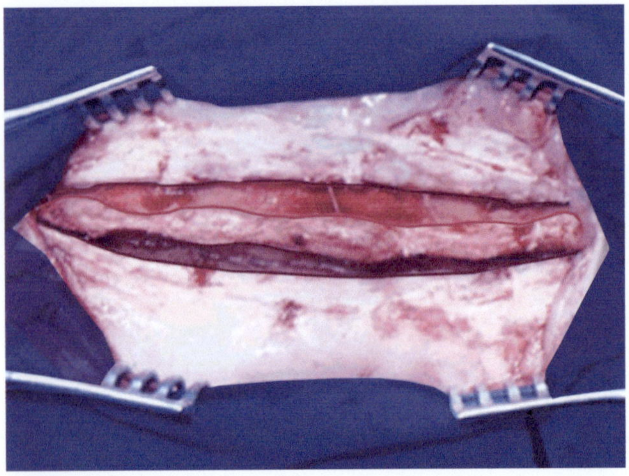

Fig. 4.6 Make a longitudinal incision along the spinous processes, preserve the ossified and ankylosing spinous processes and lamina for final internal fixation

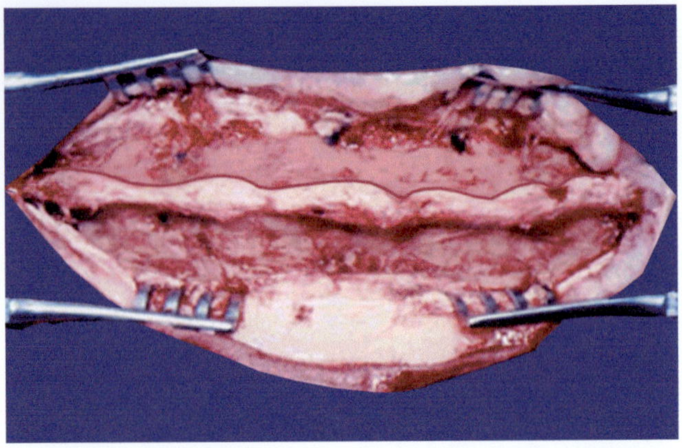

Fig. 4.7 Elevate the periosteum on lamina bilaterally to the tip of the transverse process to select the level of osteotomy

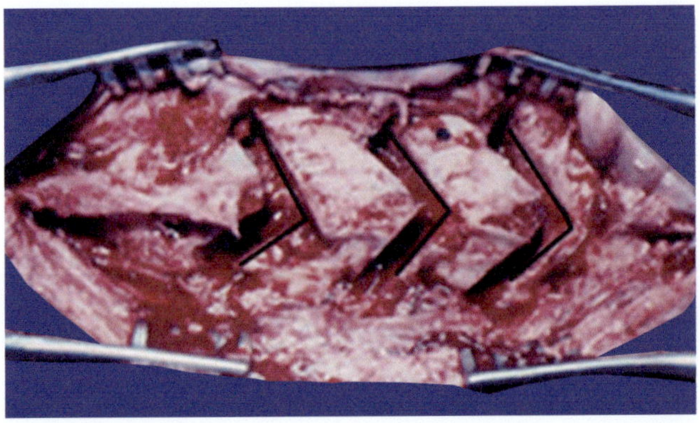

Fig. 4.8 After V-shape osteotomies of three levels were completed, the osteotomy gap was automatically closed to a certain extent

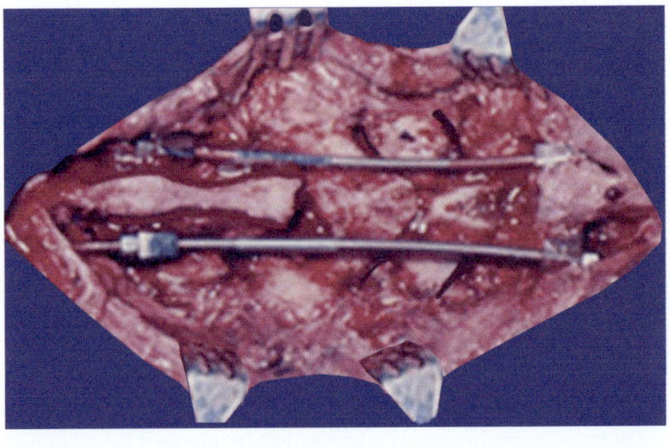

Fig. 4.9 After manual correction, the osteotomy gap was completely closed and fixed with a hook rod system

dura mater (Fig. 4.19), and separate the adhesion between the lamina and the dura mater with a nerve elevator. Then the inner bone cortex is cut through on both sides with an osteotome (Fig. 4.20). The bone chip is clamped out with a nucleus pulposus forceps. Cautions should be used in the step to avoid injury of epidural venous plexus causing hemorrhage or injury of dura mater and arachnoid causing CSF leak. In addition, it is important to remove the deep free bone debris near the intervertebral foramen (Fig. 4.21) to avoid pain caused by nerve root impingement after reduction. When the first side is done, a distractor or a self-made block is placed into the osteotomy gap (Fig. 4.22) to achieve proper distraction. Osteotomy on the other side is performed in the same way. Without

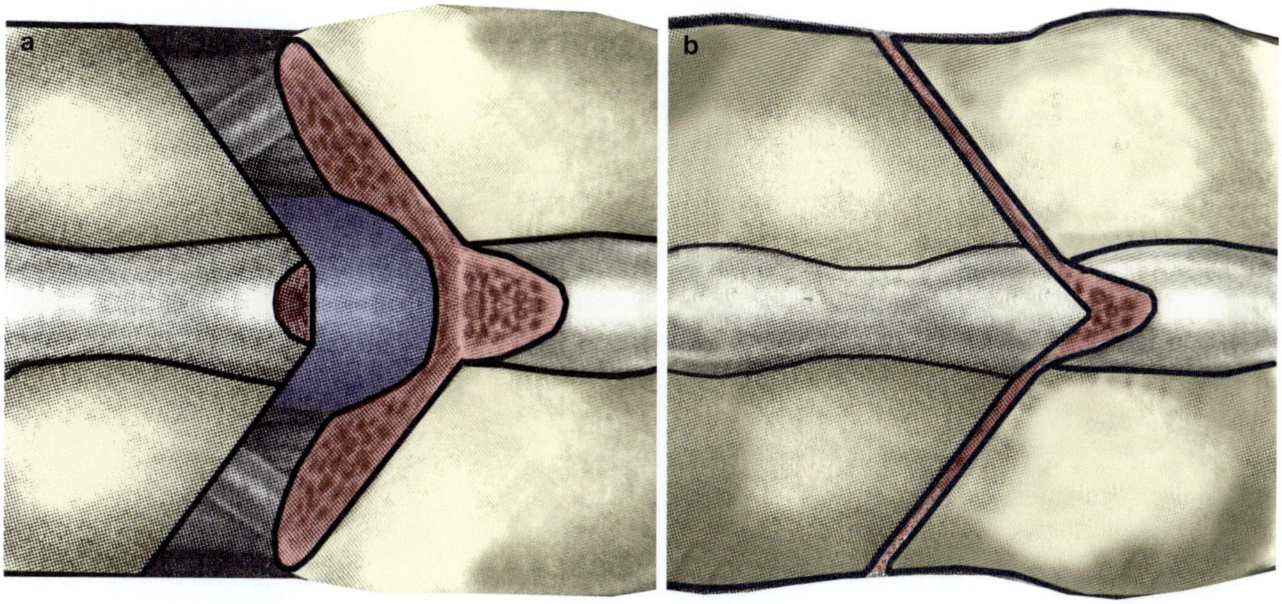

Fig. 4.10 V-shape lamina osteotomy A. V-shape osteotomy is oriented cranial. A sharp and thin osteotome should be used to make a smooth cutting surface so that the gap is to be tightly reduced, which is conducive to bone fusion. B. Once the V-shape osteotomy gap is reduced, the osteotomy surface forms an overlapping, which prevents lateral displacement. The reason is that the cancellous-on-cancellous interface has high healing potential

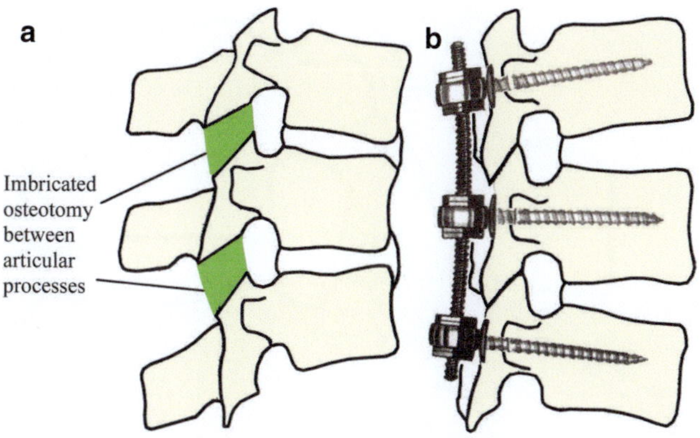

Fig. 4.11 V-shape overlapping osteotomy between multi-segmental articular processes. (**a**) Lateral view, the width of the overlapping osteotomy between multi-segmental articular processes should not exceed 8 mm. (**b**) Close and internal fixation after overlapping osteotomy

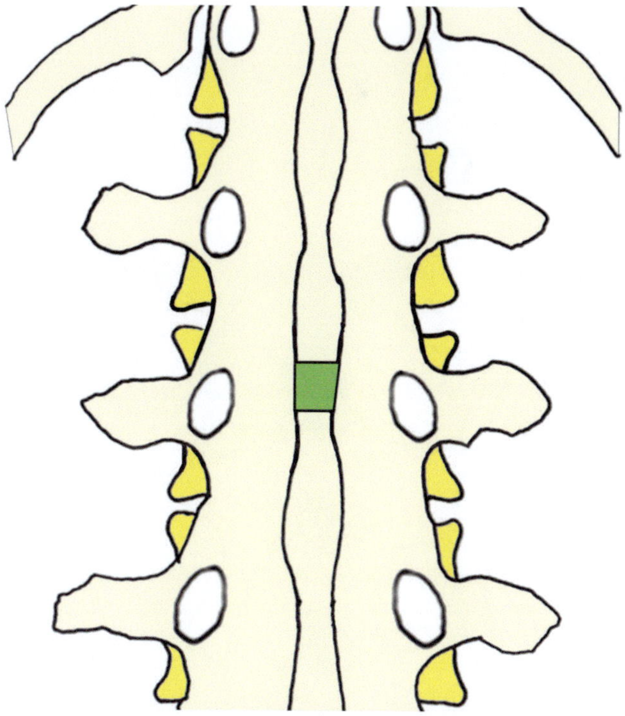

Fig. 4.12 In the center of V-shaped osteotomy, the ossified spinous process and interspinal ligament are firstly resected with a straight osteotome for 8–12 mm to access the level of the lamina

distraction by distractor or self-made block, osteotomy gap will often close by itself after both sides are done, which makes bottoming out and cleaning of remaining free bone debris difficult. After the osteotomy is completed, remove the distractor, lower the waist support, adjust the inverted V-shape bed into a flatbed, and the osteotomy gap often closes by itself to form an overlapping closure. Or the gap may be slightly compressed to close. The bone removed is shaped into a matchstick and put on top of the osteotomy gap (Fig. 4.23a, b).

Step 5: Internal fixation is chosen according to the need. For severe kyphosis, long instrumentation with a pedicles screw system is required (see Fig. 4.23). For mild kyphosis, short instrumentation with pedicles screw system, Luque rod plus wiring between spinous processes

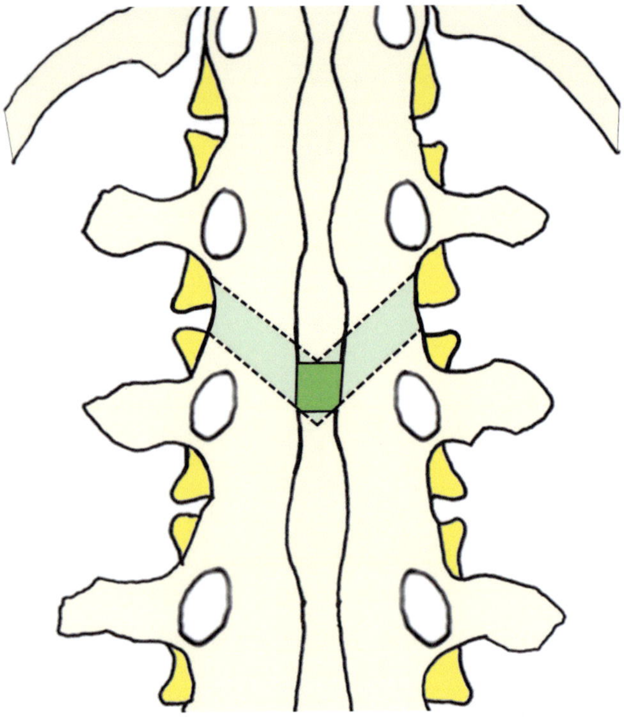

Fig. 4.13 Extend upward and outward to the intervertebral foramen and create the two ends of the V shape with a width of 8 ~ 12 mm

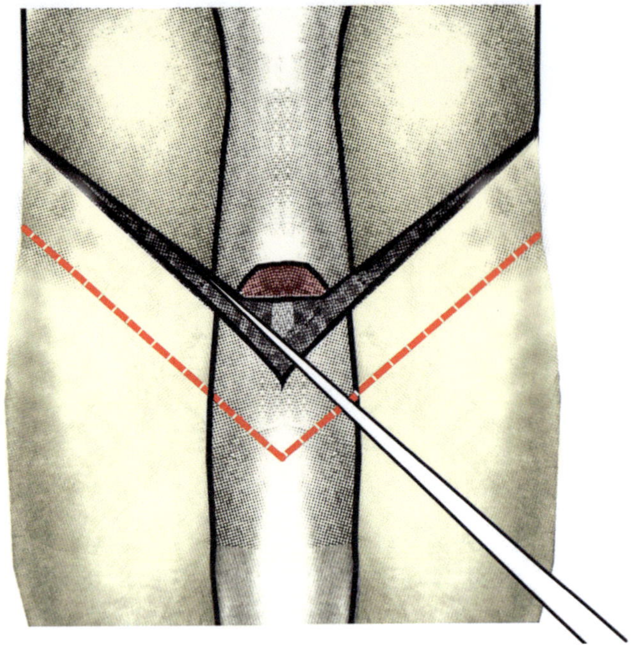

Fig. 4.15 Perform a V-shaped osteotomy with a wide straight osteotome, first on the right side and then on the left side

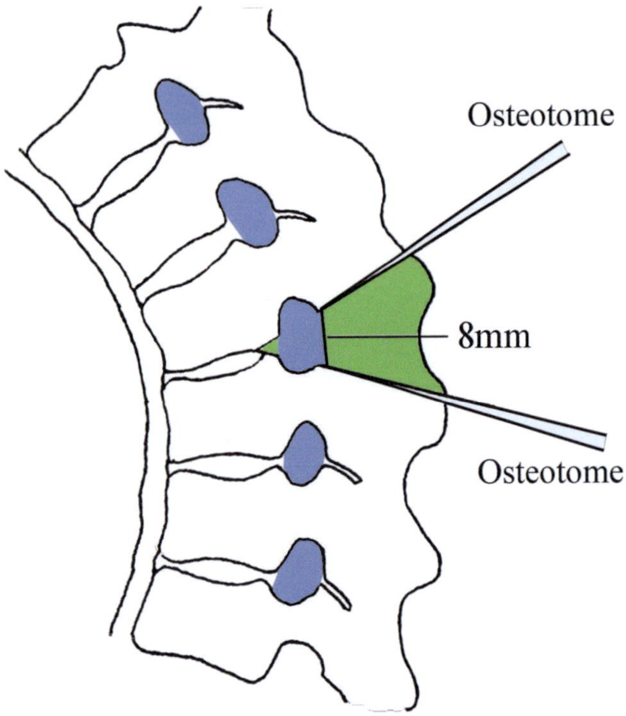

Fig. 4.14 The width of V-shaped laminectomy is 8–12 mm

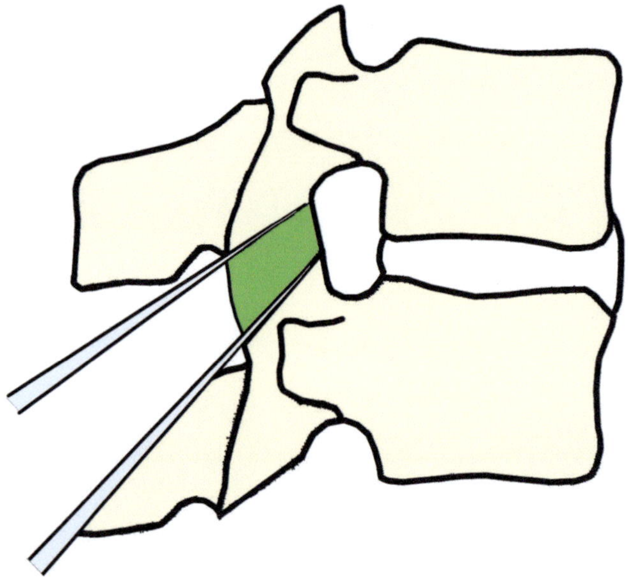

Fig. 4.16 The depth of V-shaped osteotomy is from the posterior lamina to the inner bone cortex, but not beyond

(Fig. 4.24), wiring between spinous processes (Fig. 4.25), or just external immobilization of plaster vest without internal fixation to achieve spinal stability and bone fusion.

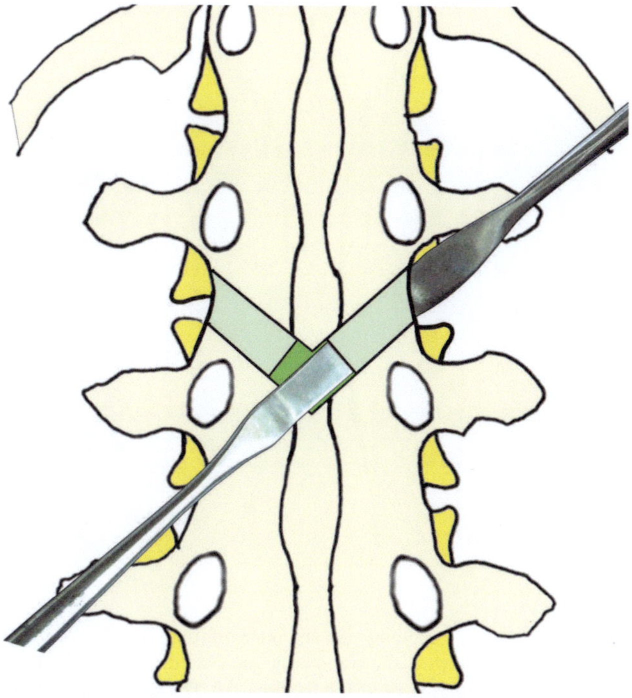

Fig. 4.17 The bone tissue between the spinous processes is excised first, and then the nerve elevator is used to dissect from lateral of neural foramen toward medial and pack with gauze. Then, the bottom is cleared with a shovel cutter to reach the inner cortex of the lamina

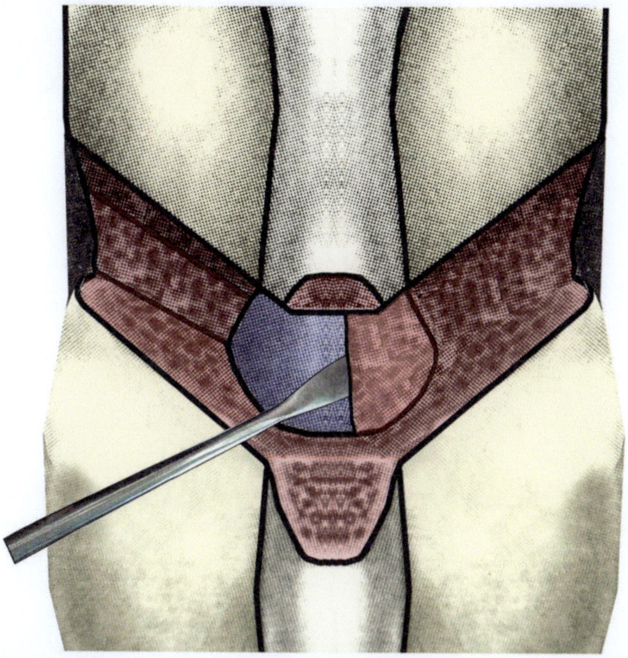

Fig. 4.18 Laminectomy between spinous processes, remove ligamentum flavum, expose dura mater and separate epidural adhesions by nerve elevator

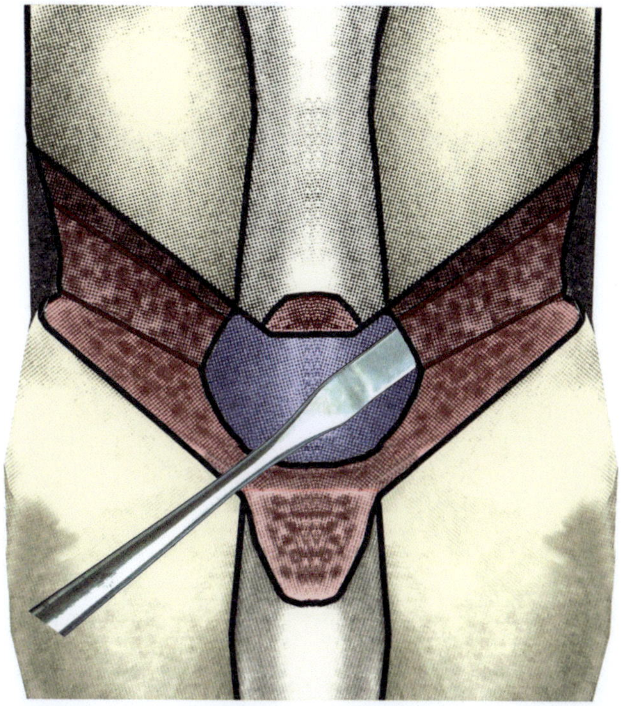

Fig. 4.19 Bottom out with a shovel, leaving only the inner cortex

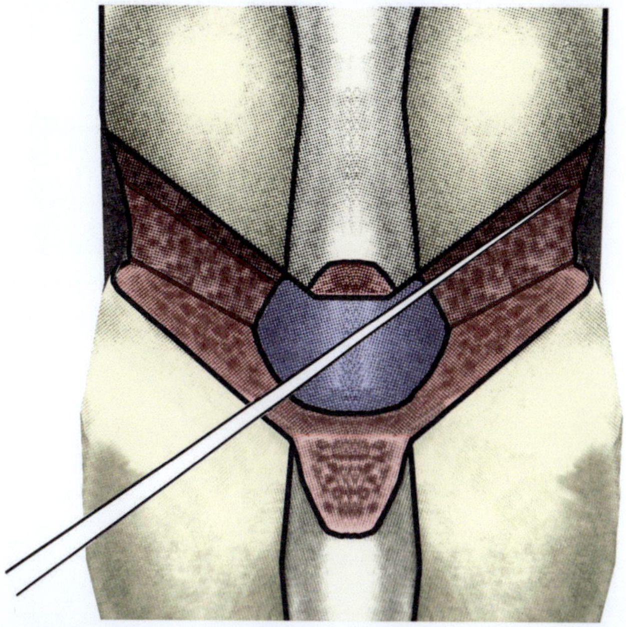

Fig. 4.20 Cut through the inner bone cortex with osteotome, but pay great attention not to injure the dura mater and avoid CSF leakage

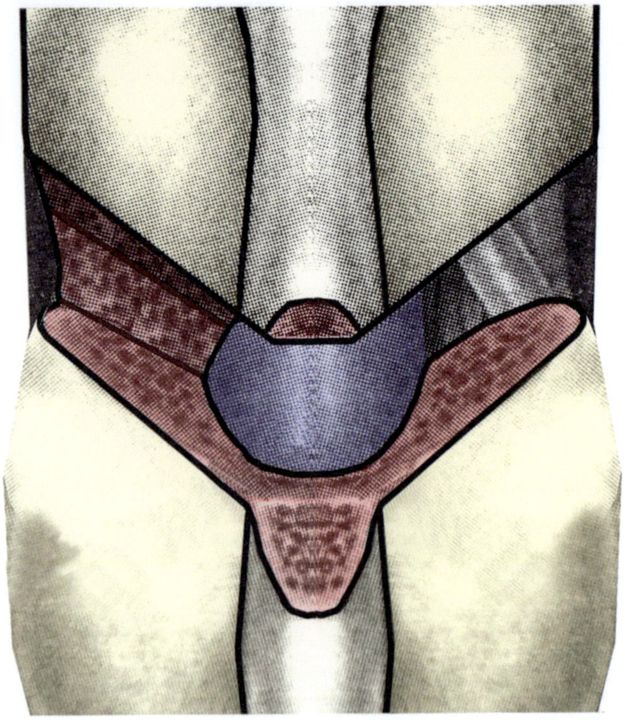

Fig. 4.21 The inter cortex of the right lamina has been removed, the dural sac and nerves are thoroughly exposed, and the deep fragments have been removed

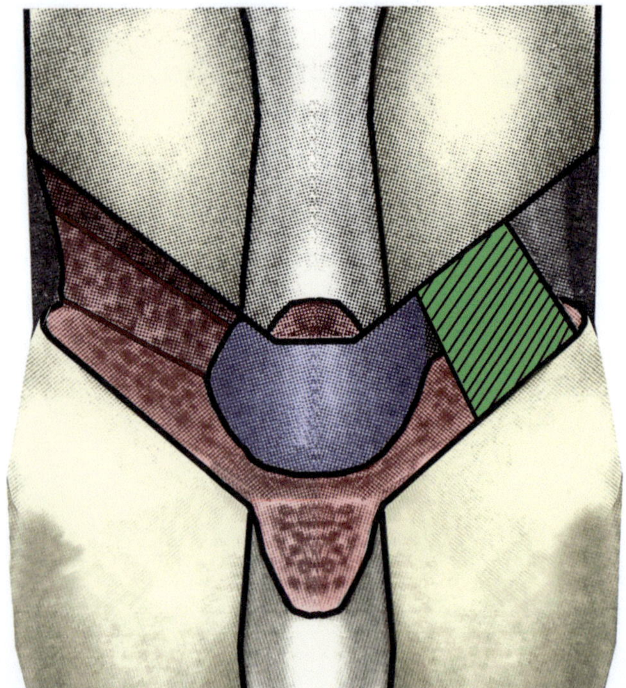

Fig. 4.22 After the osteotomy on the right side, distract the space with a blocker before repeating the osteotomy on the left side

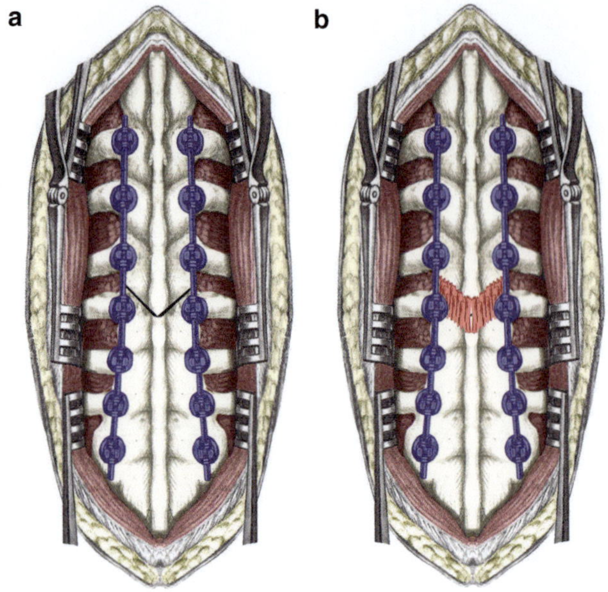

Fig. 4.23 Closing osteotomy gap and bone grafting. (a) After V-shape osteotomy is completed, the osteotomy gap closed smoothly and the pedicle screw system is used for fixation. (b) The bone resected are shaped as matchsticks and put on top of the osteotomy gap

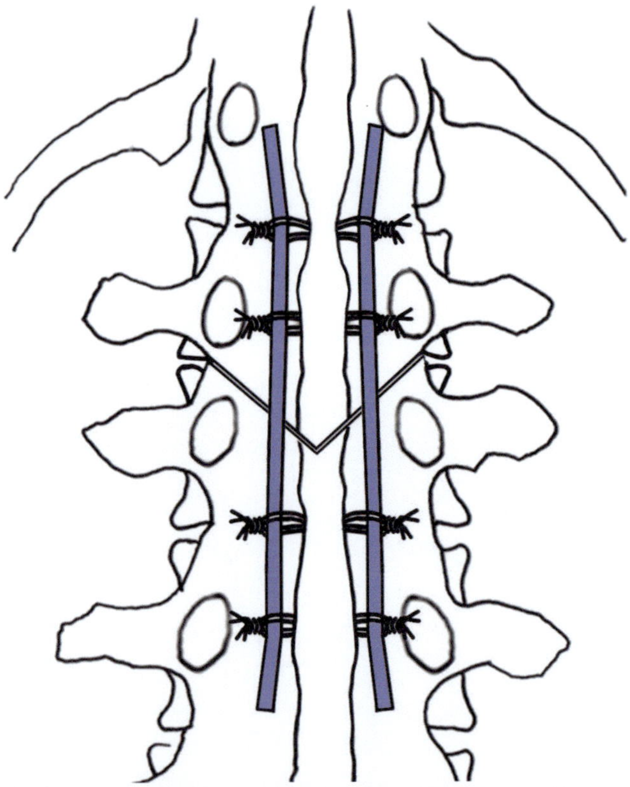

Fig. 4.24 Dynamic compression internal fixation: Luque rod plus steel wiring between the spinous processes can allow sliding between the Luque rod and the wire, and can produce self-correction when returning to the ward supine position after surgery

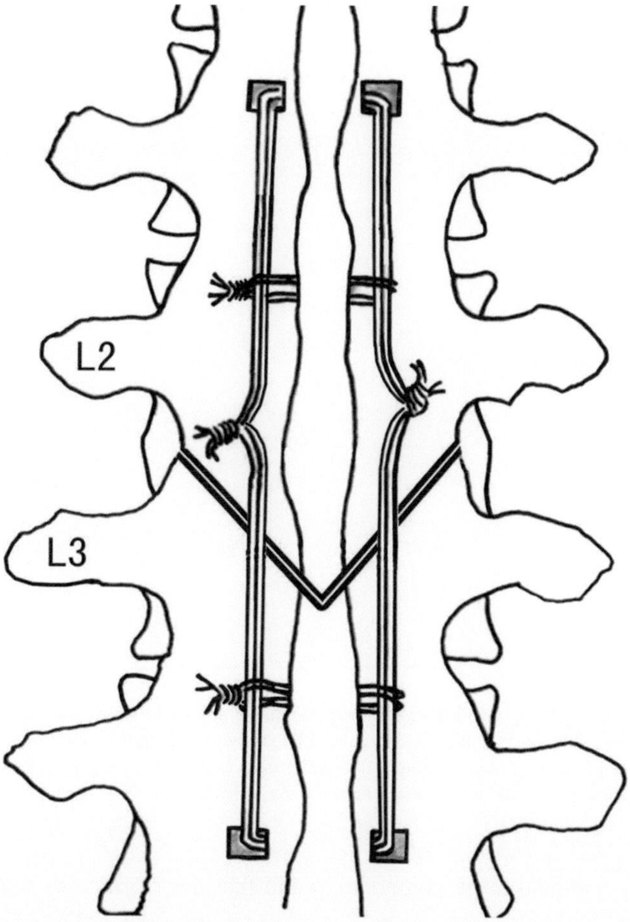

Fig. 4.25 After closing V-shape osteotomy, interspinous wiring for self-correction after operation

Step 6: To finish the procedure, remove the muscle retractor, thoroughly electrocoagulate hemostasis, place T-tube for drainage bilaterally and close by layers.

5. Postoperative management

Upon closure, a negative pressure drainage tube is placed on each side of the spinous process for negative pressure drainage after the patient is returned to the ward. A drainage tube is removed in 24–48 h, suture stitches are removed on Day 10. A plaster vest is given for external immobilization upon suture removal and maintained after discharge. In 3 months, patients should have more bed rest and less mobilization. However, patients should still mobilize joints of limbs to avoid hip or shoulder ankylosis. After 3 months, patients are encouraged to have more ambulation and outdoor activity. Patients should come back for follow-up in 6–8 months. The surgeon should decide whether to remove the plaster. After removing the plaster, X-rays should be taken to observe the healing of the bone graft.

4.3 Key Points and Precautions

1. The width and depth of osteotomy should be well controlled to avoid overcorrection or undercorrection. According to the angle of kyphotic deformity, the width of laminectomy is generally 8–12 mm.
2. It is critical to prevent the contact and friction between the instrument and the dura during operation. Repeated friction of the instrument on the dura will cause irreversible spinal cord injury.
3. Resecting lamina with a lamina rongeur bears the highest risk as the jaw of the rongeur always is always too thick for this procedure. When inserting under the lamina for biting the bone, there is a possibility of squeezing the dura mater and spinal cord. Secondly, the forceps of the rongeur may bite a very small part of the dura mater, causing dural tear and the complication of cerebrospinal fluid leakage, which brings great pain to the patient after the operation. The osteotomy surface made with the lamina rongeur is not as smooth as that made with the osteotome.
4. After osteotomy is completed on one side, a distractor or a self-made block must be placed in the osteotomy gap for proper distraction, and osteotomy on the other side with the same technique. Without the distractor or self-made block, the osteotomy gap often closes after osteotomy on both sides, which causes difficulty in bottoming out and makes it difficult to remove the remaining bone debris.
5. According to the magnitude of kyphosis angle, V-shape osteotomy can be done for 1–3 levels. The width of laminectomy is usually 8–12 mm.
6. Interspinous dynamic compression and internal fixation: it is suitable for cases with Cobb angle less than 90°. As the spinous processes, interspinous ligament and supraspinal ligament of patients of ankylosing spondylitis are the first to ossify, there forms a wide and thick longitudinal bone wall, which has a thicker and stronger bony structure than the spinous process of the general population, and is very suitable for using it for internal fixation with double Luque rod and wiring technique. This technique is simple and effective and is better than after biting the spinous process. Internal fixation with a screw–rod system is more mechanically effective. Especially double Luque rod plus wiring technique can allow the rod to slide longitudinally under the control of wire loops, without hindering the self-correction produced by the patient when lying in the flatbed after surgery with opening in anterior and close in posterior. This is the greatest advantage of Interspinous dynamic internal fixation. Its effect will last until the corrected spine is maintained by external immobilization with an overextended plaster vest, resulting in a solid osseous fusion.

7. Static pedicle screw system-internal fixation: suitable for severe ASK cases with Cobb angle above 90°. Such patients have developed severe kyphosis, high contracture of soft tissues involving rectus abdominis, mesentery, and vascular nerve tissue are also shortened in tension. To correct this deformity, spine shortening surgery is required to resect 1–2 vertebrae, open the anterior, close the posterior and apply a pedicle screw system. Rigid static internal fixation is indispensable for such patients, while strut grafting, autogenous bone grafting on lamina, and postoperative external immobilization are also critical points.
8. No internal fixation replaces the role of external immobilization. Thus, external immobilization with plaster vest or brace is indispensable after operation. The duration should not be less than 6–8 months; otherwise, there is a possibility of deformity recurrence.

4.4 Typical Case Presentation

4.4.1 Case Summary

Patient Chen X, male, 32 years old, businessman of Tianhe District, Guangzhou City. Chief complaint: at the age of 20, he developed lower back pain and general weakness. Symptoms were attenuated during the day while the pain stopped the patient from sleeping at night. He often sat up in bed throughout the night. He was extremely tired after getting up early the next morning, slightly relieved after activity, and sweated a lot. After 25 years of age, the pain was slightly improved, but the kyphosis of the back began to appear and progressed. In the last 2 years, deep grooves were found in the upper abdomen, collapsed, and the abdomen bulged forward (Figs. 4.26 and 4.27a, b). These symptoms affect breathing, with dyspnea, stomach distention, and loss of appetite. The hunchback deformity was still progressing and the patient was not able to sleep in a supine position at night (Fig. 4.28).

4.4.2 Diagnosis

Examination after admission: The patient was a 32-year-old male with acceptable nutritional status, stooping and hunched when standing, and had to bend knees and hips to achieve a horizontal gaze. A deep groove was formed in the upper abdomen, and the lower ribs were inserted into the abdominal cavity. The abdomen bulges forward, causing difficulty in breathing and eating. The patient asked for surgery to correct the deformity. X-ray examination showed that the Cobbs angle of kyphosis was 81°, the lower ribs were inserted into the abdominal cavity, the upper abdominal organs were compressed, and the lower orifice of the thoracic cage was rested on the spine to affect abdominal breathing. This deformity caused serious effects on the respiratory, circulatory, and digestive systems. With the patient's firm request for surgical treatment, we decided to prepare for surgery and perform preoperative prone posture training (Fig. 4.29).

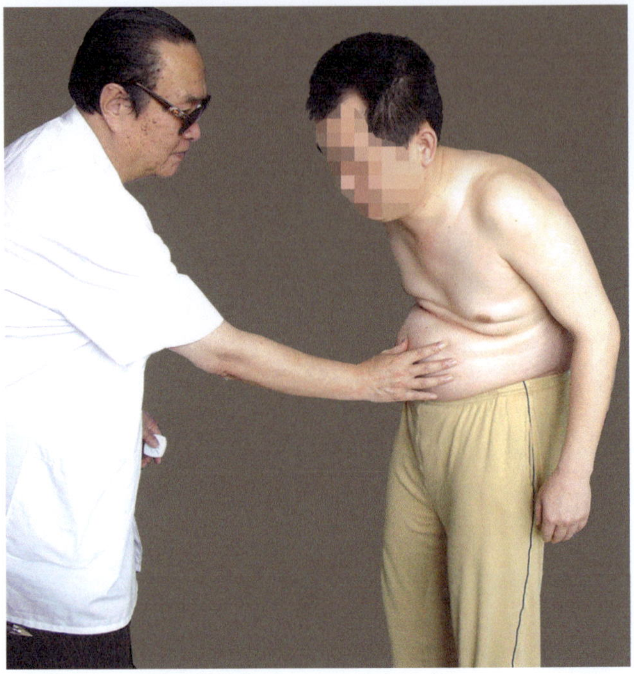

Fig. 4.26 The Cobb's angle of Ankylosing spondylitis kyphosis was 81°. The upper abdomen formed a deep groove invagination. Both sides of the ribs were inserted into the abdominal cavity, the abdomen bulged forward, so that abdominal breathing was affected

4.4.3 Surgical Plan and Postoperative Management

1. Operation Plan: It is planned to perform V-shape laminectomy under general anesthesia with tracheal intubation. The osteotomy site was between L2–3, not on the apex. The width of the osteotomy was estimated to be 1.0 cm. After the V-shape osteotomy is completed, the gap was closed by manual reduction followed by internal fixation with wiring between spinous processes to achieve self-correction and then plaster vest immobilization.
2. Surgical technique: Please refer to Section II Surgical Technique for details.
3. Postoperative treatment: When kyphosis is corrected by osteotomy, the patient can fully lie flat in bed (Fig. 4.30), with free movement of lower limbs

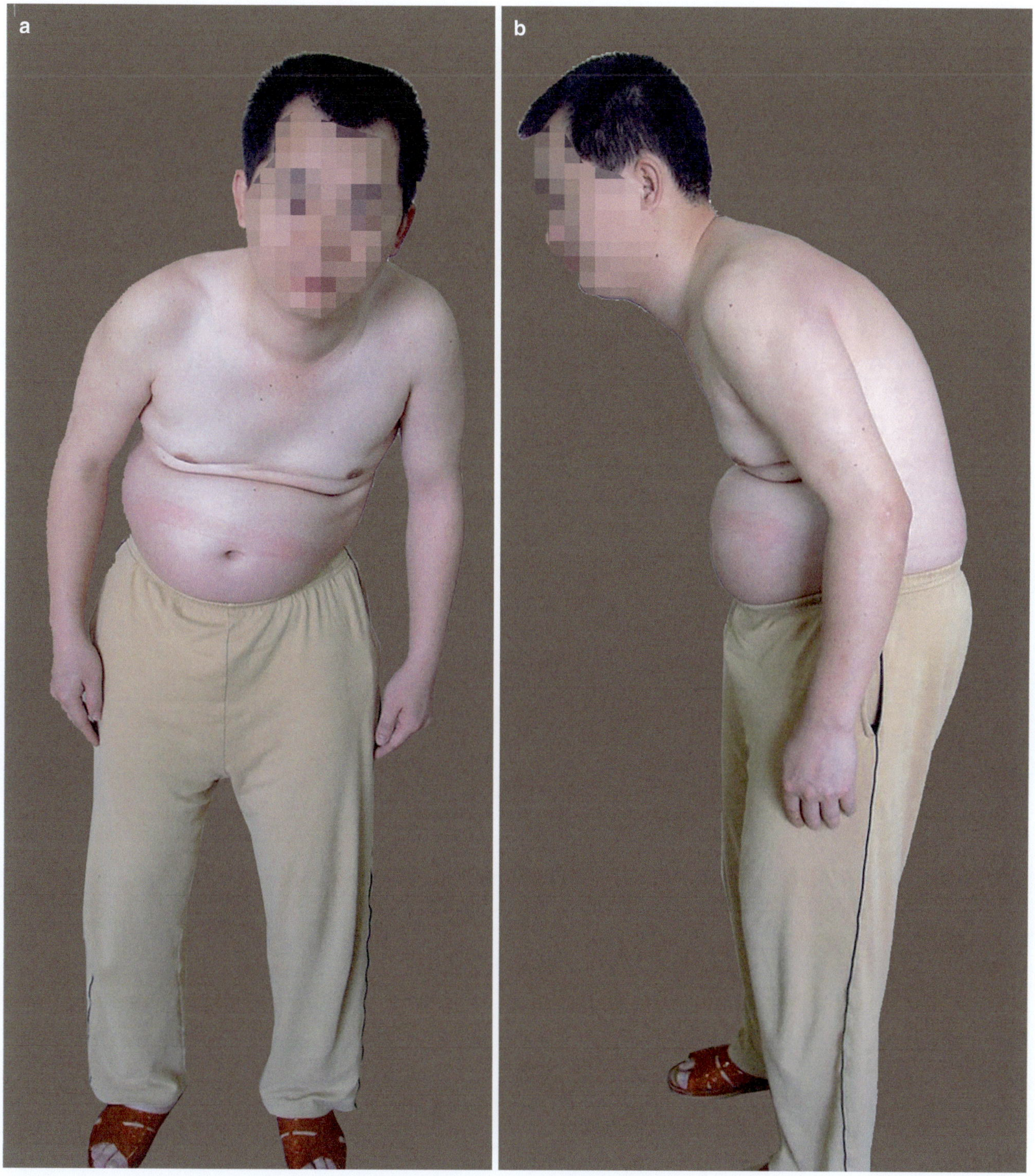

Fig. 4.27 Frontal and lateral view appearance before and after surgery

(Fig. 4.31). The preoperative deep recess of the upper abdomen has been flattened. The shining part in the photo used to be the recess now unfolded (Fig. 4.32). The distance from the xiphoid to the pubic symphysis was increased by 8 cm (Fig. 4.33). Within 3 weeks after the operation, self-correction in the flatbed worked well. More lying led to more straightening, and finally, the trunk was fully extended. Upon stitch removal and plaster vest applied, the patient regained full ambulation (Fig. 4.34a–c).

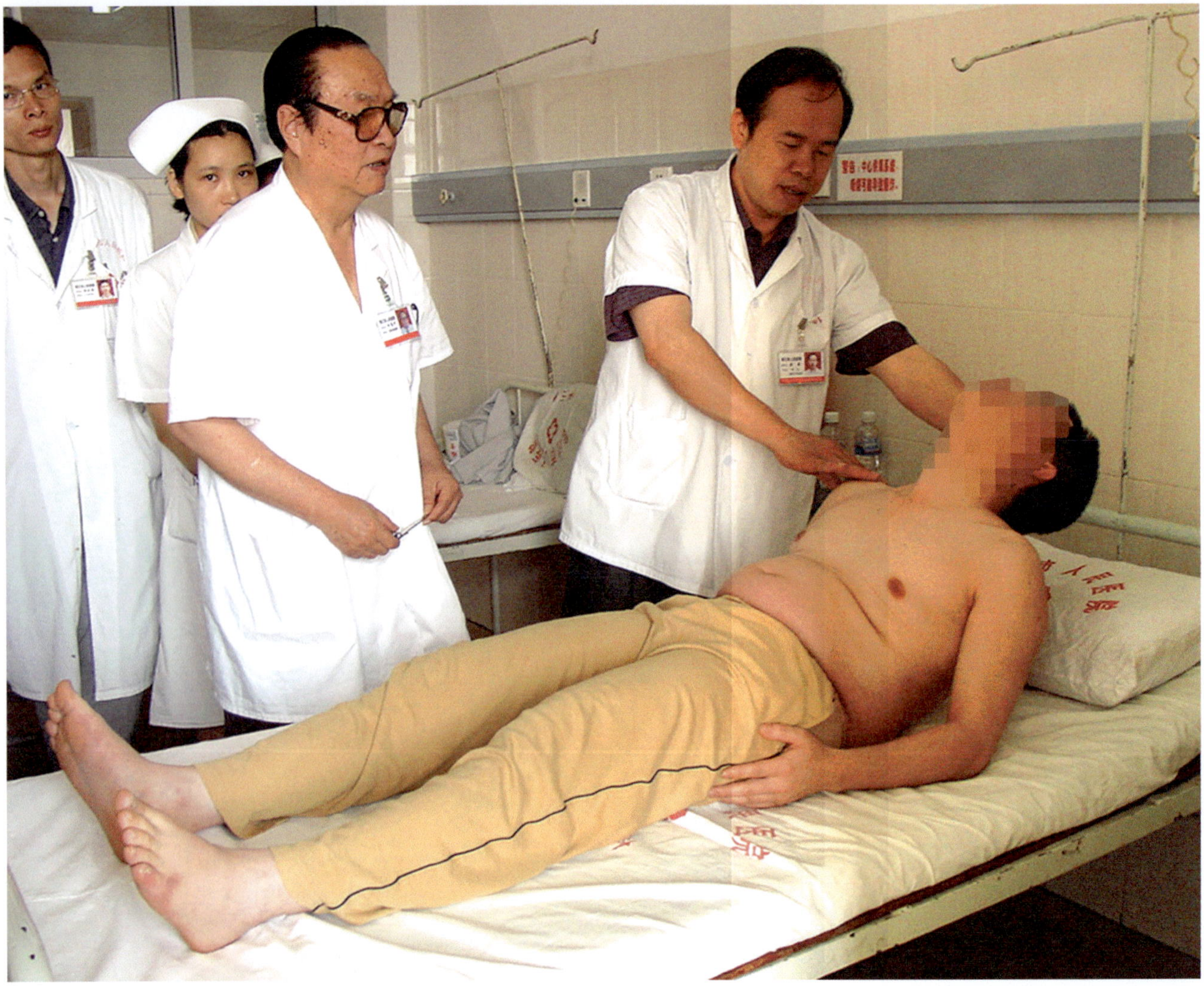

Fig. 4.28 Before the operation, the patient was not able to lie on his back. The distance between his head and pillow was more than 15 cm

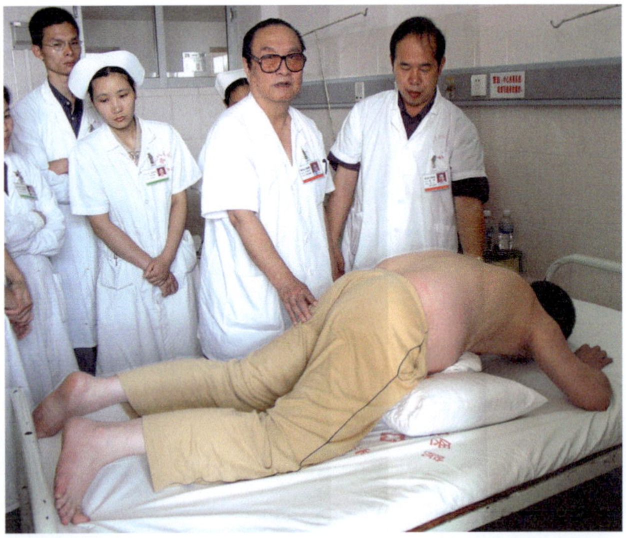

Fig. 4.29 Training of patients in surgical position (prone) before operation

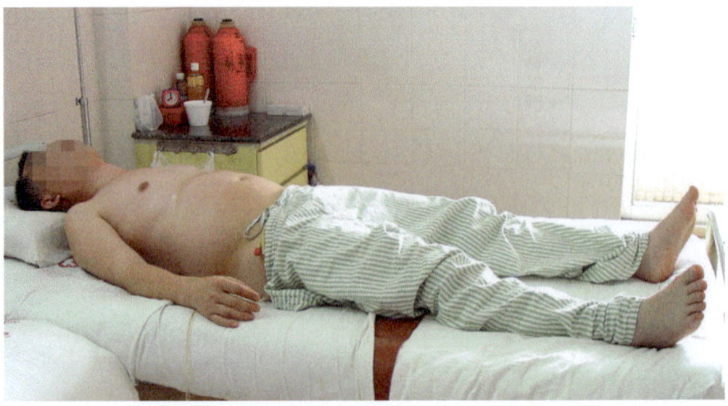

Fig. 4.30 The patient was able to lie flat immediately after surgery

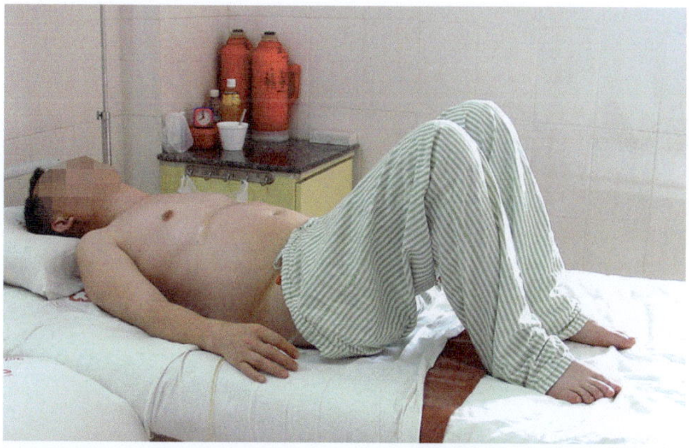

Fig. 4.31 Self-correction in flatbed with free movement of both legs

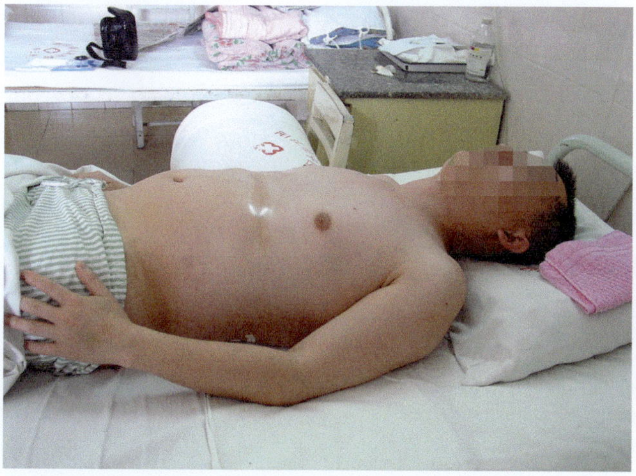

Fig. 4.32 The deep recess of the upper abdomen flattened after operation, and the shining part was the original deep recess

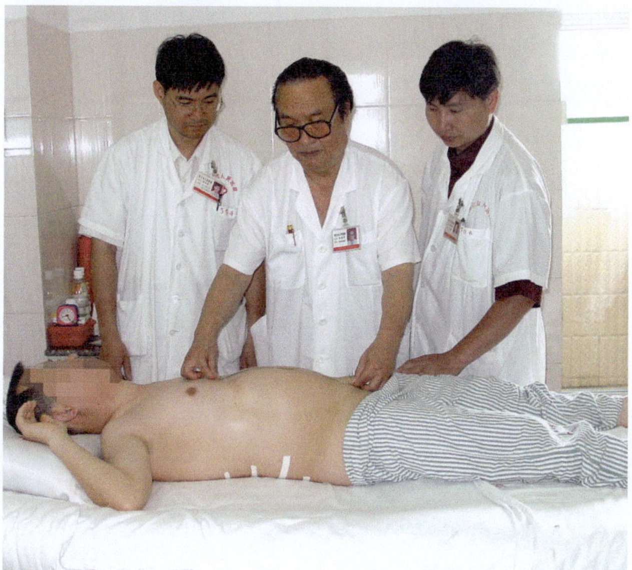

Fig. 4.33 Measuring the distance from the xiphoid to the pubic symphysis increased by 8 cm versus preoperative

4. Postoperative follow-up: 1.5 year follow-up (Fig. 4.35a, b). Two-year X-ray film follow-up (Fig. 4.36), the patient started his business in Guangzhou, and took a photo with Professor Tian during follow-up (Fig. 4.37).

4.4.4 Outcome Evaluation

Outcome evaluation of typical cases of non-apical vertebral osteotomy: Mr. Chen's kyphotic deformity had a Cobbs angle of 81°. The apical vertebra was in the lower thoracic spine. The clinical manifestations include groove like groove recess of the upper abdomen, compression of upper abdominal organs, difficulty in eating, poor appetite, and impaired abdominal breathing. To solve the above conditions, non-apical osteotomy between L2 and L3 was the most sensible choice. After correction of kyphosis deformity by non-apical osteotomy between L2 and L3, the diaphragm did not contract vertically anymore and abdominal breathing was restored to improve hypoxia. Once upper abdomen compression was lifted, gastrointestinal tract was improved, the general condition of patients, nutrition, breathing was smooth and mental state were significantly improved. Owing to the correction of kyphosis, the center of gravity was moved back, while gait and walking stability obviously improved. The patient was very satisfied with the operation, returned to normal work, and carried forward his business.

4.4.5 Expert Comments

In patient Chen X, the main symptom of ASK is a horizontal deep recess in the upper abdomen caused by kyphosis deformity. The ribs on both sides are inserted into the abdominal cavity. The lower orifice of the thoracic cage was resting on the spine, which compromised abdominal breathing, compresses the stomach, affects appetite, causing harm to digestion and food intake.

Non-apical simple laminectomy was chosen because the anterior margin of the vertebral body was not ossified, the superior-inferior diameter of the intervertebral foramen was larger, and the intervertebral space was wider than the apex level. Therefore, after osteotomy, the gap was closed automatically. Simple interspinous wiring alone was sufficient to maintain the correction of kyphosis, while postoperative self-correction in supine bed rest produced further correction effect. Conversely, if the osteotomy method was not properly selected or the osteotomy was not thoroughly performed, a long-segment pedicle screw system instrumentation, despite its reduction force, would be difficult to achieve the goal of true correction of kyphosis deformity. Therefore, osteotomy is the critical step in treating ASK. Internal fixation technique should be adaptive to the different osteotomy tech-

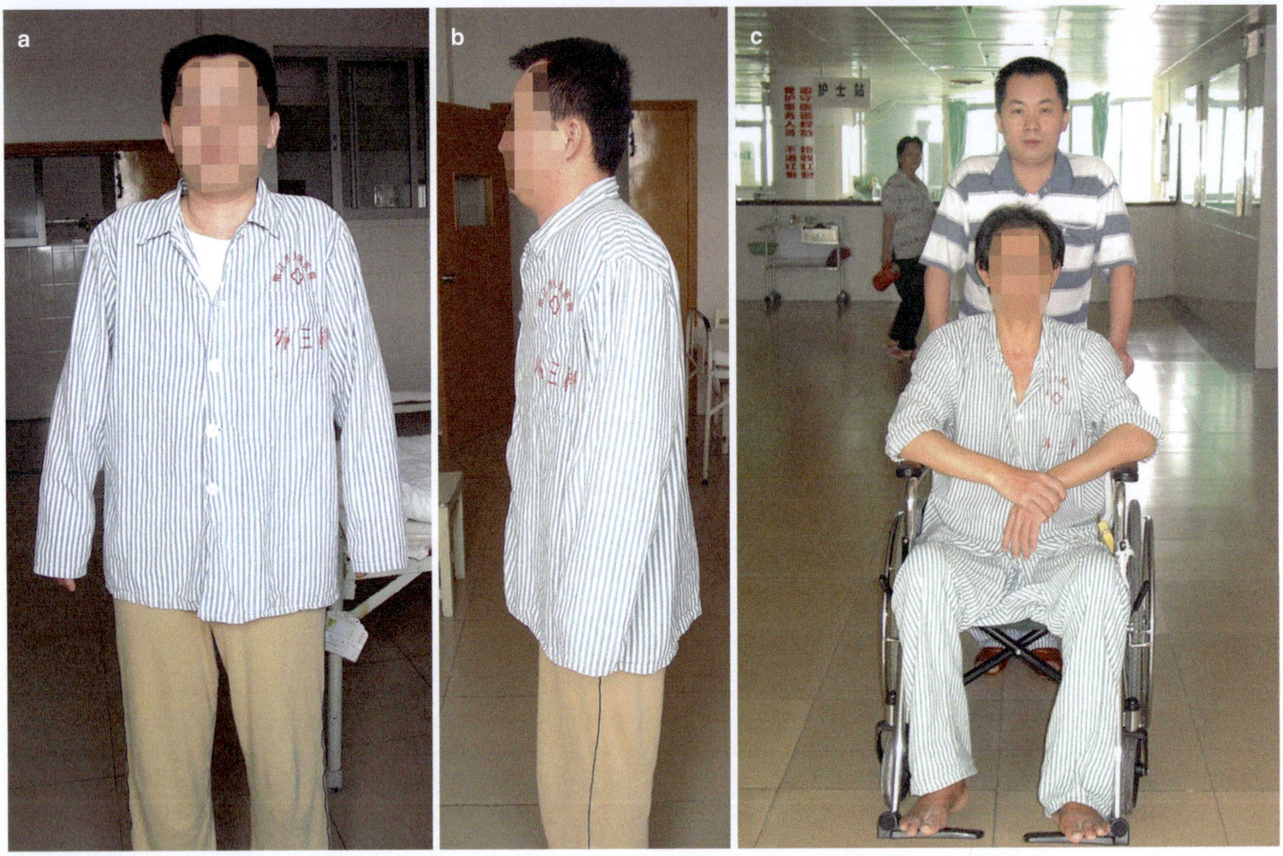

Fig. 4.34 The patient walked with a plaster vest, refreshed and delighted. 22 cm height gain. (**a**, **b**) Frontal and lateral view of postoperative plaster vest application; (**c**) the patient moved other patients around as an exercise postoperatively

niques. It is not always sensible to use a pedicle screw system for rigid internal fixation, as the rigid pedicle screw system prevents self-correction from happening after surgery.

Static internal fixation, dynamic internal fixation, or osteotomy relying on postoperative immobilization without internal fixation are the options to achieve correction for kyphosis deformity. Pedicle screw system, as a rigid fixation concept, should not be the only choice as it excludes the opportunity of self-correction and fractional manual correction after surgery, thus resulting in a suboptimal correction rate and outcome. This is an unrecognized and remarkable issue for beginners.

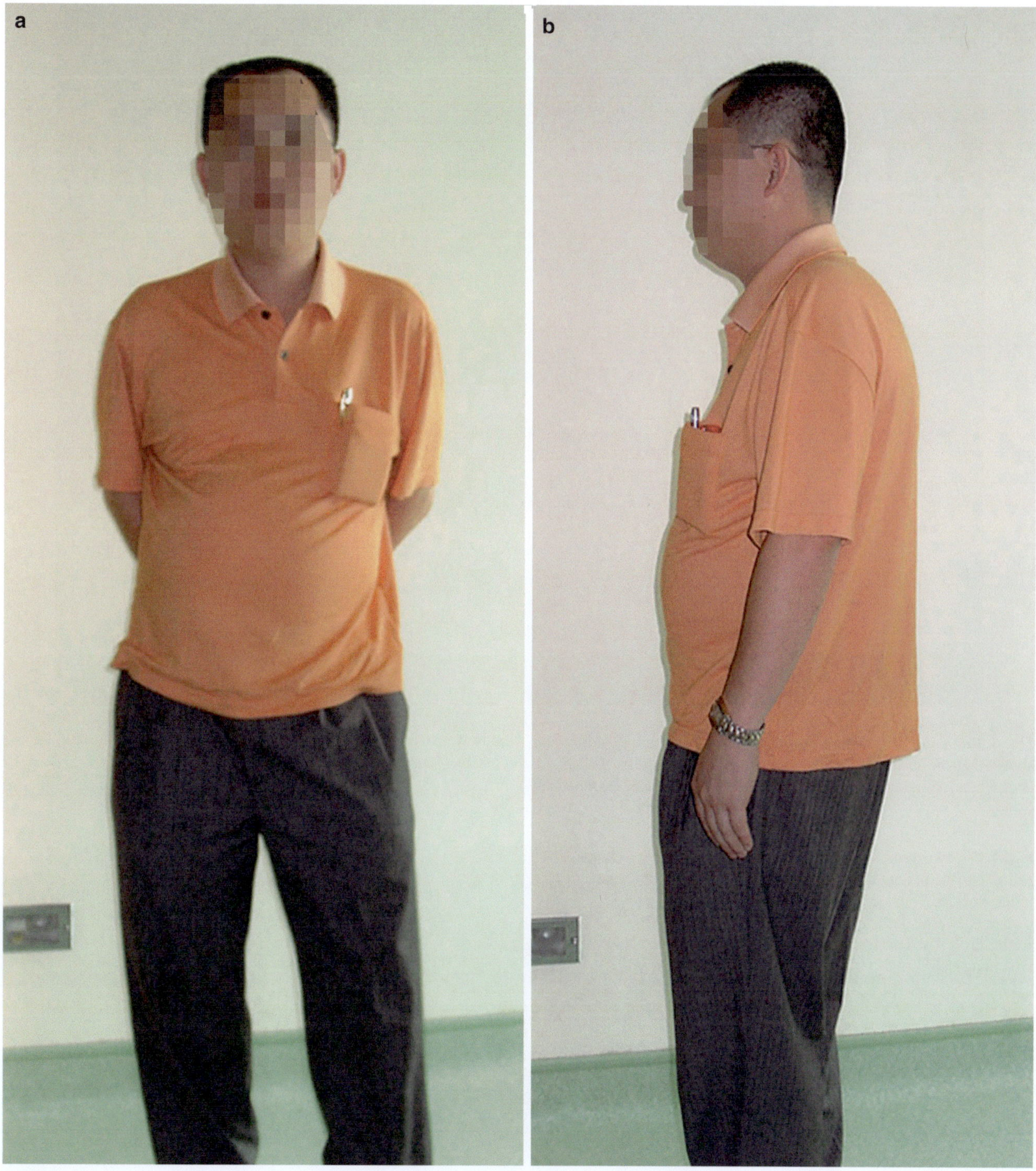

Fig. 4.35 One-and-a-half-year follow-up after operation. (**a**) Frontal body shape; (**b**) side profile

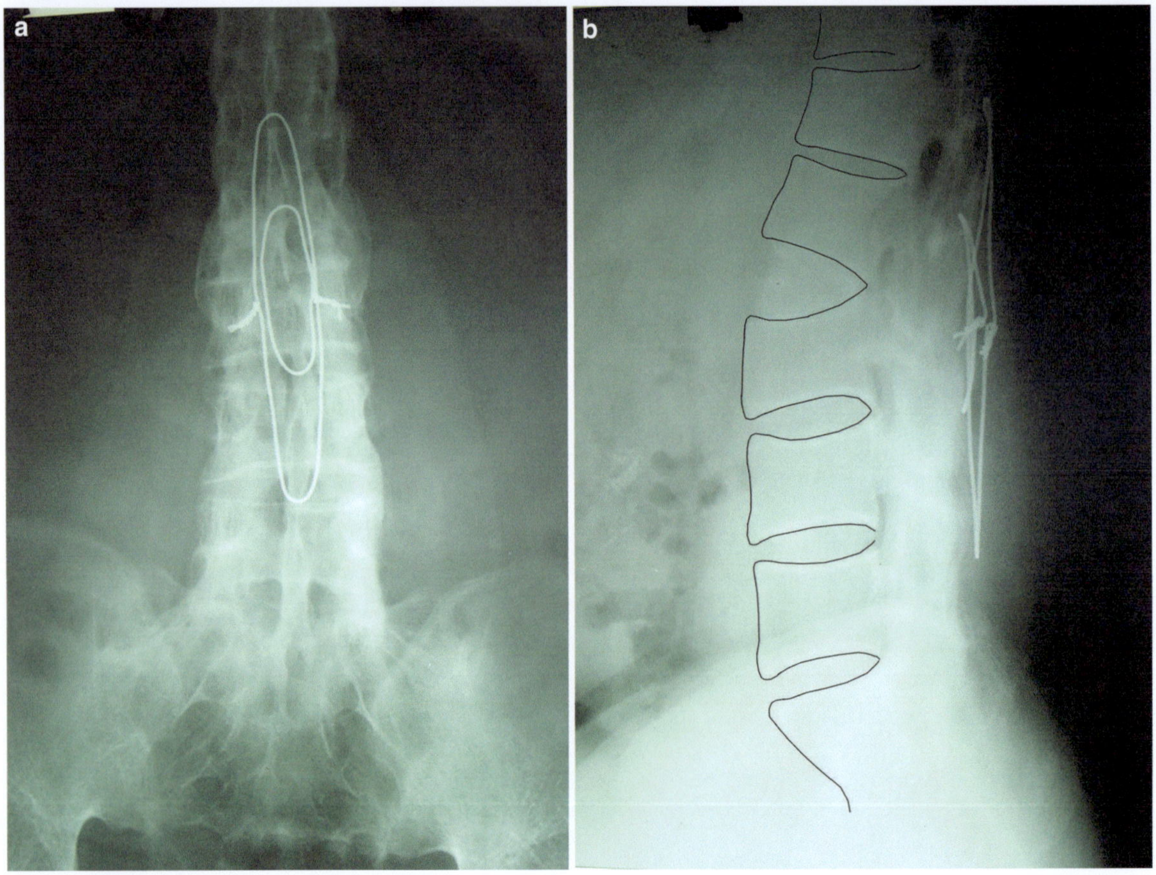

Fig. 4.36 X-ray film after 2 years operation. (**a**) Positive radiograph shows that the internal fixation wire is not broken and is well fixed. (**b**) Lateral radiographs showed that the anterior margin of the vertebral body was opened between. L2 and L3, new bone was blurred, and the posterior lamina graft was healed

Fig. 4.37 Two-year follow-up, the patient returned to his work as a business owner. (Left: the patient, Right: Professor Tian Huizhong)

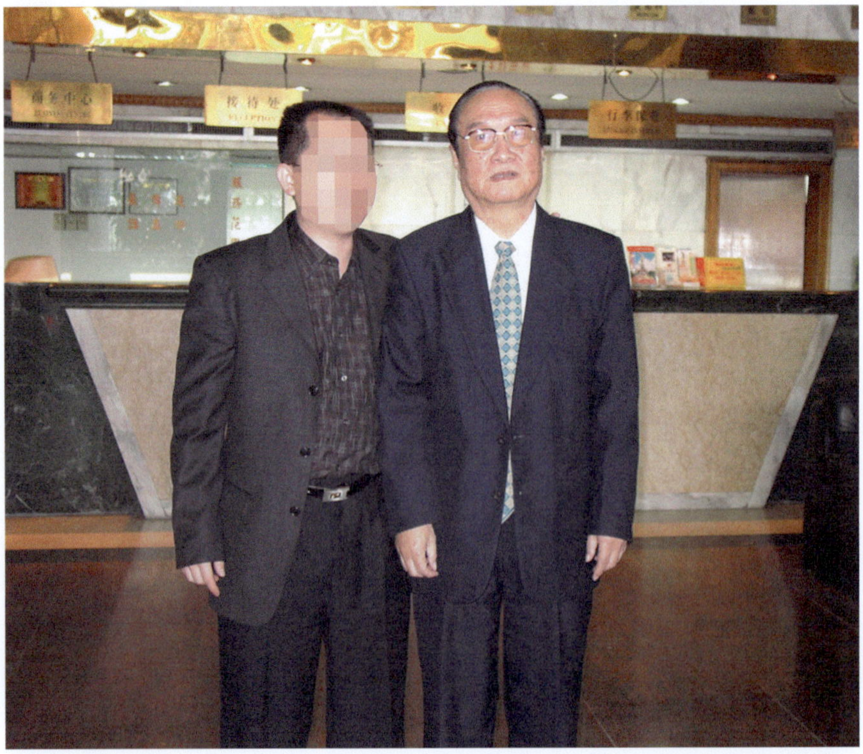

Suggested Reading

1. Tian H, Lin Q, Tan Y. Therapeutics of ankylosing spondylitis. Guangzhou: World Book Publishing Company; 2005. p. 165–95.
2. Liang Z. Transpedicular osteotomy for the treatment of kyphosis caused by ankylosing spondylitis. Chinese Journal of Orthopaedics. 1997;17(6):351–2.
3. Leong JCY, Ma A, Yau A. Spinal osteotomy for fixed flexion deformity. Journal of Orthopaedic Translation. 1978;2:271.
4. Chen A, Xu W. Spinal surgery atlas. Beijing: People's Medical Publishing House; 2001. p. 181–273.
5. Tian H, Wang B, Lv X, et al. Correction and fixation of ankylosing kyphosis and osteotomy. Chinese Journal of Orthopaedics. 2005;13(7):509–12.
6. Tan J, Feng J. Orthopedic unpadded plaster technique. Shanghai: Second Military Medical University Press; 2000. p. 126–46.
7. Tian H. Application of the "Tian's spinal osteotomes" in orthopaedic surgery. Chinese Journal of Orthopaedics. 1994;14(4):236–40.
8. Chen Q. Programmed surgical treatment of ankylosing spondylitis deformity. U.S. Chinese Journal of Orthopaedics. 2001;7: 85–7.
9. Ma Y. Clinical analysis of 200 cases of ankylosing kyphosis treated by posterior column resection. Xinjiang Medical Science. 2001;31(3):180–2.
10. Tian H, Lv X, Tian B. Correction of osteotomy of cervical and thoracic kyphosis with ankylosing spondylitis. Chinese Journal of Orthopaedics. 2006;14(7):522–3.
11. Tian H, Liu S, Ma Y. Practical spine surgery illustration. Beijing: People's Military Medical Press; 2008. p. 316–21.
12. Chen L, Li F. Diagnosis and treatment of ankylosing spondylitis complicated with stress fracture. Chinese Journal of Surgery. 1994;32(8):512.
13. Dang G. Surgical techniques for the spine. Beijing: People's Medical Publishing House; 2004. p. 246–52.
14. Tian H. Total spinal osteotomy for the treatment of kyphosis and kyphoscoliosis. Japanese Scoliosis Society program of the 25th Annual Meeting. 1991;25:23.
15. Tian H, Ma Y, Lv X. Minimally invasive V-shaped osteotomy for correction of ankylosing kyphosis. Chinese Journal of Orthopaedics. 2008;16(5):349–52.
16. Tian H, Liu S, Ma Y. Practical spine surgery. Guangzhou: Guangdong Science and Technology Press; 2008. p. 195–409.
17. Tian H, Zhang H, Liang Y. Surgical treatment of spinal deformity. Guangzhou: Guangdong Science and Technology Press; 2012. p. 1–482.
18. Tian H. Application of "Tian's spinal bone knife" in orthopaedic surgery. Chinese Journal of Orthopaedics. 2003;11(15):1073–5.
19. Tian H, Liang Y. Ankylosing spondylitis spinal deformity osteotomy and orthopedic surgery skills. Beijing: People's Medical Publishing House; 2014. p. 1–328.

5 Pedicle Subtraction Osteotomy for Ankylosing Kyphosis Deformity

Huizhong Tian, Tao Li, and Zhibo Song

5.1 Overview

In most cases of ankylosing kyphosis, a simple laminectomy can be used to close the gap between the posterior arches and open the anterior vertebral body space to achieve deformity correction. However, in a few cases, due to disc space fusion and the ossification of the anterior longitudinal ligament (Fig. 5.1), Pedicle Subtraction Osteotomy (PSO) should be used in cases where it is difficult to open the vertebral body space with simple laminectomy and manual reduction. The surgical method of PSO involves the posterior wedge resection of the spinous process, lamina and bilateral pedicles, bypassing the dural canal to remove the posterior edge of the vertebral body with Tian's osteotome (the tip of the wedge resection reaches the anterior 1/4 of the vertebral body). After manual correction, the anterior 1/4 of the vertebral body is fractured. The osteotomy gap between the vertebral arch and the posterior 3/4 of the vertebral body is closed to correct the kyphotic deformity (Fig. 5.2a, b). This is the surgical method of PSO for ankylosing kyphosis.

PSO applies for both round kyphosis and angular kyphosis, especially in cases of ankylosing kyphosis with large curves or cases with bony connections on the anterior edge of the vertebral body. The scope of osteotomy includes the lamina and pedicle. The tip of the wedge resection includes the posterior 3/4 of the vertebral body. After the osteotomy space is reduced, the anterior 1/4 of the vertebral body is compressed and fractured, and the posterior osteotomy space is closed. It is a closed osteotomy with strong stability.

5.1.1 Selection of Osteotomy Site

1. Non-apical osteotomy is performed generally between L2 and L3. As the spinal canal between L2 and 3 contains cauda equina, it is less likely to cause paraplegia.

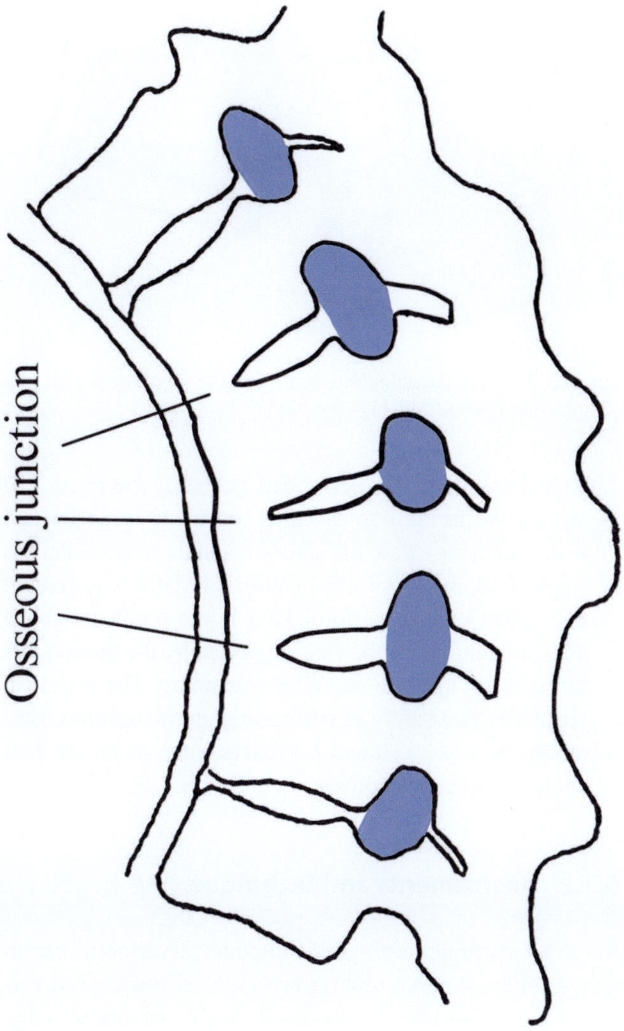

Fig. 5.1 Bony connection anterior to the anterior edge of three continuous levels is the indication of PSO

H. Tian (✉)
The Sixth Affiliated Hospital of Xinjiang Medical University, Urumqi, China

T. Li · Z. Song
Department of Orthopedics, The 2nd Affiliated Hospital of Kunming Medical University, Kunming, China

H. Tian et al. (eds.), *Spinal Osteotomy Orthopaedics*, https://doi.org/10.1007/978-981-16-1387-6_5

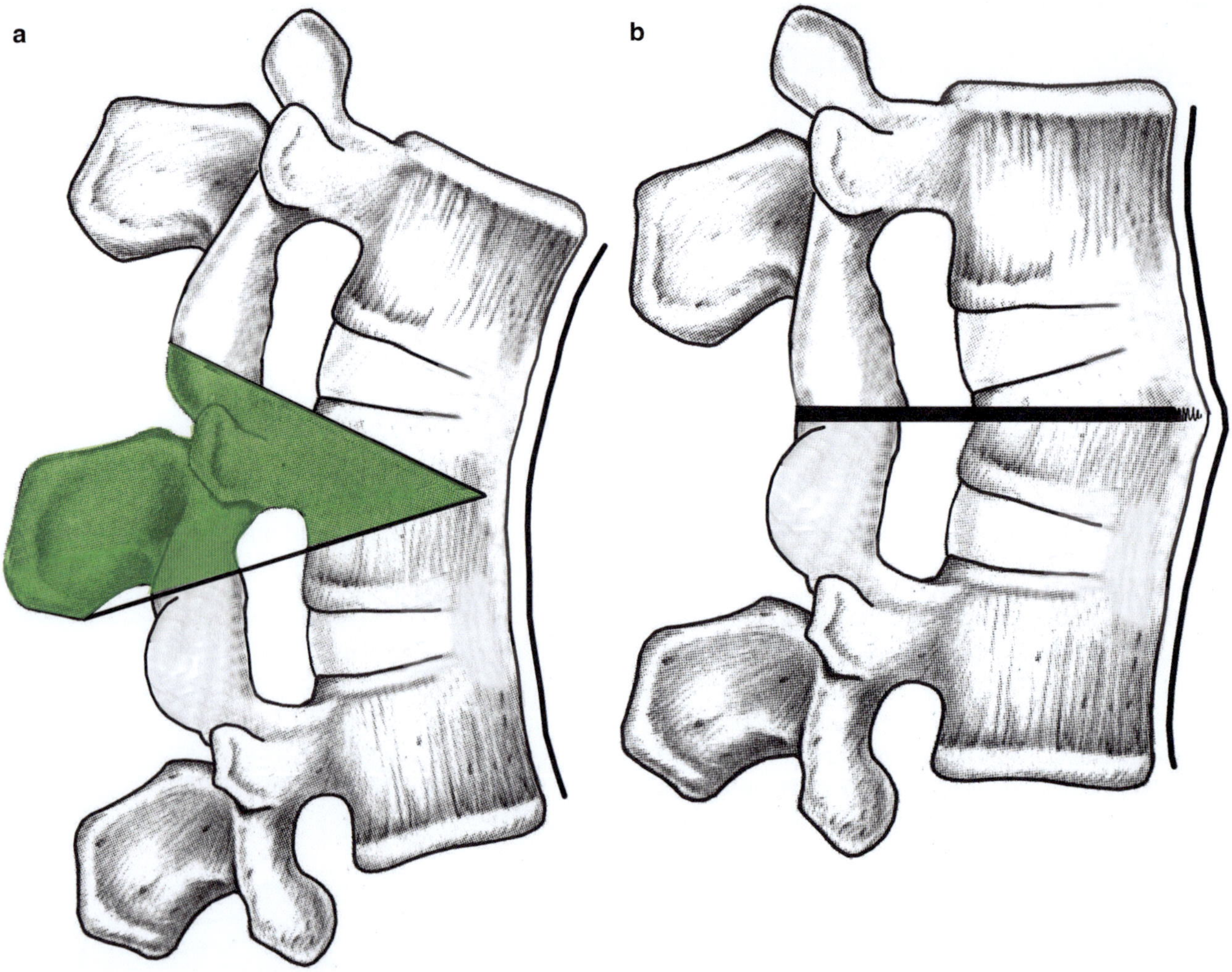

Fig. 5.2 Pedicle subtraction osteotomy. (**a**) The tip of the wedge should reach anterior 1/4 of the vertebral body. (**b**) Reduction creates anterior compression fracture with high stability

2. Apical osteotomy is performed generally between T10 and L4. As the bony spinal canal above T10 is narrow and is the segment where the anterior spinal artery enters the spinal cord, the possibility of spinal cord injury is greater. It is ideally not to perform PSO in the segments above T10. In addition, as they are supported by the thorax, it is difficult to close the gap after osteotomy. The technical feasibility and safety of performing apical vertebra osteotomy between T10 and L4 makes them to be the best choice of apical osteotomy.

5.1.2 Instruments and Technique

Surgical instruments for PSO include: 2 vertebral elevators, 2 levers, 2 nerve root retractors, 6 various curved vertebral osteotomies, 1 vertebral body posterior edge elevator, 1 posterior edge osteotome, 2 posterior edge shovels, 2 push-down osteotomes, and 2 ring curettes, summing up to 20 (Fig. 5.3). Large, medium, and small thin-blade straight osteotomes are also included, one for each (Fig. 5.4).

The vertebral body elevator is mainly used to strip the side and anterior and lateral sides of the vertebral body under the periosteum. After elevation, the lever is inserted between the vertebral body and the anterior longitudinal ligament to expose the vertebral body for osteotomy. The nerve root retractor is used to pull apart the spinal nerve roots that exit from the upper and lower intervertebral foramen, with compression hemostasis effect. Various curved osteotomes are mainly used to bypass the dural canal and perform wedge osteotomy on the vertebral body. The posterior elevator, the posterior osteotome and the push-down osteotome are basically used to resect the thin bone fragments closed the dural tube at the posterior edge of the vertebral body. Use a shovel and forceps to remove the fragment. Three thin-blade straight osteotomes of different widths are indispensable tools in spinal osteotomy. They are used for vertebral arch, vertebral

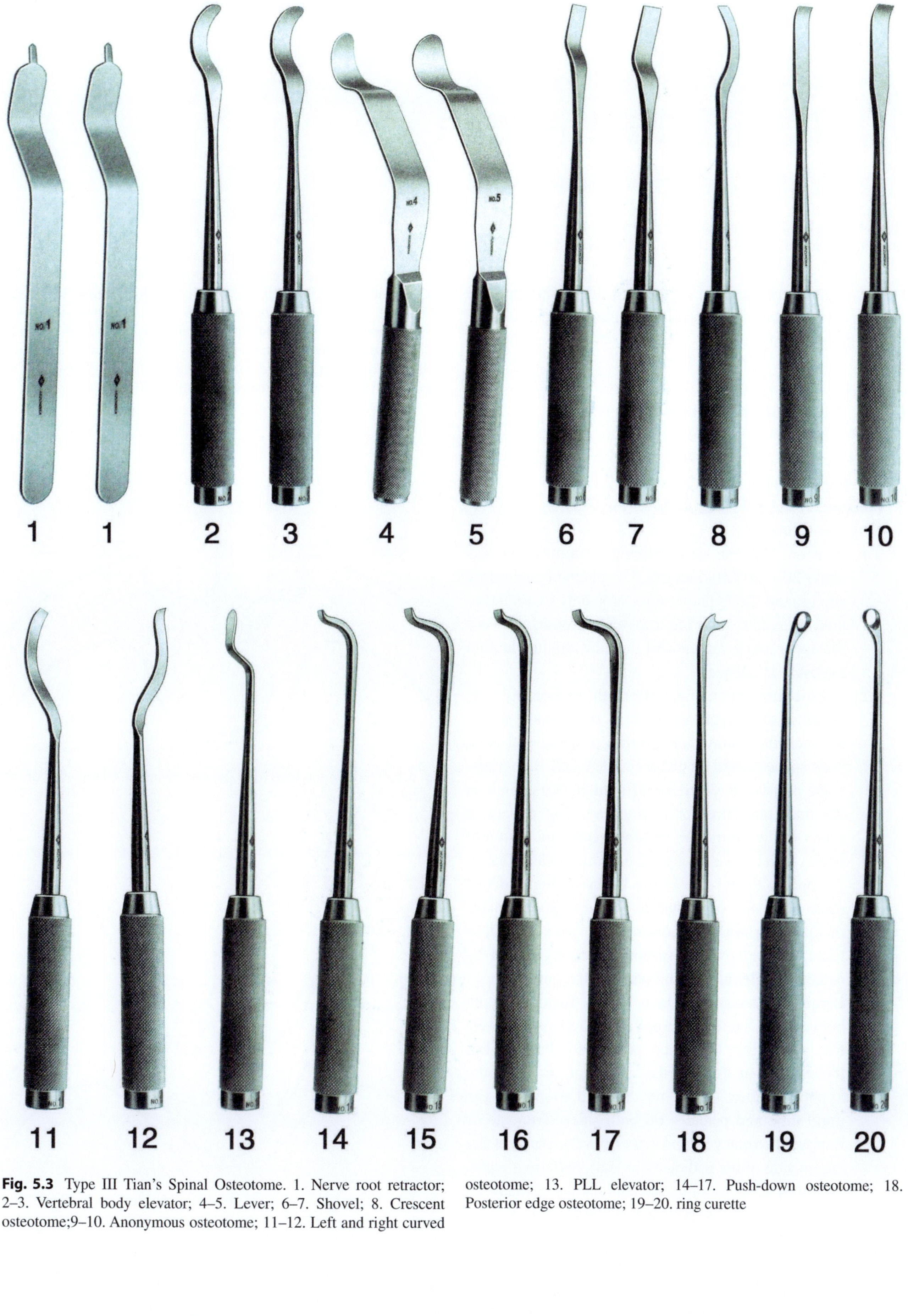

Fig. 5.3 Type III Tian's Spinal Osteotome. 1. Nerve root retractor; 2–3. Vertebral body elevator; 4–5. Lever; 6–7. Shovel; 8. Crescent osteotome;9–10. Anonymous osteotome; 11–12. Left and right curved osteotome; 13. PLL elevator; 14–17. Push-down osteotome; 18. Posterior edge osteotome; 19–20. ring curette

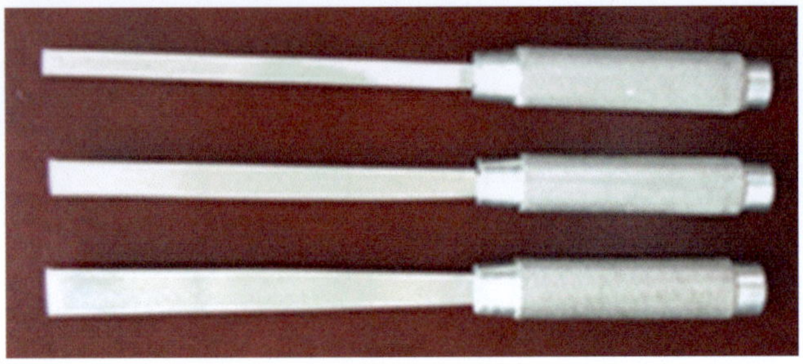

Fig. 5.4 Thin-blade straight osteotome of different with of three different widths, one for each. They are essential for spinal osteotomy

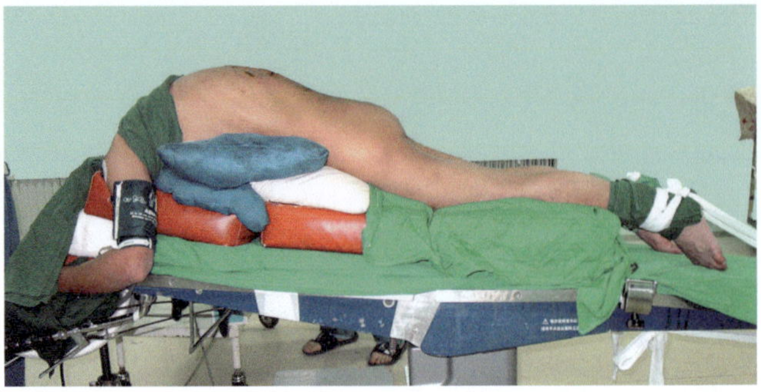

Fig. 5.5 When a patient with severe kyphosis is in the prone position, the shoulder pad should be placed to support the shoulder. The patient's head extends out of the table and is placed under the table level. The forehead is placed on a round stool with auto-adjustment. Adjust the bed into a reverse V shape and provide firm support to the abdomen and the two anterior superior iliac spines. The feet are fixed at the end of the table with bandages to prevent the patient from sliding forward. The traction belt is placed under the armpits for traction after the osteotomy is completed

body wedge osteotomy, and excision of the lamina and the lateral part of the vertebral body; interlaminar fenestration or partial laminectomy.

5.2 Surgical Procedure

1. Anesthesia: local infiltration anesthesia or tracheal intubation anesthesia.
2. Position: Prone or lateral position (Fig. 5.5).
3. Surgical technique
   3.1. Incision: Make an incision along the spinous process about 20 ~ 30 cm in length. The planned osteotomy site around the kyphotic apex is widely dissected to both sides to expose the transverse process. Toward the upper and lower ends of the incision, just lamina exposure is adequate.
   3.2. Expose the lamina to determine the osteotomy gap. In ankylosing kyphosis, there is often bony fusion between the lamina and spinous process, and facet joint space cannot be clearly recognized. The transverse process, intervertebral foramen, and pedicle is the only reference for positioning. Use a pedicle finder to determine the vertebral arch and vertebral body to be covered by osteotomy under C-arm. According to the size of the kyphotic angle, determine the width of the lamina to be removed, mark the predetermined osteotomy line with an osteotome, and remove the spinous process covered by osteotomy planning to the plane of the lamina.
   3.3. Lamina osteotomy. Once bone fusion occurs between the vertebral lamellae at the kyphotic vertex, osteotomy should be performed directly. For those without fusion, the vertebral arch of the kyphotic vertex should be removed to expose the dural tube and pedicles on both sides. Truncate or remove the transverse process from the plane of the lateral side of the pedicle (Fig. 5.6), and use a vertebral body elevator along the lateral edge of the pedicle to elevate subperiosteally anteriorly to the anterolateral edge of the vertebral body (Fig. 5.7).

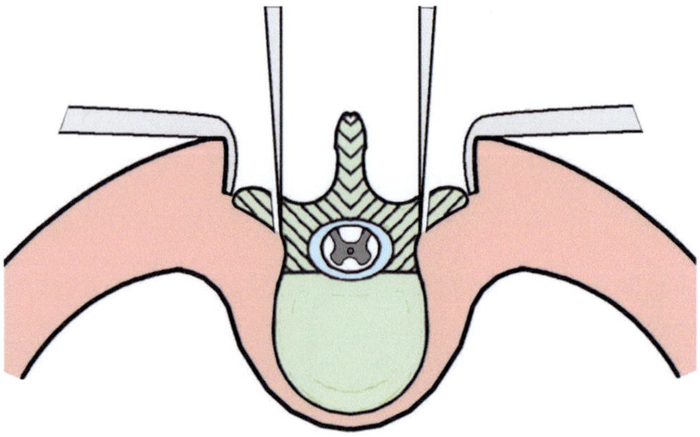

Fig. 5.6 Truncate the transverse process along the lateral edge of the pedicle

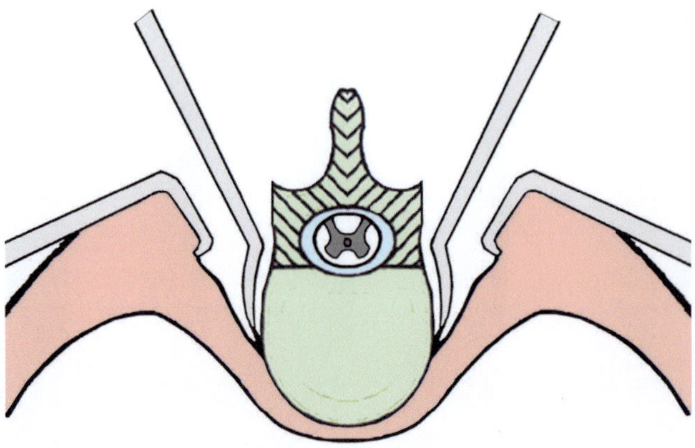

Fig. 5.7 Use a vertebral body elevator along the lateral edge of the pedicle to elevate the subperiosteally anteriorly to the anterolateral edge of the vertebral body

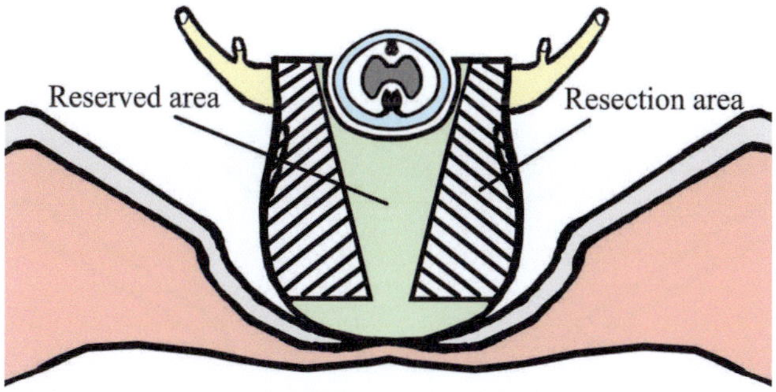

Fig. 5.8 Insert levers from both sides, expose the vertebral body, and ready for subtotal vertebral osteotomy

Fig. 5.9 After resection of posterior arch and exposure of dural canal, nerve roots, bilateral pedicles, and residue transverse process

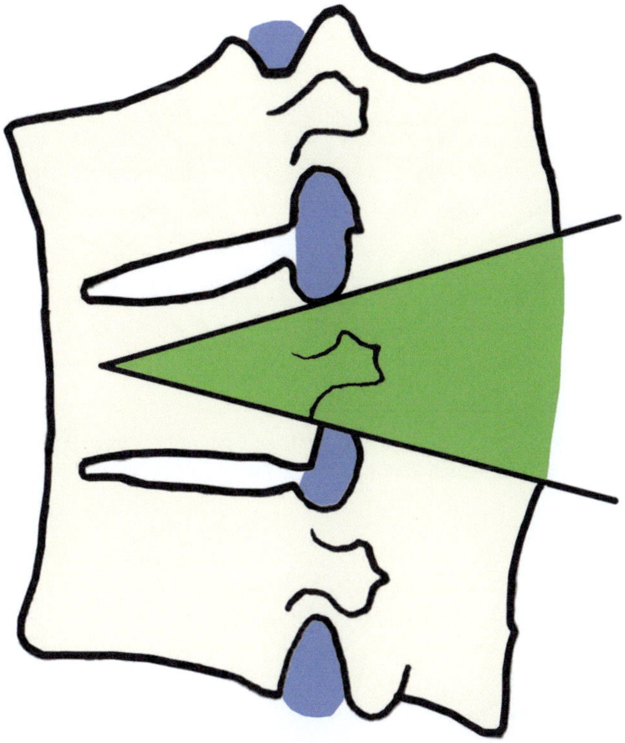

Fig. 5.10 The scope of PSO. The tip of the wedge resection is in the anterior 1/4 of the vertebral body

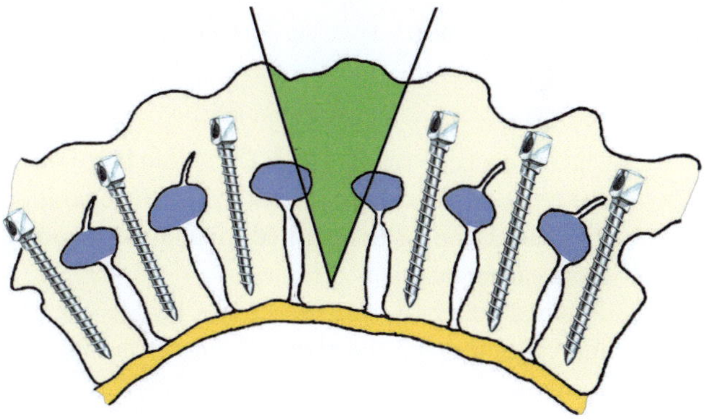

Fig. 5.11 Before osteotomy, the pedicle screws should be inserted

Push away the periosteum and anterior longitudinal ligament, insert a lever (Figs. 5.8 and 5.9). Expose the lateral aspect of the vertebral body, prepare for the next step of subtotal vertebral osteotomy (Fig. 5.10).

3.4. Insert pedicle screws and temporary fixation. Before subtotal vertebral osteotomy, the pedicle screws above and below the osteotomy gap should be inserted to be ready for fixation after reduction (Fig. 5.11). Make a temporary fixation with rod or wire, so as to avoid the spinal cord and dural tube free in the osteotomy space after the vertebral body osteotomy and correction are completed. Any displacement or stretching force can cause spinal cord injury and paralysis of both lower limbs (because after corrective steps, the anterior space of the vertebral body may open, making both ends of the truncated spine unstable). Prevent the displacement of the bony spinal canal which may cause compression of the spinal cord.

3.5. Use a straight osteotome to perform osteotomy of the pedicle and the lateral edge of the vertebral body (Fig. 5.12a, b): Temporarily save the thin bone sheet of the medial edge of the pedicle and the posterior edge of the vertebral body, and remove most of the pedicle, and the posterior 3/4 of the vertebral body,

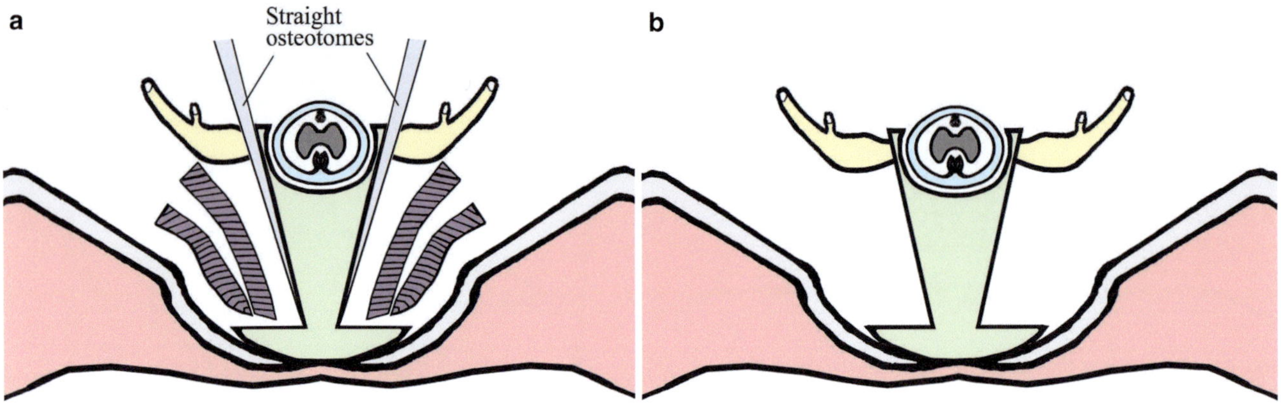

Fig. 5.12 Osteotomy of pedicle and lateral part of the vertebral body. (**a**) Resect pedicle and lateral part of the vertebral body with straight osteotome. (**b**) After resection of pedicle and lateral part of the vertebral body

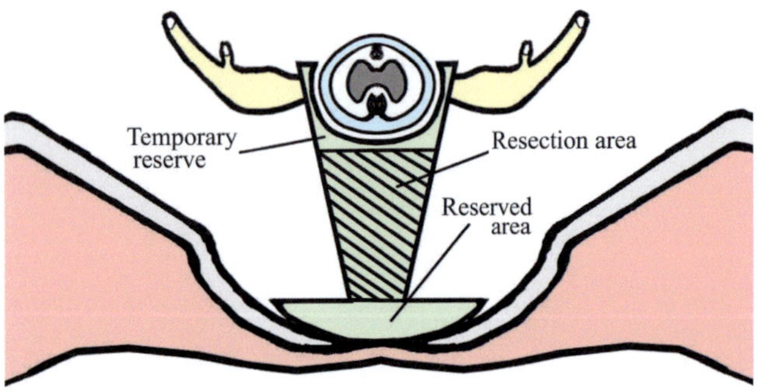

Fig. 5.13 The diagonal area indicate the central part of the vertebral body to be resected

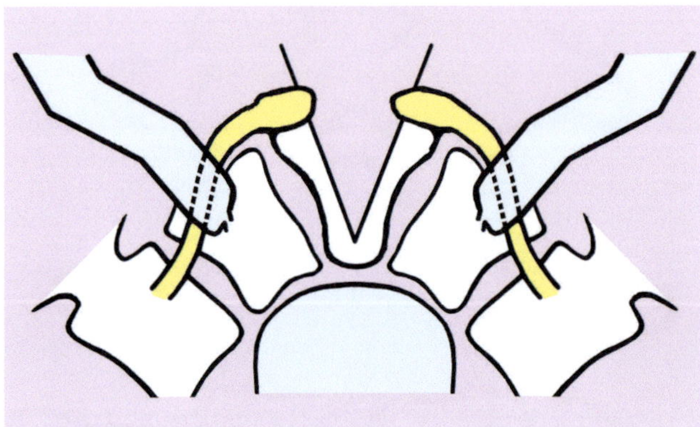

Fig. 5.14 Retract the exiting nerve roots with the nerve retractor. The tip of the nerve retractor should insert into the bone to protect the nerve roots from slipping into the field

leaving a wedge space (Fig. 5.13). Avoid bleeding of the epidural venous plexus and make the operation difficult. Bone wax is applied to stop the bleeding from cancellous sinus.

3.6. Subtotal vertebral body osteotomy. Bypass the spinal canal through the posterior approach and performing subtotal vertebral body osteotomy is the key step of this operation. Bleeding of the soft tissues in front of the vertebral body stops spontaneously due to the compression of the lever. Thus, intercostal vessel or lumbar vessel ligation is spared. The spinal nerve roots exiting from the upper and lower intervertebral foramen are retracted with a special nerve root retractor (Fig. 5.14). With adequate exposure, a subtotal osteotomy of the vertebral body is performed, and a thin layer of cortical bone at the posterior edge of the vertebral body is retained to avoid bleeding from the epidural venous plexus. For the bleeding of the cancellous sinus in the vertebral body, bone wax can be applied to stop the bleeding. After most of the vertebral body osteotomy is completed, pack the osteotomy site with a gelatin sponge and gauze to stop the bleeding. Then, use the special instrument to cut off the thin bone sheet on the posterior edge of the vertebral body as fast as the operator can (Figs. 5.15 and 5.16). At this time, there will be active bleeding from the epidural venous plexus. After the osteotomy of the posterior edge of the vertebral body is completed, the osteotomy gap is immediately closed to shorten the spine, expand and widen the dura, and compress the epidural venous plexus to stop bleeding (Fig. 5.17). After the osteotomy gap is completely closed, bleeding from the deep wound can be completely stopped.

4. Postoperative management:

After the operation, a negative pressure drainage tube is placed on each side of the spinous process and the patient is sent back to the ward for vacuum drainage. The drainage tube is removed in 24 ~ 48 h. The sutures are removed on the 10th day. After the sutures are removed, the plaster vest is applied for external immobilization upon discharge. Within 3 months, the patient should have more bed rest, less ambulation, and move the joints of the limbs

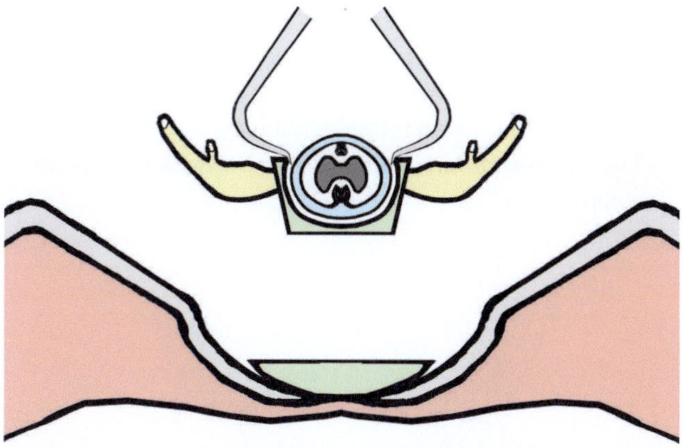

Fig. 5.15 The posterior 3/4 of the vertebral body is resected followed by resection of the medial edge of the pedicle with push-down osteotome

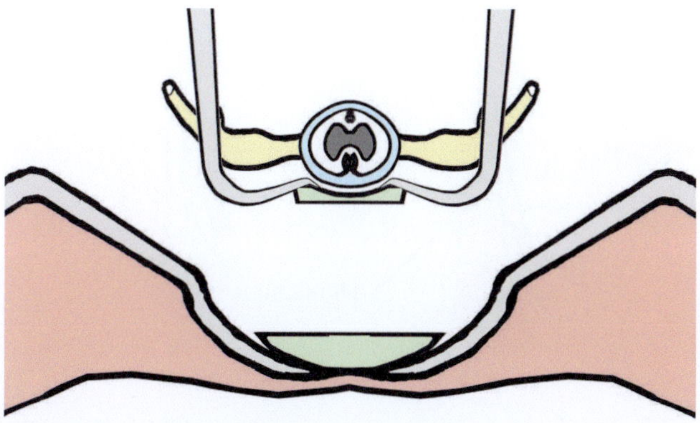

Fig. 5.16 Resection of thin sheet of bone of the posterior edge of the vertebral body with push-down osteotome

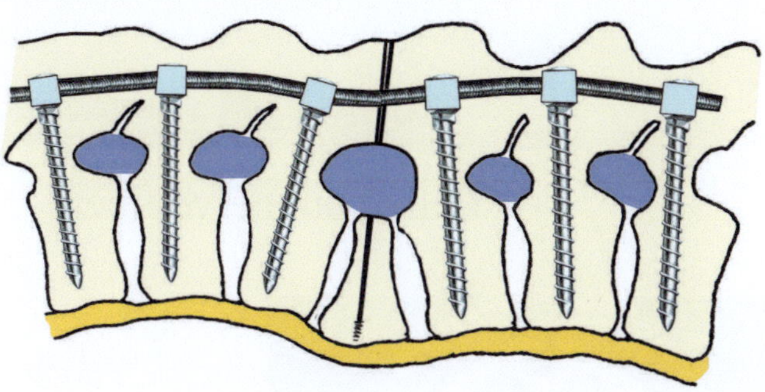

Fig. 5.17 Completion of closing reduction and internal fixation. The dural canal is expanded and widened in the osteotome level to compress the epidural venous plexus leading to hemostasis

while lying in the bed to avoid stiffness of the hip or shoulder joint. After 3 months, the patient can have more ambulation outdoor activities. After 6–8 months, the patient should come to the hospital for follow-up. The surgeon will decide whether to remove the plaster. After the plaster is removed, X-rays are taken to evaluate bone graft healing.

5.3 Key Points and Precautions

5.3.1 Key Points and Precautions

1. PSO for ankylosing kyphosis is a wedge-shaped osteotomy including spinous process, lamina, bilateral pedicles, and posterior 3/4 of vertebral body along the lateral edge. The anterior 1/4 of the vertebral body and the anterior longitudinal ligament are not truncated, and the compression fracture will be generated when the osteotomy space is closed in the final correction. This method is more stable than vertebral column resection, and it is not easy to cause dislocation of the osteotomy gap. However, sometimes the 1/4 vertebral body and the anterior longitudinal ligament left by PSO are ossified and hard. When being reduced, compression fractures cannot be produced. Instead, they will be completely broken. The anterior longitudinal ligaments are also torn at the same time, resulting in a complete bony discontinuation. So, the temporary internal fixation should be properly prepared before the osteotomy and correction.
2. When correcting the kyphotic deformity, attention should be paid to correct any accompanying scoliosis. In this case, the osteotomy gap should be made with different widths on the two sides to correct the scoliosis at the same time.
3. Before performing PSO, the pedicle screws above and below the osteotomy gap should be placed and fixed with temporary rods or wires to prevent the osteotomy from being unstable, dislocation of the spinal canal, and compression of the spinal cord.
4. When closing the osteotomy gap, the force should not be too strong or too aggressive, so as to avoid the occurrence of paraplegia due to the dislocation of the osteotomy end.
5. For severe kyphosis cases, due to the shortening of the rectus abdominis, it is difficult to straighten the patient's trunk at one time. It is best to perform elastic internal fixation (wire fixation) after osteotomy and lie in a flatbed after the operation. The soft tissue is released gradually, and finally, the purpose of straightening the trunk is achieved.
6. When reducing the rod into the screw, the closure of the osteotomy gap should be monitored at any time. If there is a malalignment of the osteotomy gap before and after or lateral dislocation, it should be adjusted immediately (ensure that the spinal canal can be aligned) to prevent compression of the dural tube and spinal cord.

5.3.2 Complications and Prevention

1. Superior Mesenteric Artery Syndrome (Fig. 5.18). For severe kyphosis, the method of shortening the trunk by vertebral body resection or the method of fractional manual correction after osteotomy should be used to prevent superior mesenteric artery syndrome.

2. Paraplegia due to compression of spinal cord and nerves. Avoid damage to the spinal cord or nerve roots with instruments during osteotomy. Avoid excessive force during manual reduction causing the translation of the osteotomy gap.
3. Dura tear and CSF leak. When performing an osteotomy close to the dural tube, special care should be taken not to damage the dura mater (Fig. 5.19). Once a CSF leak occurs, repairs can be performed during the operation. Those irreparable are covered with gelatin sponge. After the operation, mannitol dehydration must be performed. The patient should lie in a prone position with local compression.

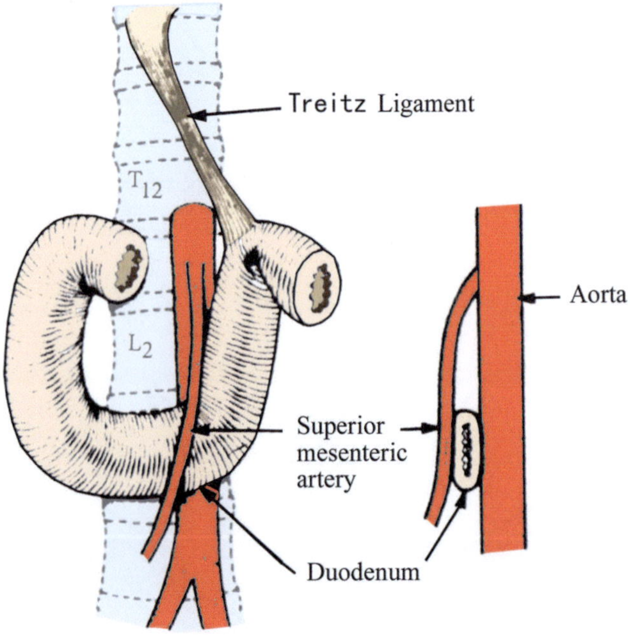

Fig. 5.18 Pathogenesis of superior mesenteric artery syndrome

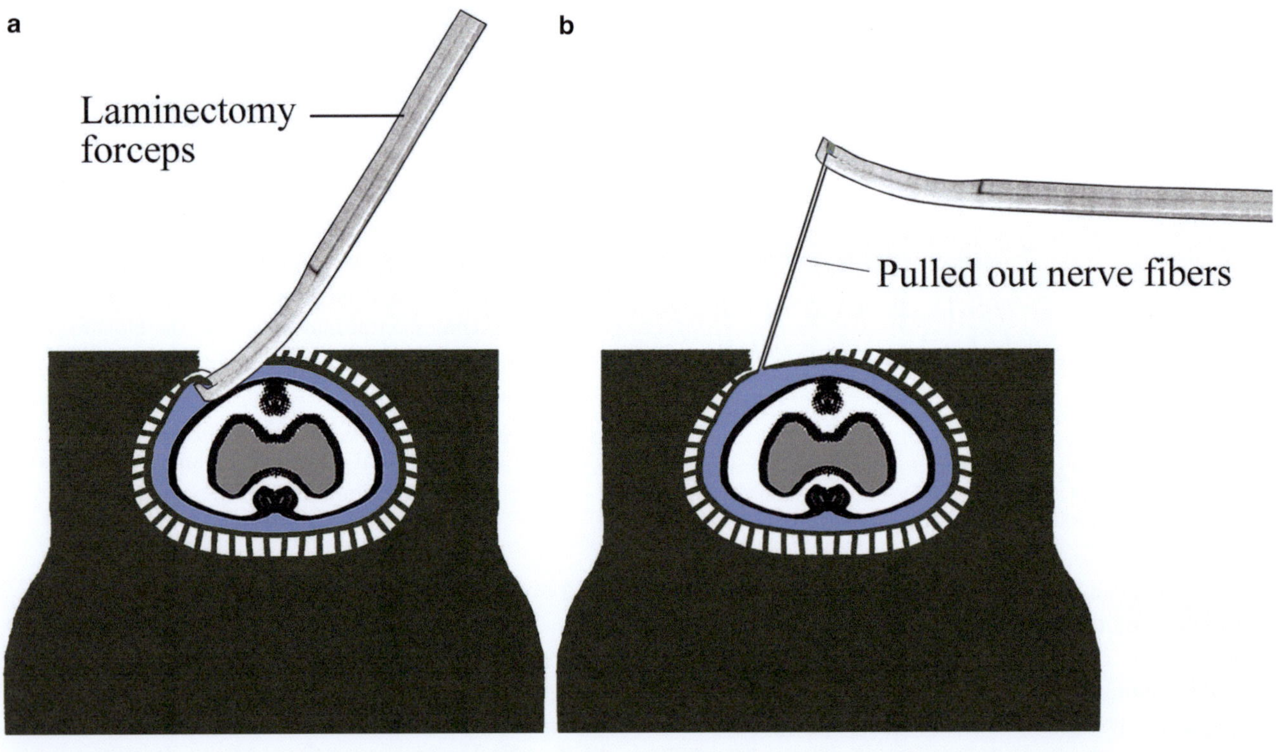

Fig. 5.19 When resection bone tissue close to the dura canal with rongeur, it is likely to have dura tear and "thread pulling." (**a**) The jaw of a rongeur may capture a tiny part of the dura. (**b**) A nerve fiber is pulled out from the dura for a significant length have dura tear and "thread pulling"

Suggested Reading

1. Leong JCY, Ma A, Yau A. Spinal osteotomy for fixed flexion deformity. Journal of Orthopaedic Translation. 1978;2:271.
2. Tian H. Total spinal osteotomy for the treatment of kyphosis and kyphoscoliosis. Japanese Scoliosis Society program of the 25th Annual Meeting, 1991;25:23.
3. Tian Huizhong, Tian Y, Zheng X, Tian S. Posterior invasion and vertebral osteotomy. Spinal Deformation. 1992;7(1):4–11.
4. Liang Z. Transpedicular osteotomy for the treatment of kyphosis caused by ankylosing spondylitis. Chinese Journal of Orthopaedics. 1997;17(6):351–2.
5. Tian H. Surgical treatment of kyphosis kyphosis. Chinese Journal of Orthopaedics. 1992;12(3):162–5.
6. Tian H, Li F. Spinal deformity and osteotomy. Xi'an: World Book Publishing Company; 2001. p. 377–741.
7. Tian H. Spinal surgeons should be good at using rongeurs and osteotome. Chinese Journal of Modern Operative Surgery. 2002;6(1):67–8.
8. Tian H, Liu S, Ma Y. Practical spine surgery illustration. Beijing: People's Military Medical Press; 2008. p. 189–385.
9. Chen A, Xu W. Spinal surgery atlas. Beijing: People's Medical Publishing House; 2001. p. 77–300.
10. Tian H. Application of "Tian's spinal bone knife" in orthopaedic surgery. Chinese Journal of Orthopaedics. 2003;11(15):1073–5.
11. Hou S. Spinal surgery. Beijing: People's Military Medical Publishing House; 2005. p. 444–610.
12. Xu S, Ge B, Xu Y. Practice of orthopaedics. 2nd ed. Beijing: People's Military Medical Publishing House; 2003. p. 598–636.
13. Tian H, Lin Q, Tan Y. Therapeutics of ankylosing spondylitis. Guangzhou: World Book Publishing Company; 2005. p. 165–235.
14. Tian H, Liu S, Ma Y. Practical spine surgery. Guangzhou: Guangdong Science and Technology Press; 2008. p. 195–409.
15. Tian H, Wang B, Lv X, et al. Correction and fixation of ankylosing kyphosis and osteotomy. Chinese Journal of Orthopaedics. 2005;13(7):509–12.
16. Ma Y. Clinical analysis of 200 cases of ankylosing kyphosis treated by posterior column resection. Xinjiang Medical Science. 2001;31(3):180–2.
17. Dang G. Surgical techniques for the spine. Beijing: People's Medical Publishing House; 2004. p. 102–252.
18. Chen Q. Programmed surgical treatment of ankylosing spondylitis deformity. U.S. Chinese Journal of Orthopaedics. 2001;7:85–7.
19. Chen L, Li F. Diagnosis and treatment of ankylosing spondylitis complicated with stress fracture. Chinese Journal of Surgery. 1994;32(8):512.
20. Tian H, Lv X, Tian B. Correction of osteotomy of cervical and thoracic kyphosis with ankylosing spondylitis. Chinese Journal of Orthopaedics. 2006;14(7):522–3.
21. Tian H, Ma Y, Lv X. Minimally invasive V-shaped osteotomy for correction of ankylosing kyphosis. Chinese Journal of Orthopaedics. 2008;16(5):349–52.
22. Tian H, Li M, Wang Z. Key points and diagrams of thoracolumbar surgery. Beijing: People's Medical Publishing House; 2012. p. 375–417.
23. Tian H, Liang Y. Ankylosing spondylitis spinal deformity osteotomy and orthopedic surgery skills. Beijing: People's Medical Publishing House; 2014. p. 1–328.

6 Vertebral Column Resection for Ankylosing Spondylitis Kyphosis

Huizhong Tian, Yuan Ma, and Jingming Xie

6.1 Overview

Radiographic findings of ankylosing spondylitis including ankylosis of sacroiliac joints and facet joints of the spine, progressive sclerosis, ossification of annulus fibrosus, anterior longitudinal ligament, interspinous ligament, and interlaminar ligament. With the progression of disease, back pain gradually fades away while interspinous and interlaminar bony ankylosis forms. Finally, the spine presents a "bamboo segment," indicating ankylosis of the vertebral body and vertebral arch of multiple levels. At this time, pathological changes cause severe loss of motion as well as lumbar lordosis. Meanwhile, compensatory kyphosis of thoracic and cervical segments occurs, forming a long curve of kyphosis which looks like a wheel on the lateral X-ray (Fig. 6.1). The ankylosing deformity keeps the head in flexion. The patient is forced to maintain balance and look straight ahead by a compensatory knee and hip flexion (Fig. 6.2). With kyphosis, the patient has to lie in a lateral position instead of a supine position (Fig. 6.3). As explained earlier, structural spinal deformity of ankylosing spondylitis affects patients' physiological function and even causes psychological depression.

Radiological sacroiliac joint arthritis is the characteristic of ankylosing spondylitis. The word Ankylosing Spondylitis (AS) is derived from Ankylos Spondylos in Greek. Ankylos means "bend," Spondylos means "spine." However, modern studies demonstrated that a "bent" spine just present in the late stage of AS among just a few severe patients. Radiological sacroiliitis is the objective marker to indicate the disease in the early stage. The first diagnostic criterion of the disease was set in 1961, which is the Rome Criteria. It includes five clinical criteria and one radiological criteria: (1) lower back pain and stiffness, lasting for more than 3 months, no relief from rest, (2) chest pain and stiffness, (3) limited range of motion of the lumbar spine, (4) limitation of thoracic expansion, (5) iritis, or history of iritis, and (6) characteristic X-ray findings of sacroiliac arthritis of AS. Diagnosis of AS is established if the patients meet the radiological criteria and one of the five clinical criteria, or four clinical criteria. Five years later in 1966, the New York

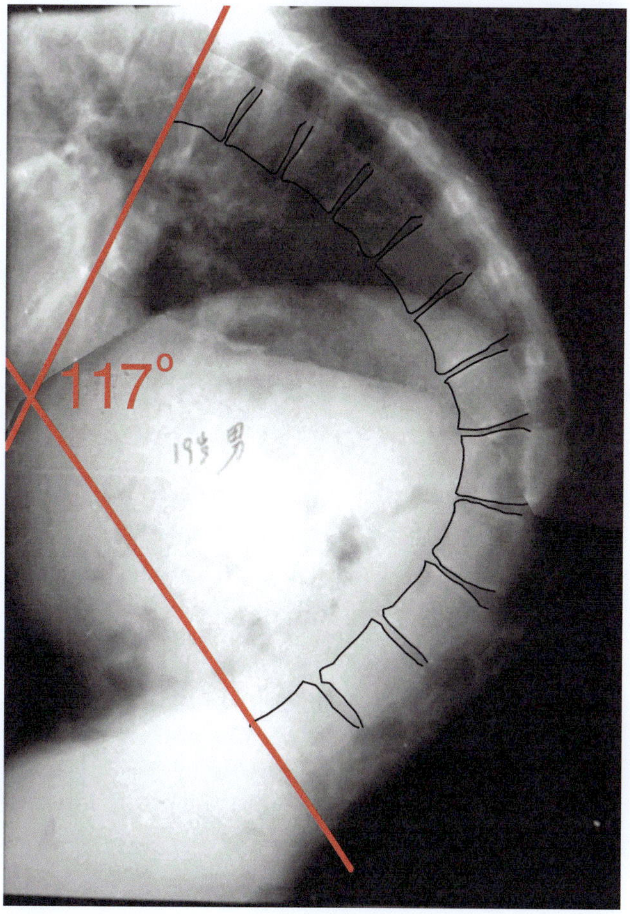

Fig. 6.1 A long C-shaped kyphosis like a bicycle wheel

H. Tian · Y. Ma (✉)
The Sixth Affiliated Hospital of Xinjiang Medical University, Urumqi, China

J. Xie
Department of Orthopedics, The 2nd Affiliated Hospital of Kunming Medical University, Kunming, China
e-mail: xiejingming@vip.163.com

H. Tian et al. (eds.), *Spinal Osteotomy Orthopaedics*, https://doi.org/10.1007/978-981-16-1387-6_6

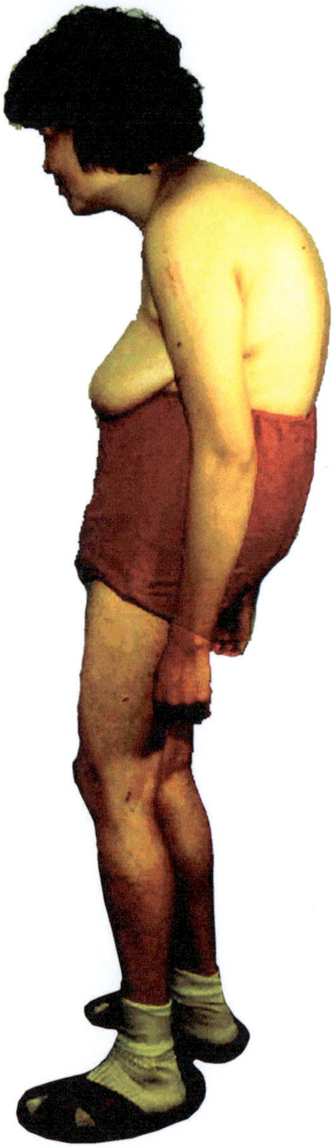

Fig. 6.2 The standing posture of long curve kyphosis in ankylosing spondylitis. The patient's head leans forward and knee hip flexion are flexed to compensate for the standing balance and achieve the purpose of looking straight ahead

Criteria requires radiological sacroiliac arthritis plus other criteria as follow: (1) limitation of lumbar mobility in all directions (flexion, lateral bending, extension), (2) history of pain or pain in the thoracolumbar or lumbosacral region, and (3) limitation of thoracic expansion and the expansion measured at the level of the 4th intercostal space is less than 2.5 cm. AS diagnosis is established by meeting the above four criteria. The New York Criteria describes and classifies the radiological features of sacroiliac arthritis to different grades. The requirements of the New York Criteria are relatively strict, which does not facilitate early diagnosis. New diagnostic criteria were proposed later, such as Vander Linden's modification on New York Criteria. But the essential element of radiological sacroiliac arthritis remains unchanged.

Smith Petersen is the first surgeon to correct ankylosing kyphosis (in 1945) by osteotomy which is named as "spinal osteotomy" and actually means translaminar osteotomy and deformity correction. From 1961 to 1980, Professor Tian Huizhong from the Xinjiang Institute of Spinal Surgery of China began to perform spinal osteotomy in ASK patients following Smith Petersen's surgical technique. The age of the patient was around 30 years and the kyphotic Cobb angle was less than 80°. Under general anesthesia with endotracheal intubation, the translaminar osteotomy, either transverse or V-shape osteotomy were performed. The osteotomy gap was closed by traction and manual press. Bone debris harvest was grafted around the lamina. Trunk casting was used and changed to plaster vest in 2–3 weeks after operation. He divided the patients with AS into two types: mild (Fig. 6.4) (Cobb angle <80°) and severe (Figs. 6.5 and 6.6) (Cobb angle >80°). Mild cases were treated with V-shape osteotomy with plaster vest instead of internal fixation. The latter was reserved only for severe cases. Subtotal vertebral body osteotomy or vertebral column resection was used in the cases which exist rigid bony fusion that cannot restore the spinal alignment after osteotomy. During the 30 years from 1981 to 2011, a total of 2400 cases of mild and severe ankylosing kyphosis were treated in Tian's center.

Osteotomy for ankylosing kyphosis was first performed by Smith Petersen in 1945. In China, Tian Huizhong in Xinjiang began to treat ankylosing kyphosis by osteotomy in 1961. Later, Liu Runtian from Tianjin, Ma Jingkun from Shanxi, Wu Zhikang from Beijing, and Wan Nianyu from Qingdao applied this technique to treat AS at early times as well. After 1980, more and more large centers in the Northeast of China, Guangdong, Shandong, Fujian, Shanghai, Tianjin, etc. carried out this work.

The principle of spinal osteotomy is identical to that for limbs. It requires a wedge osteotomy with an osteotome and then closes the wedge to correct the deformity to restore normal spinal alignment. But the difference is that the spinal cord locates in the spinal canal and two spinal nerve roots exit from the intervertebral foramen. This brings great difficulty to spinal osteotomy compared with the simpler procedure of osteotomy for long bone, where just straight osteotomes are needed. However, without specific instruments, it is impossible to keep spinal cord and nerve roots intact while making circumferential vertebral osteotomy and wedge resections around the dural sac, especially in vertebral column resection for kyphosis. Thus, spinal osteotomy receives special attention in spinal deformity correction.

Spinal osteotomy for ankylosing spondylitis kyphosis can be divided into the following grades: transverse translaminar osteotomy, V-shape translaminar osteotomy, subtotal vertebral arch and body osteotomy and vertebral column osteot-

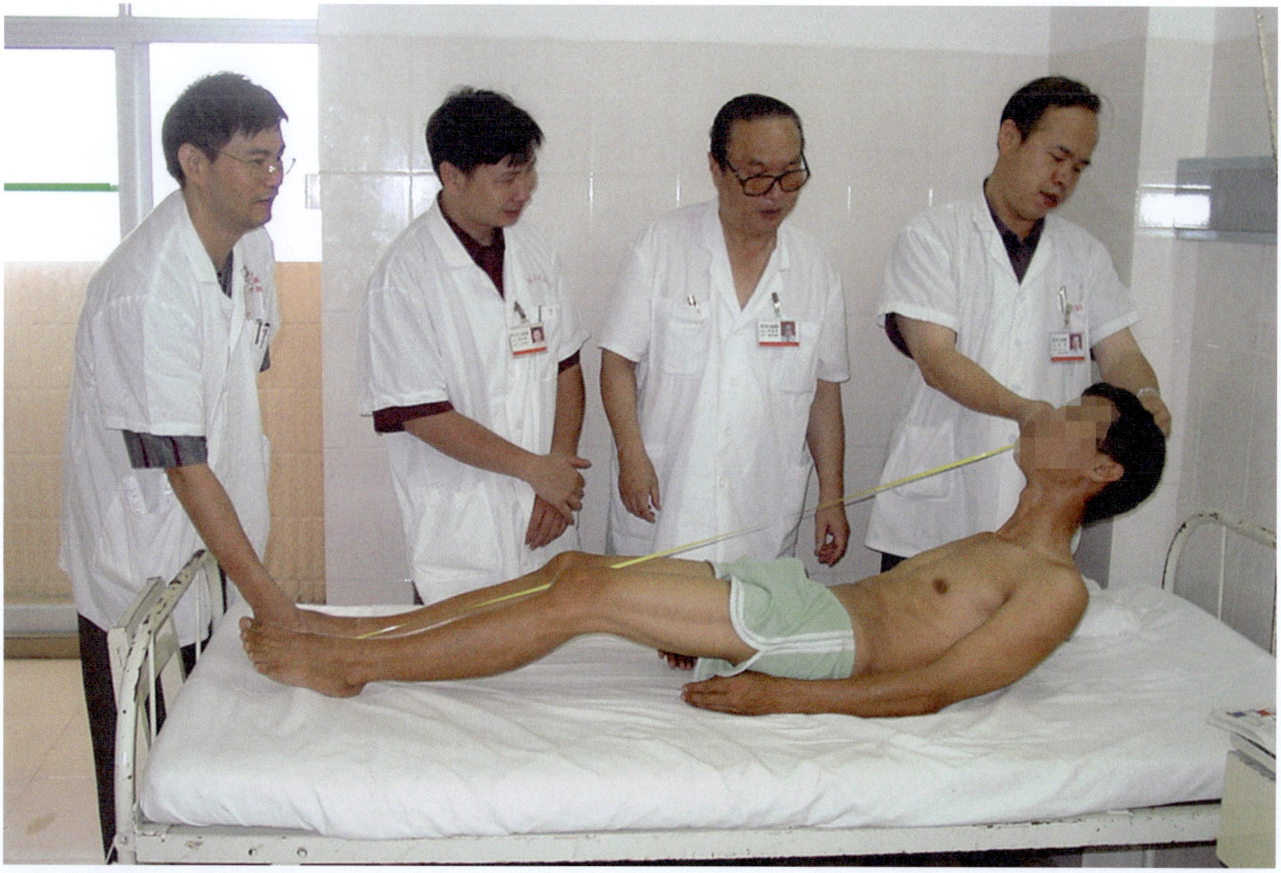

Fig. 6.3 Patient with ankylosing spondylitis kyphosis lie on the bed with their heads cocked up, he needs the support of thick pillows to keep a supine position

omy. According to the relation between the apical segment of kyphosis and osteotomy segments, procedures can be divided into apical vertebral osteotomy and non-apical vertebral osteotomy.

Application of VCR for ankylosing kyphosis: when the anterior edge of the vertebral body and anterior longitudinal ligament of the kyphotic segment with a large Cobb angle is completely ossified, it will be difficult to correct deformity radically by using translaminar osteotomy or subtotal vertebral arch and body osteotomy. In this circumstance, VCR should be considered. The wedge of VCR (involving one or two intervertebral spaces) is greater than subtotal osteotomy (Fig. 6.7a–c). The anterior margin of the wedge resection is the anterior longitudinal ligament. This will make the spine shorten and better straightened upon closing the wedge (Figs. 6.8 and 6.9). Sometimes by compressing on the posterior instrumentation, the anterior side of the osteotomy level will be even opened (Fig. 6.10). This explains why VCR corrects more than subtotal osteotomy. When VCR involves a wide scope, a strut graft in the intervertebral space with cortical bone and trabecular bone should be performed (Fig. 6.11) to prevent the spinal cord tortuosity caused by excessive spinal shortening.

The osteotomy and fixation concept of VCR for ankylosing kyphosis are different from those for tuberculous or congenital angular kyphosis. In these two conditions, the principle of internal fixation after VCR is a combination of posterior compression and anterior distraction while it often requires a long instrumentation. While in ankylosing kyphosis usually with a round curve, posterior compression only is usually enough to stabilize the spine without adding anterior distraction force. This is the difference between round kyphosis and angular kyphosis regarding internal fixation.

Apical vertebra is the only target of osteotomy for angular kyphosis while for round kyphosis non-apical vertebra is an alternative. Compare with translaminar osteotomy, VCR has the advantage of correcting both kyphosis and scoliosis by asymmetric resection of vertebra, so VCR covers a wider range of indications.

After VCR for ASK, a relatively short segment instrument is usually adequate to maintain spinal stability and there is no need for anterior strut grafting. On the contrary angular deformity requires long-segment instrumentation and strut grafting anteriorly. With bone debris grafting only on top of the lamina, sound bone healing is generally achievable upon half-year X-ray follow-up (Fig. 6.12a, b).

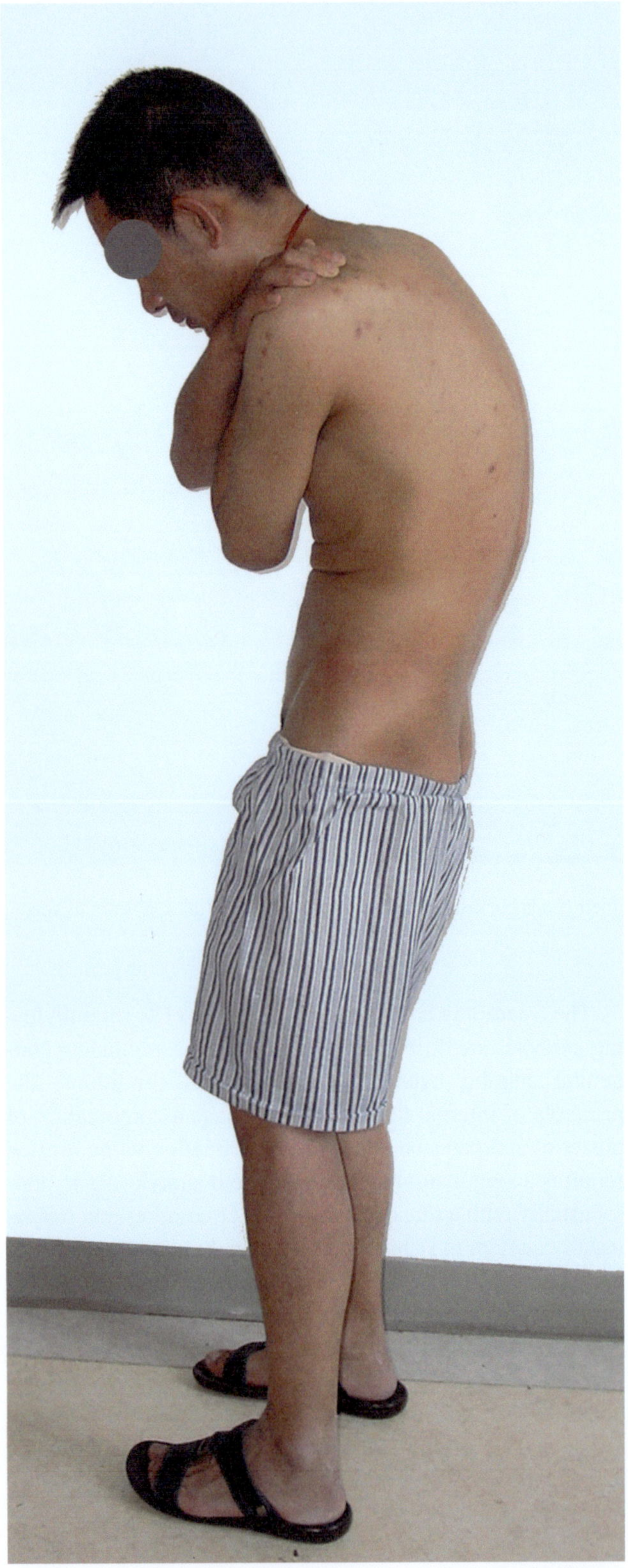

Fig. 6.4 Mild ASK (Cobb angle <80°=)

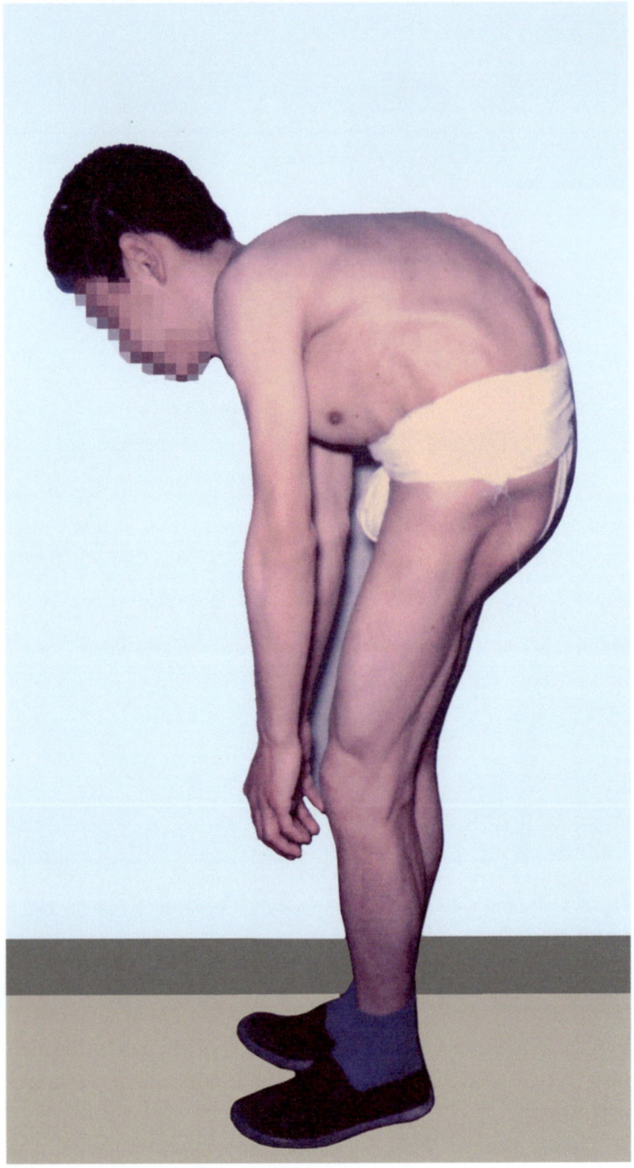

Fig. 6.5 Severe ASK (Cobb angle >80°) is the indication for vertebral column resection (VCR)

6.2 Surgical Procedure

1. Preoperative preparation
   1.1. Instruments: Specialized instruments for VCR (Fig. 6.13), internal fixation instruments, general surgical instruments.
   1.2. Osteotomy site:
   Non-apical vertebra: generally between L2 and L3 where just cauda equina is found in the spinal canal. So, it is safe to correct here and less likely to cause

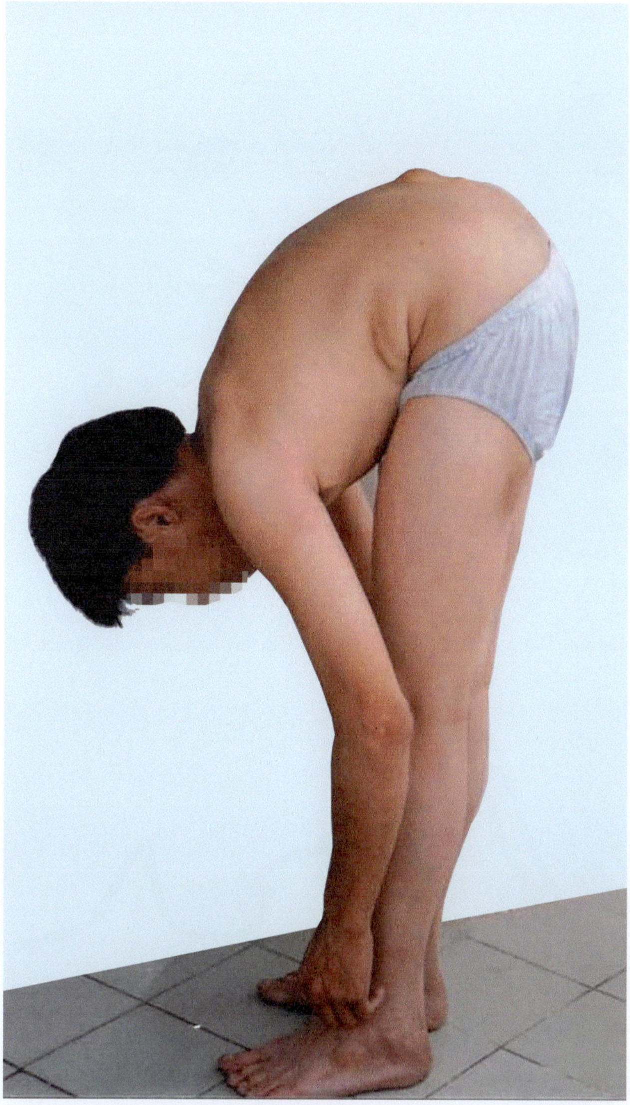

Fig. 6.6 This patient represents the most severe case of ASK. VCR and spine shortening is needed as the contracture of neurovascular structures, visceral organs and soft tissue of the trunk wall will restrict the extension of the spine

paraplegia. It is frequently used for ankylosing spondylitis kyphosis.

Apical vertebra: ideally between T10-L4 where it is relatively easy and safe to reduce the spine.

2. Anesthesia: Local infiltration anesthesia, general anesthesia with tracheal intubation or bronchoscope.
3. Patient positioning: Proper positioning plays a critical role for osteotomy and whole treatment. It requires close cooperation between surgeons and other staff in the operation room. In the prone position, the patient should be placed on the operating bed with an arch-shaped support cushion under the body (Fig. 6.14). The shoulders should be supported with a special shoulder plate. The void under the trunk should be filled with padding which is going to be removed for the trunk to straighten after the osteotomy is accomplished. The lateral decubitus position is mostly used for patients with severe ankylosing kyphosis. The cephalic and caudal traction bands should be prepared before surgery to facilitate the reduction after osteotomy. Prone position is most commonly used, as it is more controllable during reduction than lateral position (Fig. 6.15).
4. Surgical procedure:

The first step, incision and exposure: A 20–30 cm longitudinal incision is made along spinous processes, split muscles to expose the articular process, lamina, and transverse process bilaterally. In other words, exposure should be extended to the costotransverse process joint of both sides at the osteotomy segment. Toward the two ends of the incision, exposure to the lateral edge of the lamina is enough (Fig. 6.16).

The second step, cut through the transverse processes to expose pedicles and vertebral body: From the lateral edge of the pedicle (equivalent to the root of the transverse process), cutting through the transverse process on both sides (Fig. 6.17). Then the anonymous elevator (a device in the Tian's osteotome) is used to carefully elevate subperiosteally along the pedicle to the vertebral body waist (Fig. 6.18). Finally, change over to vertebral elevator and continue to elevate until the anterolateral edge of the vertebral body (Fig. 6.19).

The third step, use a lever retractor to protect segmental vessels: Removing the vertebral elevators, insert lever retractor subperiosteally to the anterior edge of the vertebral body. Apply force on the lever retractor to expose the whole vertebral body, (Fig. 6.20) and compress the segmental arteries and veins in front of the vertebral bodies. Usually, segmental vessel ligation is not needed.

The fourth step, translaminar osteotomy: This procedure should go directly ahead for osteotomy if there is interlaminar bony fusion at kyphosis apex. If not, one or two vertebral arches at the osteotomy level should be resected to expose the spinal canal, nerve roots, and pedicle on both sides (Fig. 6.21).

The fifth step, pedicle screws or sublamina hook placement: Before osteotomy, pedicle screws or lamina hooks should be applied above and below the osteotomy segment (Fig. 6.22) to avoid displacement of osteotomy site if they are applied after osteotomy.

The sixth step, vertebral body osteotomy: Expose the vertebral body from both sides, the nerve roots from upper and lower segments should be protected by a retractor and keep it out of the operative field (Fig. 6.23). Temporary rod should be placed before vertebral body osteotomy to prevent spinal cord injury from spinal instability and displacement once the spine is disconnected. From both lateral sides, cut through the vertebral body all the way to the anterior longitudinal ligament, retaining a

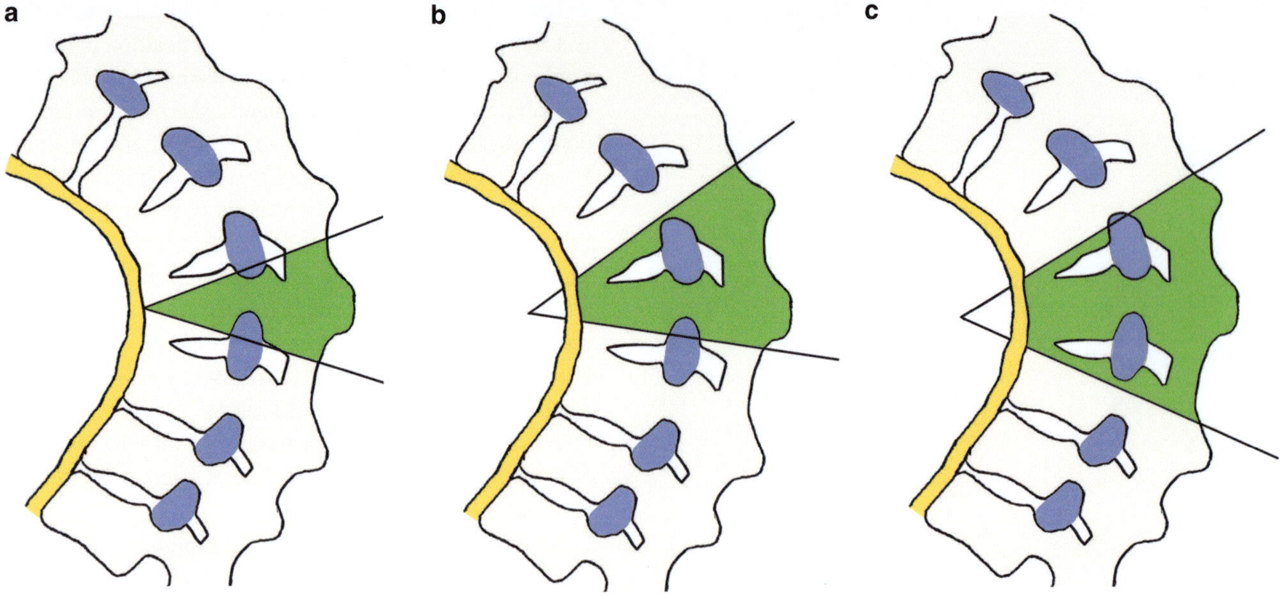

Fig. 6.7 Range of total spinal osteotomy. (**a**) Endplate-preserving VCR contained in one vertebral body. (**b**) VCR involving one disc space. (**c**) VCR involving two disc spaces

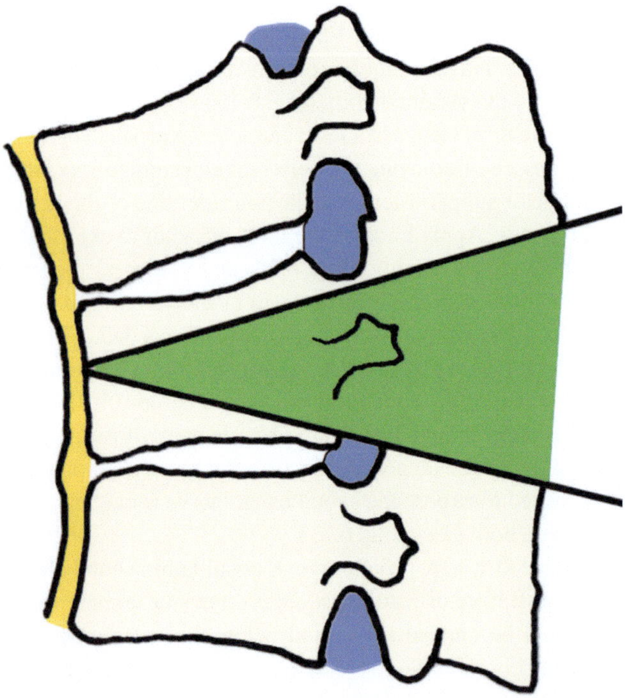

Fig. 6.8 The anterior of VCR wedge should reach anterior longitudinal ligament

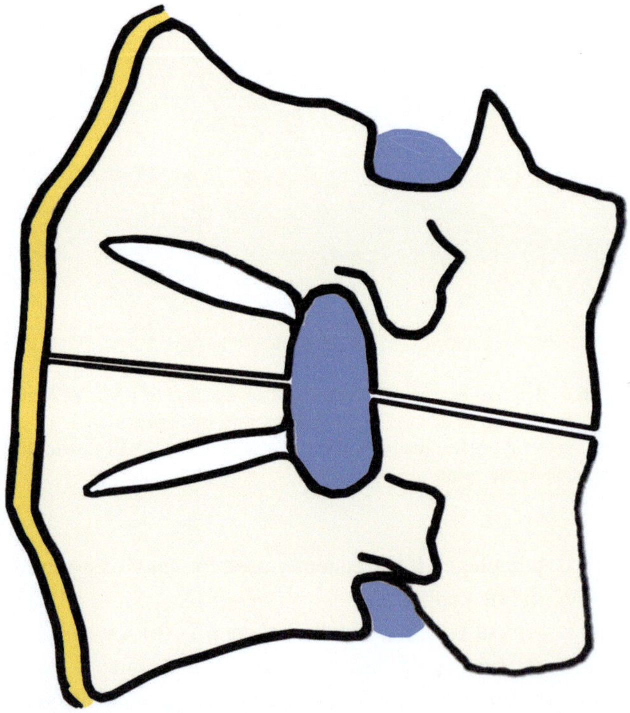

Fig. 6.9 If the osteotomy wedge is completed to have "bone on bone," grafting could be spared

thin bone sheet of the posterior edge of the vertebral body (Fig. 6.24) to prevent bleeding from epidural venous plexus. The lateral part of the vertebral body is removed with straight osteotomes (Fig. 6.25), followed by central resection with shovel osteotomes and crescent osteotomes, and temporarily preserves a thin bone sheet at the posterior edge of the vertebral body (Figs. 6.26 and 6.27).

The seventh step, resection of the posterior edge of the vertebral body: After a majority of the vertebra is

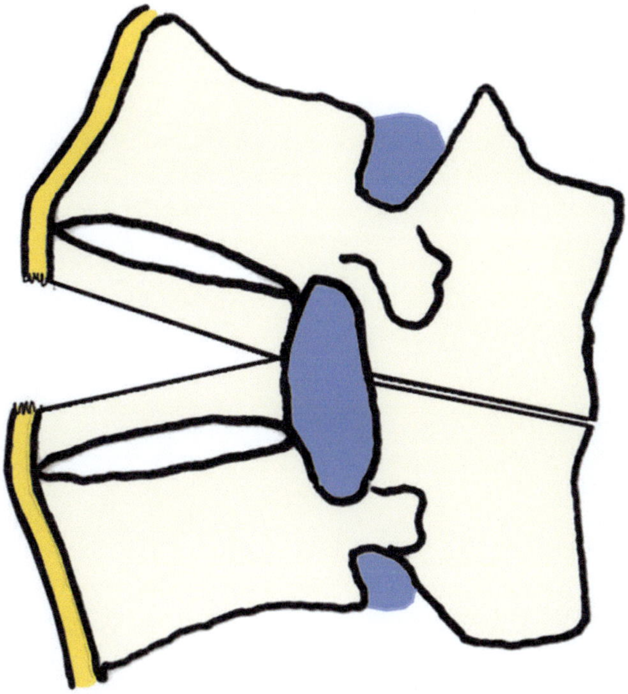

Fig. 6.10 VCR allows the anterior opening of the osteotomy segment for more correction

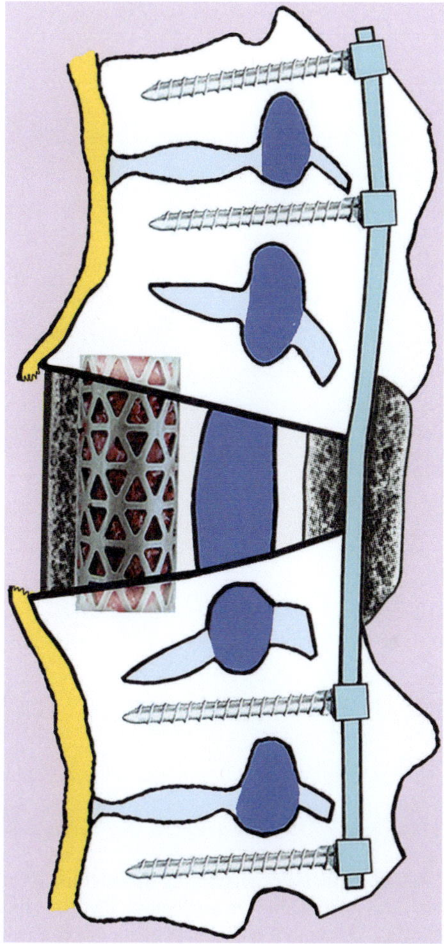

Fig. 6.11 After VCR, interbody and interlaminar grafting with rigid posterior long instrumentation

removed, the inner edge of the pedicle (Fig. 6.28) and the posterior edge of the vertebral body (Fig. 6.29) are pushed and removed as soon as possible by push osteotome. At this time, active bleeding may occur from the epidural venous plexus. Palpating the osteotomy gap to confirm free of bone fragment when the gap should be closed immediately (Fig. 6.30). Upon complete closure, the dural sac expands and widens (Fig. 6.31) to compress the epidural venous plexus and the bleeding will stop naturally.

The eighth step, internal fixation: Fixation following osteotomy for ASK can be divided into two types: (1) dynamic compression internal fixation, suitable for translaminar osteotomy for the kyphotic angle between 76° and 90°. As the ossification and hyperplasia of spinous processes, the interspinous ligament and the supraspinous ligament form a wide and thick longitudinal septum which is utilized to facilitate the dynamic compression internal fixation implantation instead of resecting it arduously. The patient can lie in a supine position in bed after the interspinous dynamic compression internal fixation by Luque rods and wiring (Fig. 6.32a, b). Keeping this position allows the spine to straighten naturally and it has the potential to further correct the kyphosis without limitation of internal fixation instruments, and more effective. However, no one internal fixation replaces the prominent role of external immobilization of hyperextended plaster vest in ankylosing kyphosis correction, as the plaster vest prevents kyphotic recurrence and accelerates firm bone fusion. (2) Static pedicle screws system. It is used for severe ankylosing kyphosis with a Cobb angle of more than 90°. With the progression of kyphotic deformity, such patients have developed severe contractures of rectus abdominis muscle and soft tissues. Mesentery and neurovascular structures are also shortened, being the source of tension upon correction. To correct this deformity, it is necessary to shorten the spine after 1- or 2-level VCR, and then close the posterior osteotomy gap and open the anterior column followed by long segmental instrumentation, anterior strut grafting, lamina grafting, and external immobilization which are all crucial and essential (Figs. 6.33 and 6.34).

The ninth step, place a drainage tube and close the incision: It is preferable to use bilateral negative pressure drainage tubes to avoid infection caused by hematoma. Electrocoagulation hemostasis should be performed carefully before the incision was closed in layers.

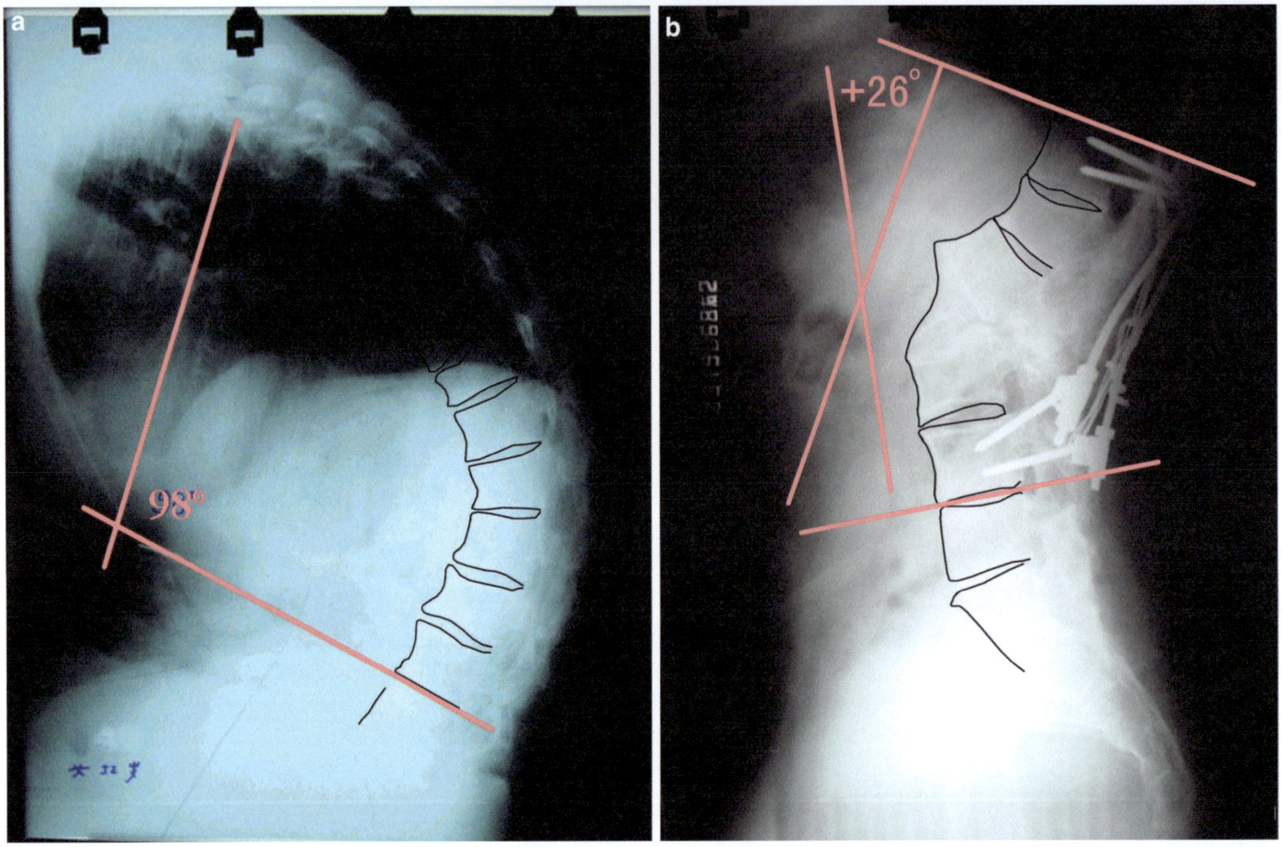

Fig. 6.12 Round kyphosis of ankylosing spondylitis. After posterior compression, short instrumentation is adequate. Dynamic fixation (with wiring or elastic rod fixation) allows secondary correction by lying in bed after an operation. Dynamic fixation also eliminates the need for bone grafting in opening anteriorly (just interlaminar bone grafting with bone debris is needed). Sound bone healing behind the lamina and between the vertebral body. (**a**) Preoperatively kyphotic angle was 98°. (**b**) Good bone fusion between the vertebral body and behind the lamina

5. Postoperative management:
   The patient should lie in the supine position with the pillow or cotton pads support according to the correction of kyphosis. In addition, alternating pillow positions between the two sides contribute to prevent pressure ulcers. Negative pressure drainage tubes should connect with suction bottles and patency should be maintained all the time. The following day after the operation, the amount of drainage fluid between 200 and 400 ml is a sign of free of blood effusion in the wound. The drainage tubes can be removed on Day 2 or Day 3 postoperatively. Once stitches are removed 10 days after surgery, external immobilization of hyperextended plaster vest is to be applied. Patients can ambulate with a plaster vest which is going to be maintained for 6–8 months.

6.3 Highlights and Considerations

1. Contracture of abdominal soft tissue in severe ankylosing kyphosis.
   With the progressing of round kyphosis, the distance between the xiphoid process and pubic symphysis decreases. This leads to contracture of abdominal skin, fascia, and muscle which stops the spine from straightening after osteotomy. The preferred technique of fixation for severe ankylosing kyphosis is dynamic compression fixation. It allows the spine to straighten spontaneously in the supine position and then abdominal soft tissues will be stretched gradually to obtain further correction.

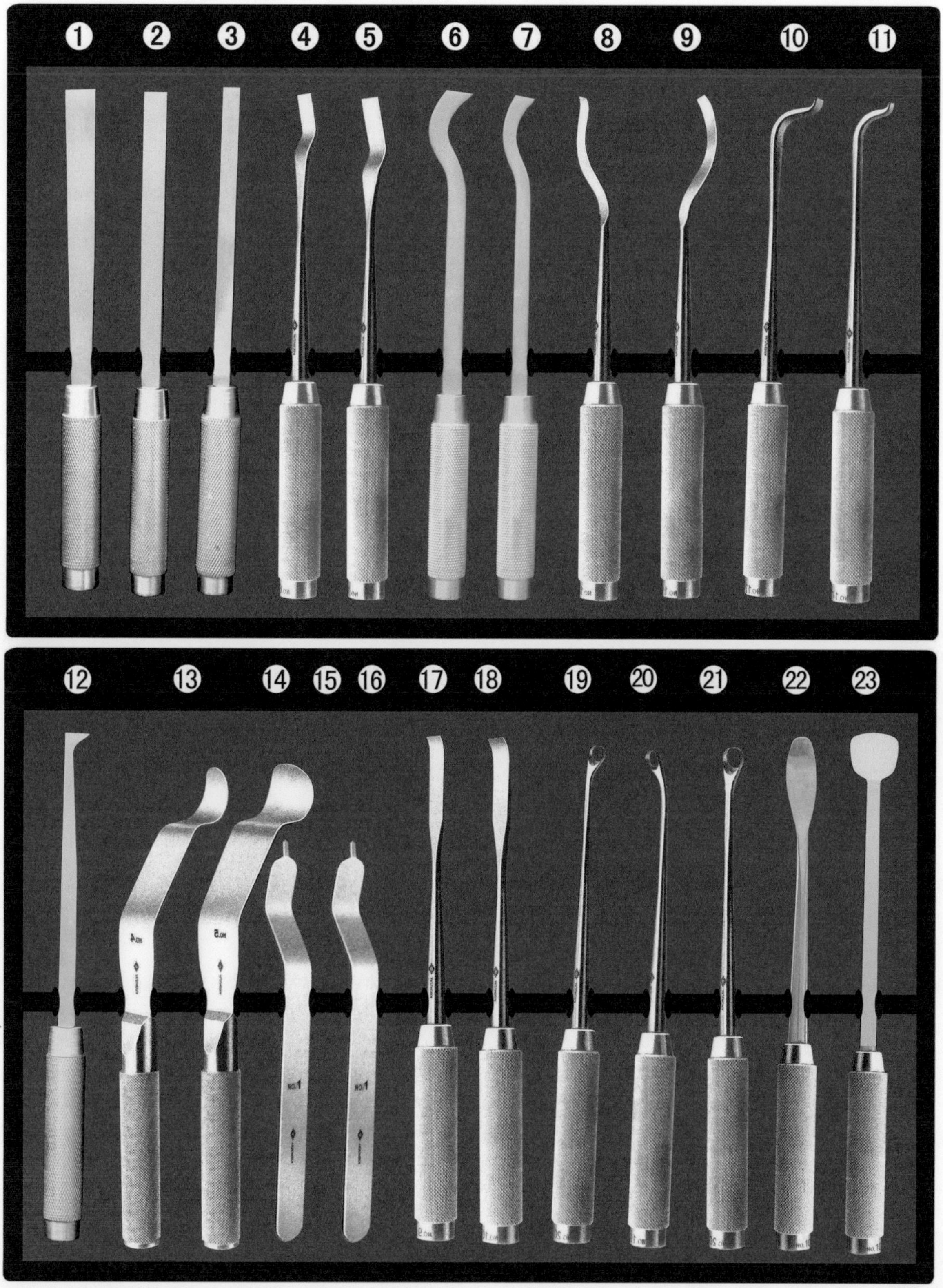

Fig. 6.13 A set of 23 Tian's osteotomes of type VII: No. 1–3 Straight osteotomes (large, medium and small), No. 4–5 Shovel osteotomes (large and small), No. 6.7 Crescent osteotomes (large and small), No. 8–9 Left and right osteotomes (left and right), No. 10–11 Push osteotomes (large and small), No. 12 Oblique tip osteotome, No. 13–14 Lever plates (wide and narrow), No. 15–16 Nerve root retractor, No. 17–18 Anonymous strippers (large and small), No. 19–21 Hollow scraper spoons (left, right, and straight), No. 22–23 Anonymous strippers (large and small)

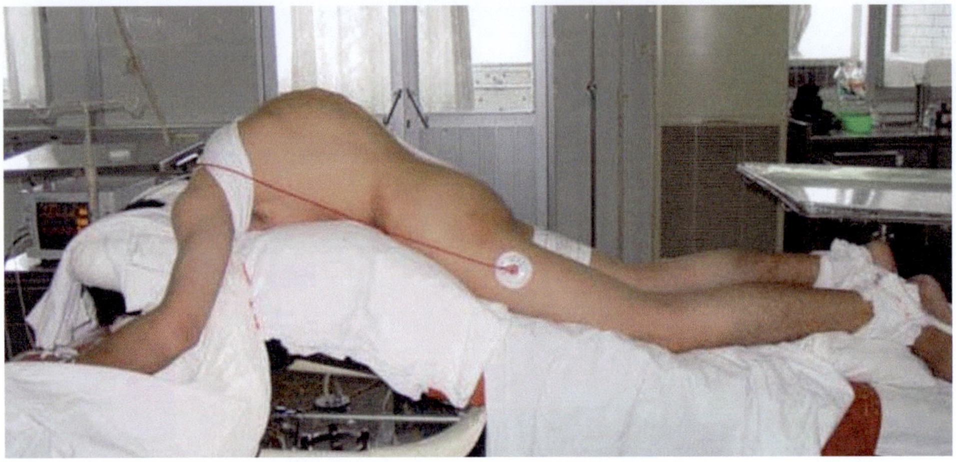

Fig. 6.14 In the prone position, the patient should be placed on the operating table with an arch-shaped support cushion under the body. The shoulders should be supported with special shoulder plates and the patient's head is placed on the adjustable stool. Adjust the operating table to V-shape with padding-filled cushion support under anterior superior iliac spines and abdomen. Fasten feet to the end of the bed with bandages to prevent the body from moving forward. Fix the traction belt under the armpits for traction after osteotomy

Fig. 6.15 In the case of a large kyphotic angle, the lateral decubitus position is an alternative. The sternal traction band and lower limb traction band should be deployed in advance for traction and reduction after osteotomy

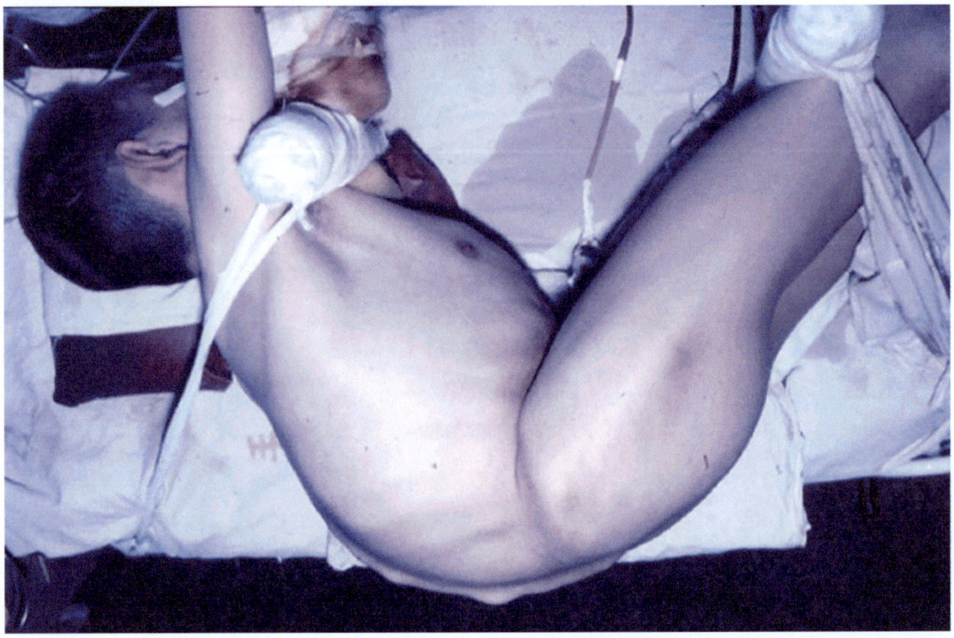

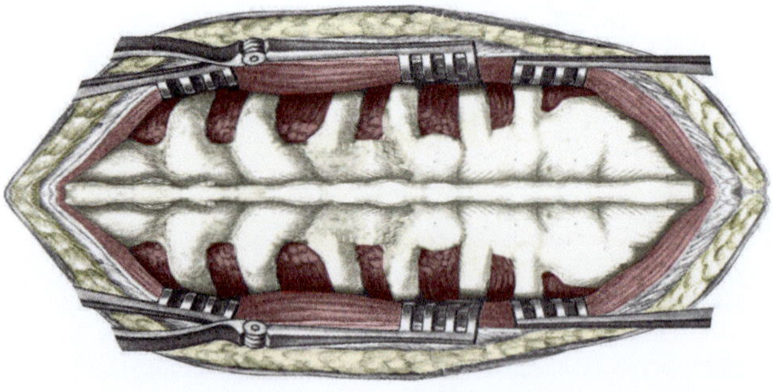

Fig. 6.16 The length of the incision is about 20–30 cm, exposing bilateral lamina, articular process, and transverse process

2. Selecting VCR for treating kyphosis.
   VCR is an option for both round kyphosis and angular kyphosis. However, many technical feasibility factors should be considered including osteotomy site, Cobb angle, age, etiology, bleeding tendency, underlying disease, and general condition. This technique is very effective, but patients should be carefully selected.
3. Bleeding and hemostasis in osteotomy.
   There are three main sources of bleeding during osteotomy: (1) bleeding from cancellous sinus vertebral bodies (Fig. 6.35a, b); (2) bleeding from epidural venous plexus (Fig. 6.36a, b); and (3) bleeding from intercostal vessels or lumbar arteries and veins (Fig. 6.37a, b). To

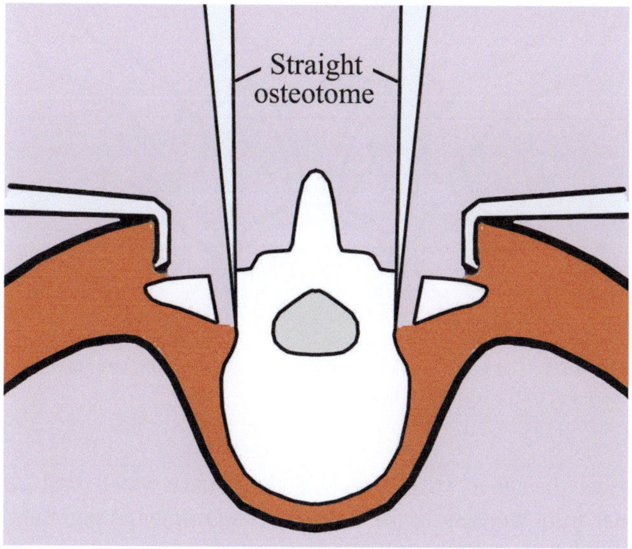

Fig. 6.17 To cut through the transverse process along the lateral edge of the pedicle with a straight osteotome

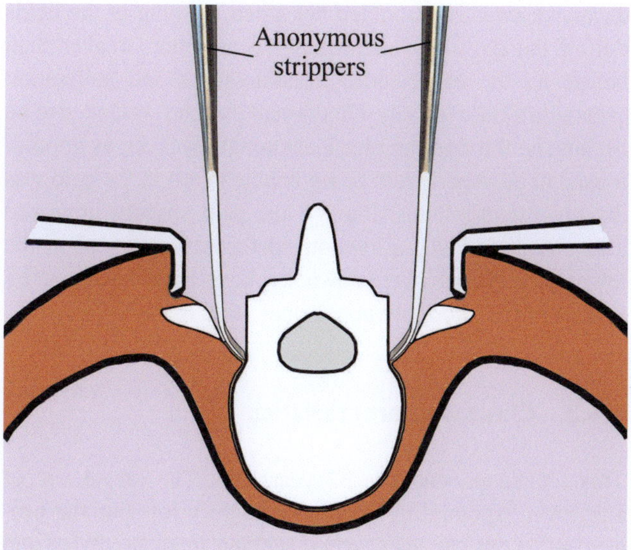

Fig. 6.18 The anonymous elevator (a device in Tian's set of osteotomes) elevates carefully subperiosteally along the pedicle to the vertebral body waist

reduce these bleedings, there are some tips we emphasize as following. Firstly, subperiosteal elevation should be carefully performed to avoid damaging the blood vessels across the vertebral body. Secondly, the osteotomy surface should be smooth to facilitate hemostasis by bone wax. Thirdly, the thin bone sheet at the posterior edge of the vertebral body should be retained for quick cutting in the last step. When the osteotomy gap is closed, bleeding from the epidural venous plexus is stopped naturally due to the compression of dilated dural sac.

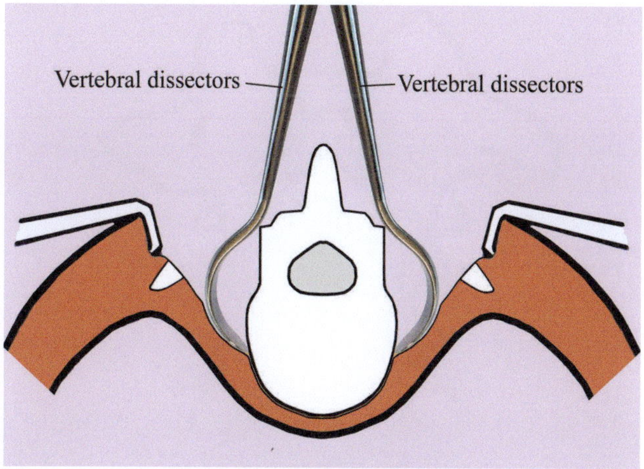

Fig. 6.19 Change over to vertebral dissectors and continue to elevate forward to the anterolateral edge of the vertebral body

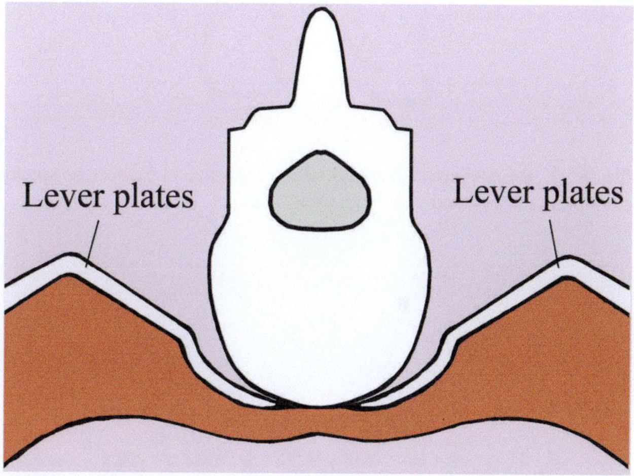

Fig. 6.20 Insert the lever retractor, to elevate segmental vessels and the paravertebral soft tissue

4. When closing the osteotomy gap with manual manipulation, use gentle force to prevent displacement and paraplegia.
5. One-stage posterior osteotomy for correcting kyphosis is very effective but there are also great risks so that careful evaluation should be carried out before operation. Specific surgical instruments are needed for posterior osteotomy to reduce the risk of paraplegia and spinal cord injury.
6. A sharp osteotome can reduce resistance and avoid spinal cord injury caused by shock. But there are some requirements for osteotomes: (1) the osteotome must have a sharp and thin blade, (2) the spine must be stabilized, and (3) the surgeon must have adequate skills.
7. When correcting the kyphosis by osteotomy, ideally the spinal cord and dural sac should be shortened with low tension. Cord distraction and tension, the major cause of paraplegia, is the last thing surgeon would have during surgery.

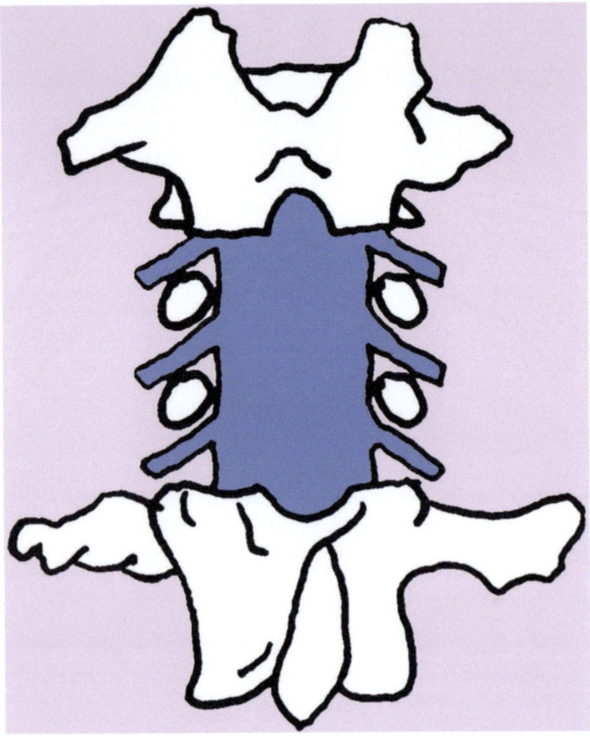

Fig. 6.21 Resect vertebral arches of two segments to expose the spinal canal, nerve roots, and pedicle of both sides

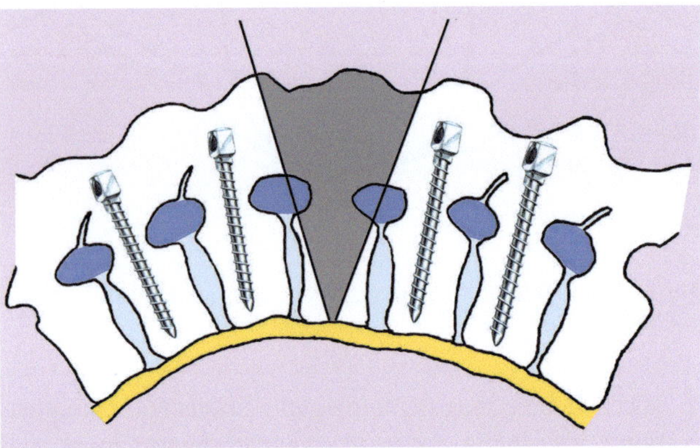

Fig. 6.22 Before osteotomy, pedicle screws or lamina hooks should be applied above and below the osteotomy segment

6.4 Typical Case

6.4.1 Case Summary

The patient, Huang XX, female, 32-year-old, is a farmer on the South China Sea coast of Yangjiang City, Guangdong Province. She was a farmer and fisher. The chief complaint: since the age of 16, she developed backache which disabled her from working in the field. Pain aggravated at night and deprived her of sleep. She often sat on the bed groaning with the hands holding her knees, sweat breaking out all over her body and trickled down her back. Symptoms slightly alleviated after activity in the morning but backache and body stiffness were very serious just after waking up. Fatigue and excessive sweating troubled her when working in the fields during the day. Physical strength was much weaker than before as she experienced breathlessness and palpitation even with a little activity. Others said that she pretended to be ill, but she felt that her physical strength was not as good as it used to be. Apart from being unable to work, the pain was the biggest problem. Although the pain slightly improved after the age of 20, a kyphotic deformity appeared in the lower back. As pain went down, kyphosis aggravated year by year to form the current appearance (Fig. 6.38a–d).

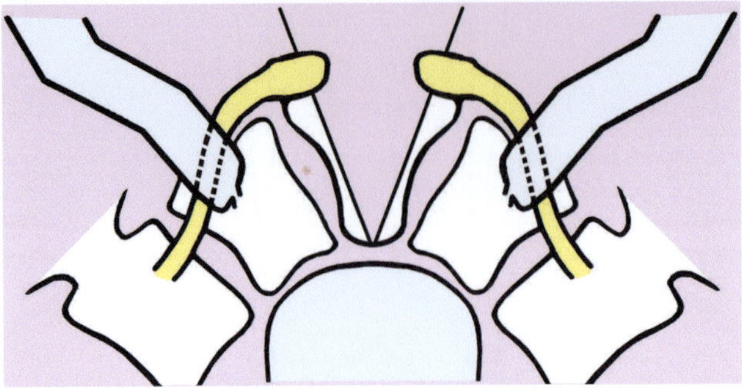

Fig. 6.23 The nerve roots should be protected by a retractor and keep them out of the operative field

6.4.2 Clinical Characteristics

This female patient was 32 years old. The prevalence of ankylosing spondylitis in females is very low but she progressed to the late stage when seeking medical advice and formed a severe thoracolumbar kyphosis. The body's center of gravity shifted forward so the trunk lost balance and leaned forward. She was unable to take a supine position during sleep and the ribs on both sides were inserted into the abdominal cavity; thus, abdominal breathing was restricted. Meanwhile, chest breathing was also compromised due to costovertebral joints ossification, so the patient's respiratory function was extremely limited with poor physical fitness. The patient's life was greatly threatened due to dysfunction of respiration, circulation, and digestion caused by severe kyphosis.

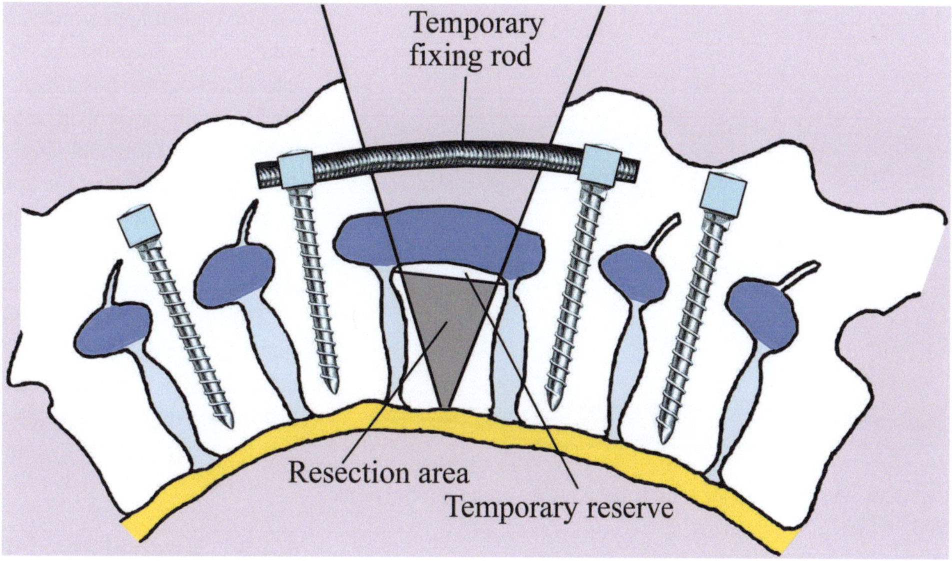

Fig. 6.24 After placing the temporary rod, the wedge resection is performed. The posterior wall of the body should be preserved temporarily for final resection

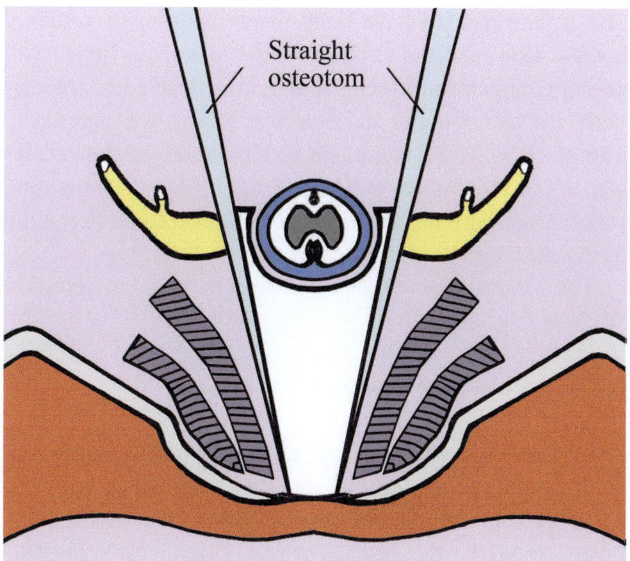

Fig. 6.25 The lateral part of the vertebral body was removed with straight osteotomes

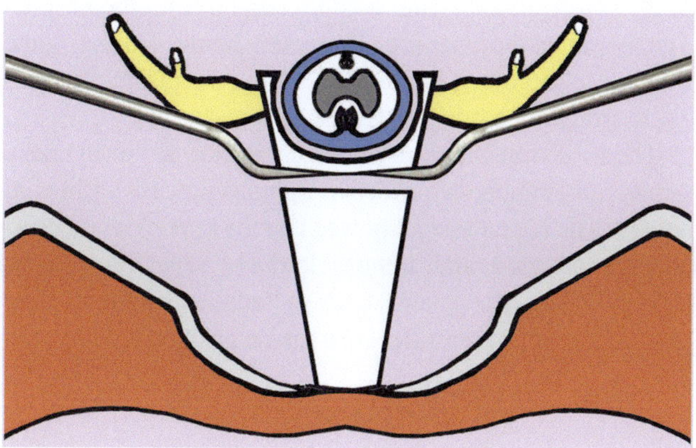

Fig. 6.26 The central part was removed with shovel osteotomes

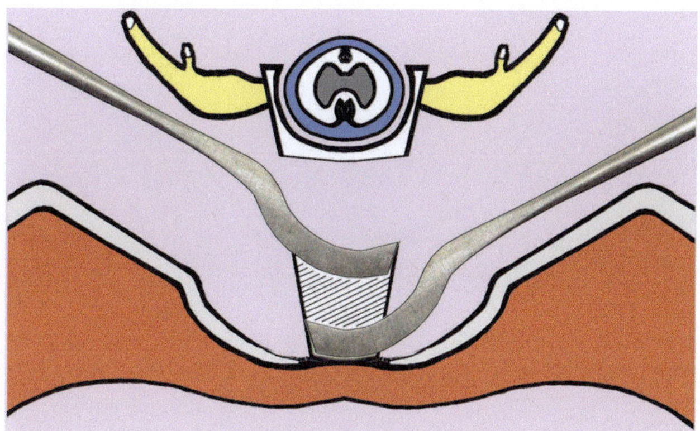

Fig. 6.27 The central part was removed with crescent osteotomes

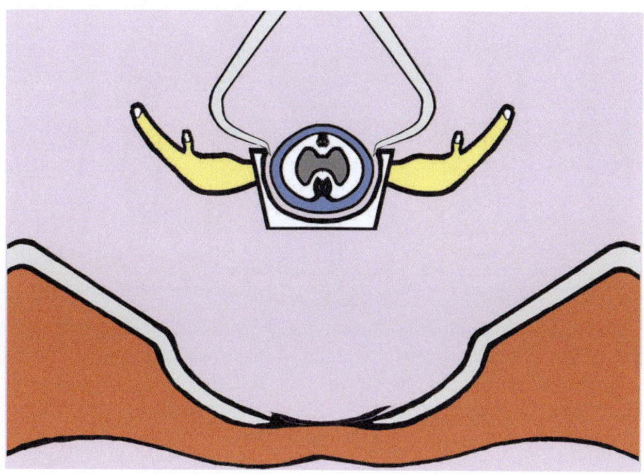

Fig. 6.28 Push osteotomes were used to cut off the inner edge of the pedicle

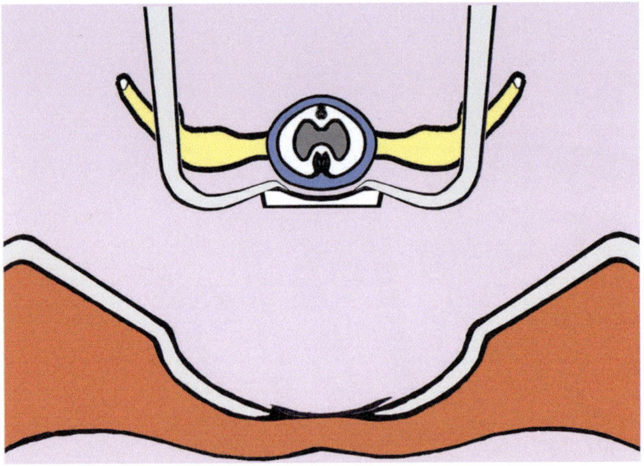

Fig. 6.29 Push osteotomes is used to cut off the posterior edge of the vertebral body

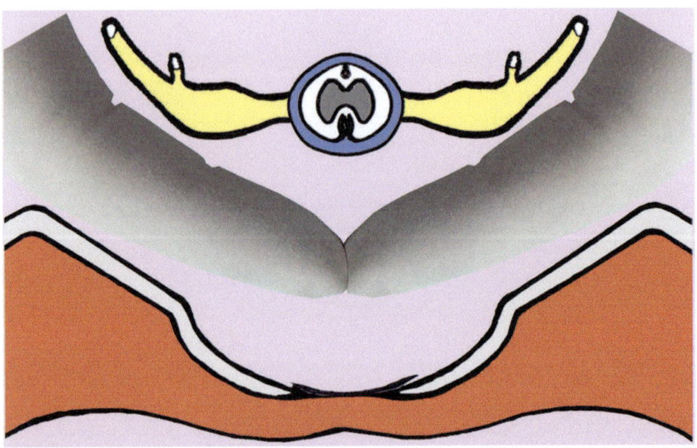

Fig. 6.30 Palpating the osteotomy gap to confirm free of bone fragment

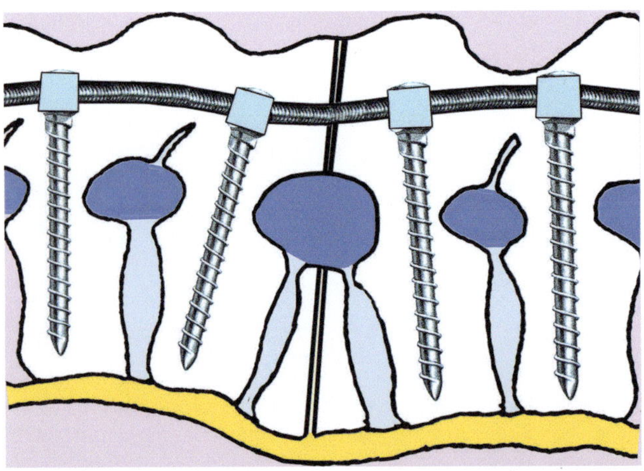

Fig. 6.31 When the gap is closed, the dural sac expands and widens to compress the epidural venous plexus and the bleeding will stop naturally

The typical appearance and X-ray findings are adequate to establish the diagnosis of AS in the late stage. A whole spine lateral radiograph has a great value in evaluating severe kyphosis. It usually presents as a large round-shaped thoracolumbar kyphosis, like a wheel (Fig. 6.39). However, the value of the AP view is limited as the spine presents in two segments due to thoracic and lumbar curve to the anterior (Fig. 6.40). Sacroiliac joint X-ray will not give more information and the HLA-B27 test is only to consolidate the diagnosis.

The focus of the examination is to determine whether patient status is suitable for surgical treatment and to identify surgical indications and contraindications. As surgery is the only effective treatment method for ankylosing spondylitis kyphosis, the role is not replaceable by non-operation therapies.

6.4.3 Surgical Plan and Postoperative Management

The patient did not have bony fusion anterior of vertebral bodies. However, the kyphotic angle was quite large, with severe contracture of rectus abdominis muscle and the distance between xiphoid and symphysis pubis was shortened. Therefore, VCR including one vertebral body and two discs was needed to shorten the spine (Fig. 6.41a–c). Shortening prevents superior mesenteric artery syndrome and stretching of the abdominal wall.

The surgical procedure of VCR can be found in Sect. 6.2.

6.4.4 Outcome Evaluation

After a series of clinical examinations, the patient underwent VCR to correct ankylosing spondylitis kyphosis with tracheal intubation and general anesthesia on October 25, 2002. Postoperatively, the kyphosis was completely corrected and the patient was able to sleep in the supine position (Fig. 6.42a, b). Ten days after operation, the stitches were removed and the trunk was immobilized by a hyperextended plaster vest. She was able to ambulate with the plaster vest freely (Fig. 6.43a, b). She was discharged from the hospital 21 days after the operation and went home. During home follow-up, she was lying in bed wearing the plaster vest and doing straight leg raising exercise (Fig. 6.44a, b).

The AP X-ray images after operation showed that dynamic screw–rod fixation was effective, spinous process wiring did not fail. The lateral image showed that the kyphosis was completely corrected and lumbar lordosis was 15° at now (Fig. 6.45a, b). The patient was very satisfied with the operation and said, "I haven't slept in a supine position for 12 years,

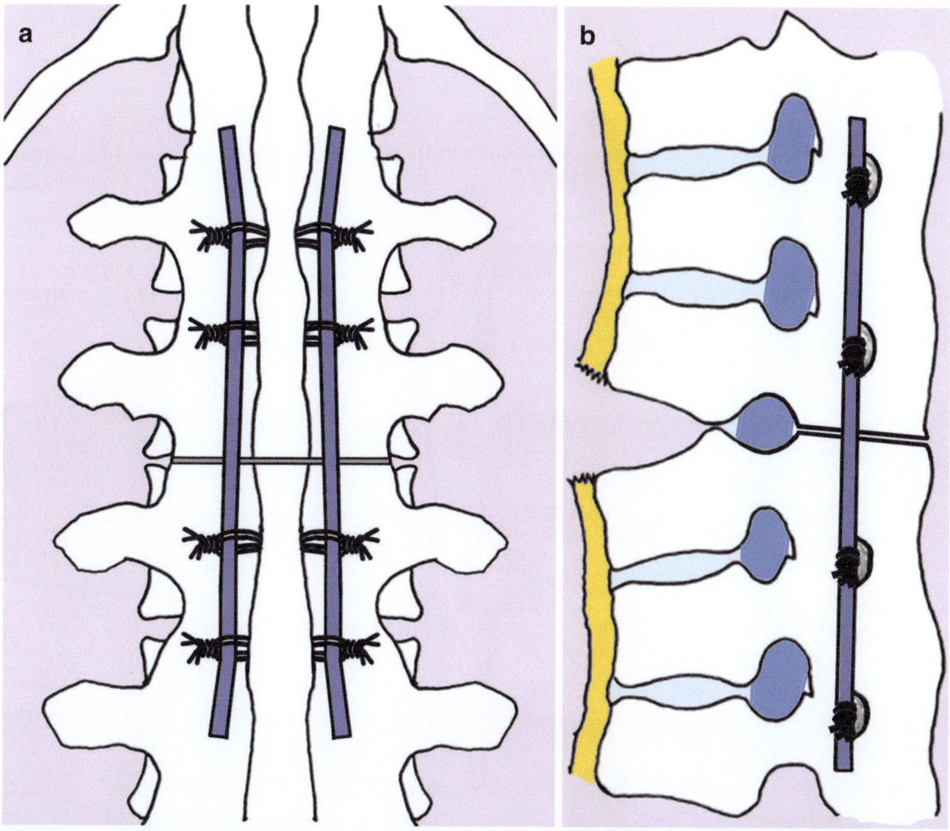

Fig. 6.32 Interspinous dynamic compression internal fixation: Luque rods and wiring allows sliding; thus, the spine straightens naturally to further correct the kyphosis when patients lie down. (**a**) Schematic frontal view. (**b**) Schematic lateral view

and now I can do it. I'm so happy!" Six months later, the plaster vest was removed and an X-ray was taken in the follow-up. With the spontaneous correction of the dynamic fixation system, lumbar lordosis further improved from 15° to 26°. It can be seen that there are a large number of indistinct new bones in the space of the intervertebral body, and there is also bony fusion behind the lamina (Fig. 6.46a, b). Compared with preoperative X-ray images, the gross correction was 124° (from 98° kyphosis to 26° lordosis) and formed a normal lumbar lordosis at last follow-up (Figs. 6.39 and 6.46b).

Compared with preoperative status as a severe ASK, the appearance was corrected completely in frontal and lateral view. With the elimination of hypoxia, the patient took a new look, just like 10 years younger (Figs. 6.38a–d and 6.47a, b).

6.4.5 Expert Comments

1. Osteotomy is the only treatment method for advanced stage ankylosing spondylitis kyphosis. It not only corrects the deformity but also improves and strengthens physical conditions. Patients tend to have cardiopulmonary and digestive dysfunction before surgery. Surgical intervention improves the dysfunction and refreshes patients' spirits with the improvement of nutrition and oxygen supply.
2. Ankylosing spondylitis kyphosis osteotomy surgery not only improves the patient's appearance but also improves the patient's general health, enhances the patient's physique, and prolongs the patient's life. It is a surgical method of great therapeutic significance.
3. However, there are some difficulties in ankylosing spondylitis kyphosis osteotomy, so we should study it carefully in order to understand its essentials.
   (a) Surgeons should have a clear concept of spinal anatomy so that they will not get lost anytime in the operation field.
   (b) Surgeons should have the basic skills of using a thin blade osteotome to operate on the spine. This requires hardworking in training.
   (c) Surgeons should be capable of dissecting the spinal nerve roots during the operation to prevent the spinal nerves from being injured.
   (d) Surgeons should mind bleeding and master the hemostasis technique.

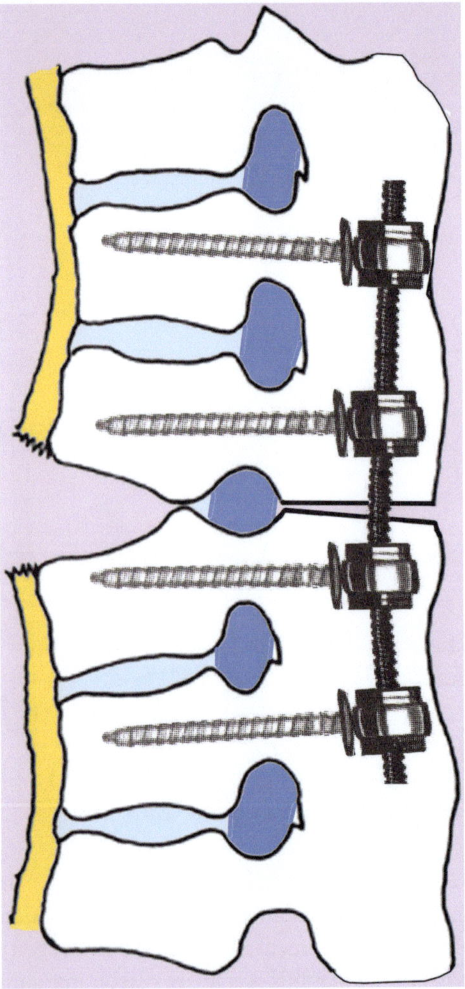

Fig. 6.33 Instrumentation with static long-segment pedicle screw system after anterior distraction and posterior compression

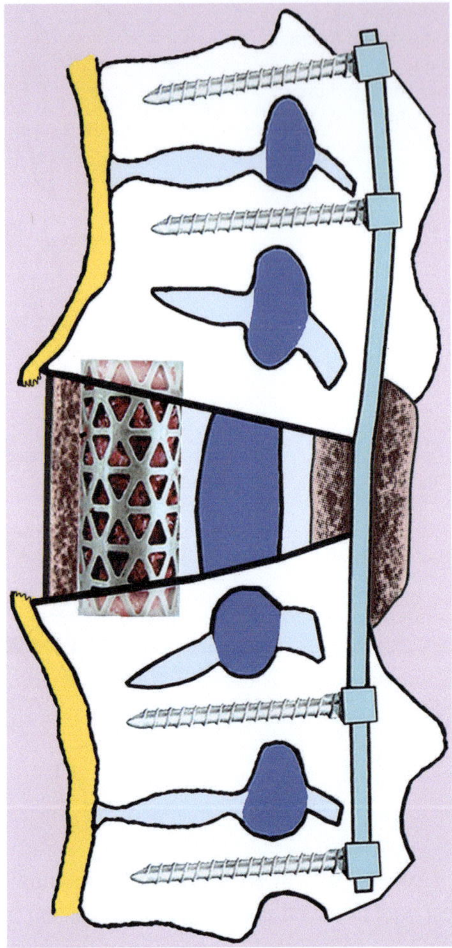

Fig. 6.34 If the extensive resection involves one or two disc spaces, the anterior column should be reconstructed with a strut graft. The posterior edge of the laminar should be totally approximated to avoid shortening of the spine and buckling of the dura

(e) Surgeons should prevent cerebrospinal fluid leakage.
(f) Surgeons should take action to prevent displacement of the osteotomy site.
(g) The spinal cord is more sensitive to distraction than shortening.
(h) The preferable type of internal fixation should be adequately evaluated, e.g., dynamic fixation versus static fixation.
(i) Indications of postoperative postural correction or step-by-step manual correction without internal fixation should be well understood.

The above principles and surgical technique must be acquired to be qualified with ankylosing spondylitis kyphosis osteotomy.

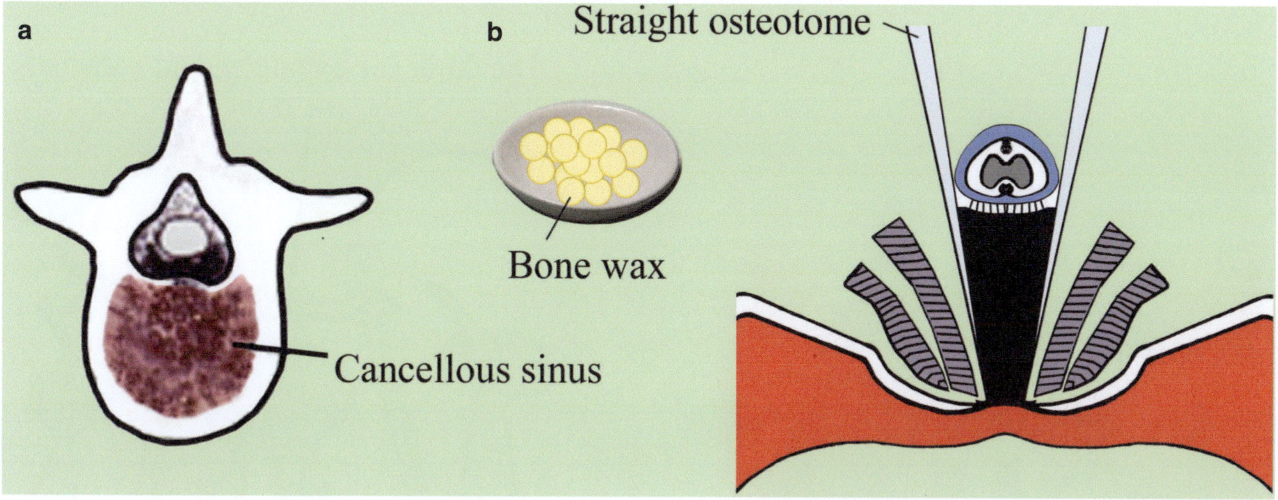

Fig. 6.35 (**a**) Bleeding from cancellous sinus. (**b**) Keep osteotomy surface smooth and apply bone wax

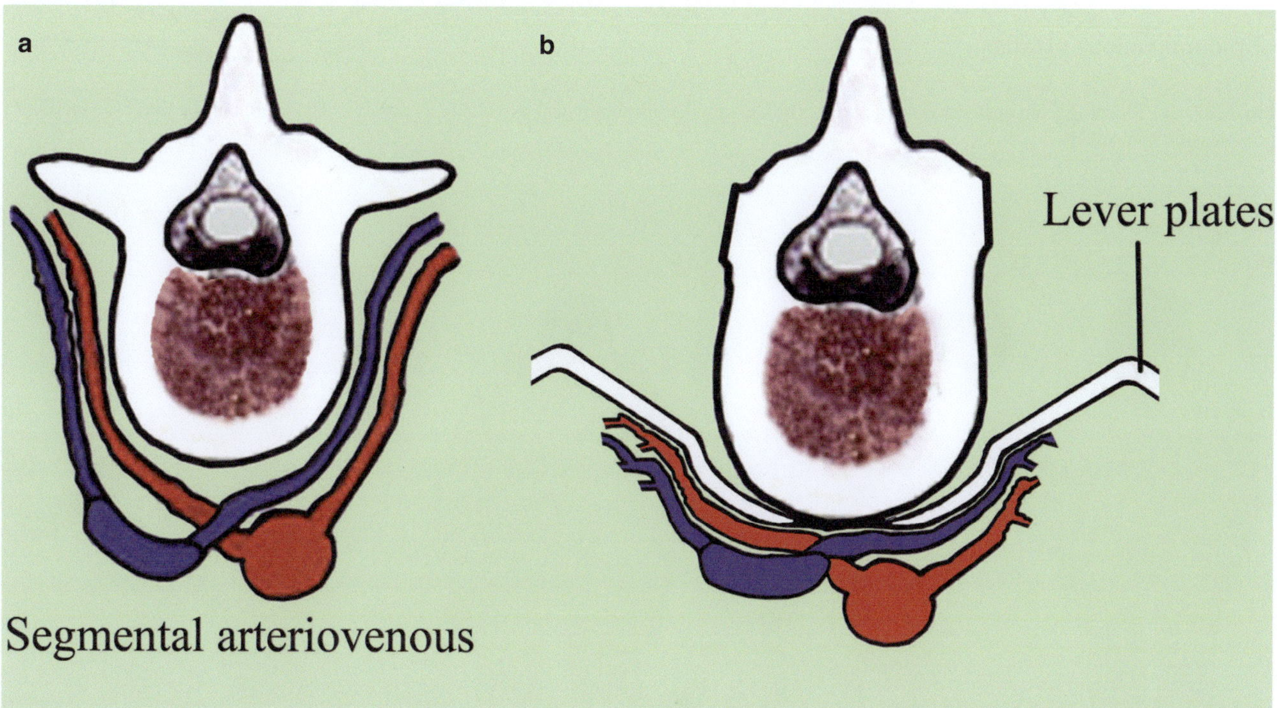

Fig. 6.36 (**a**) Bleeding from intercostal vessels or lumbar arteries and veins. (**b**) Subperiosteal elevation only, protection with lever retractor

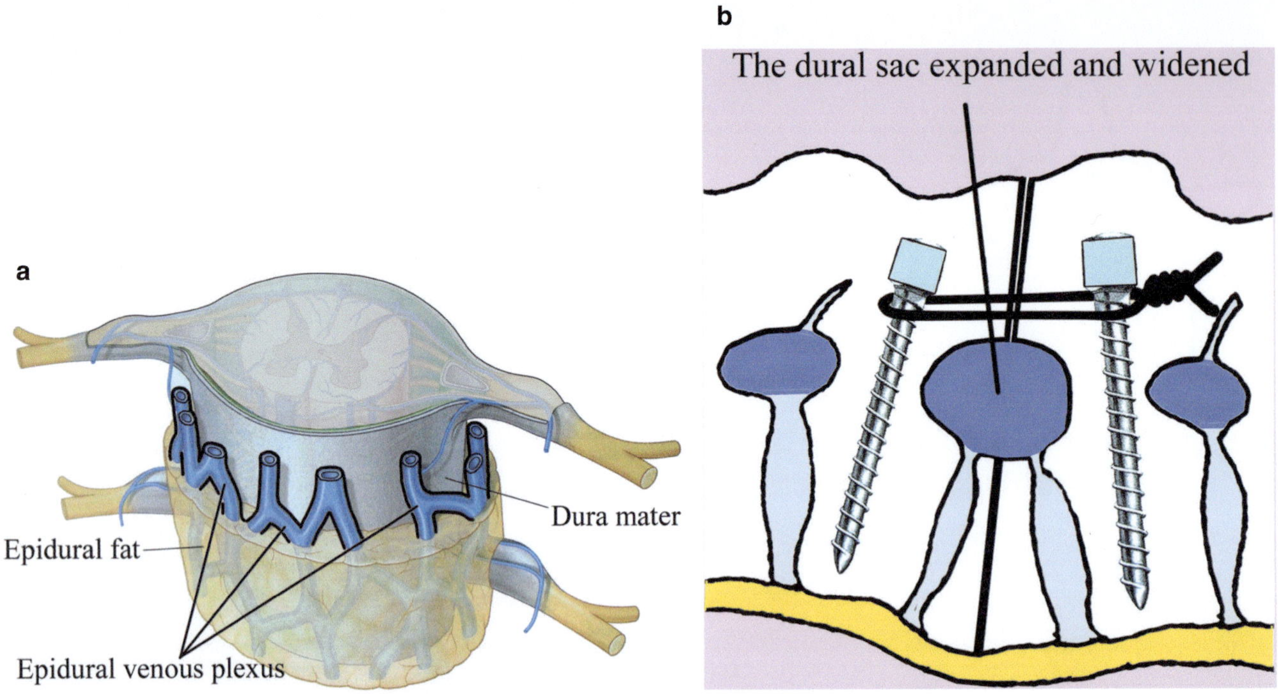

Fig. 6.37 (**a**) Bleeding from epidural venous plexus. (**b**) Closing the osteotomy gap as quickly as possible. Expansion of the dural sac facilitates compression hemostasis

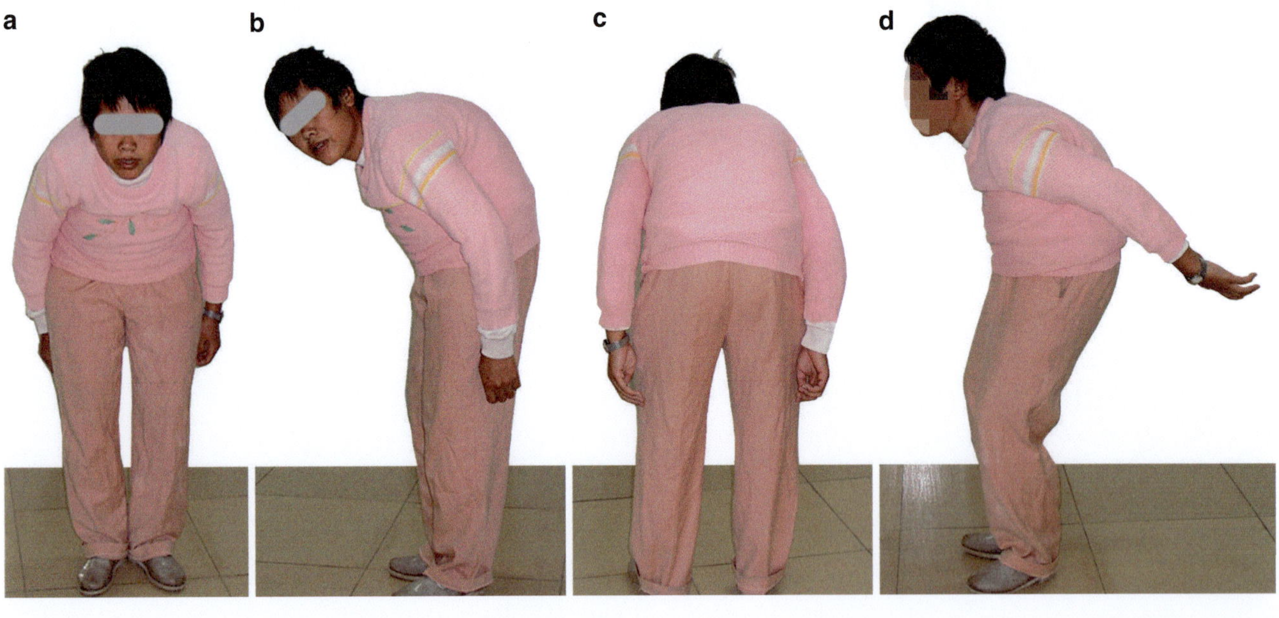

Fig. 6.38 Patient, female, 32 years old, severe ankylosing spondylitis with 98° kyphotic angle. Appearance in various positions before operation. (**a**) Frontal view. (**b**) Lateral view. (**c**) Back view. (**d**) In activity

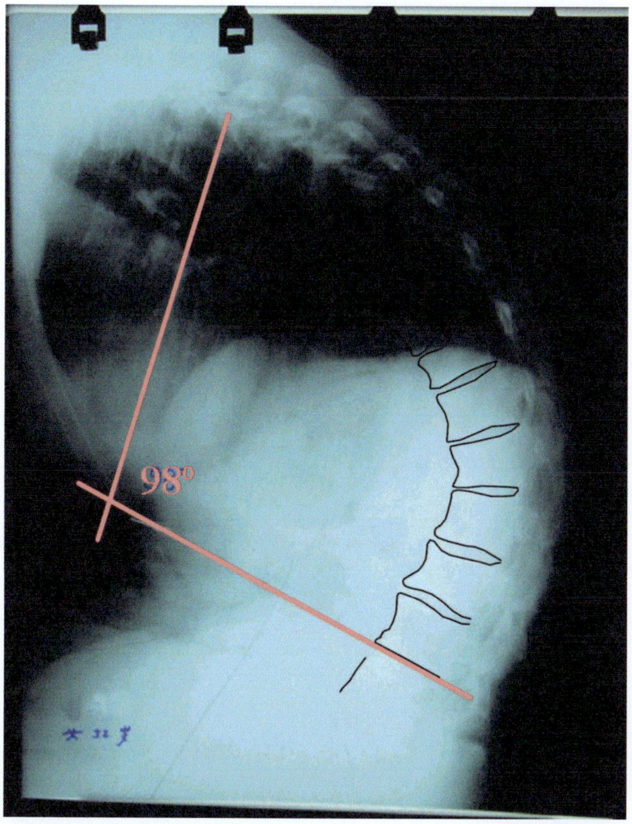

Fig. 6.39 The lateral radiograph

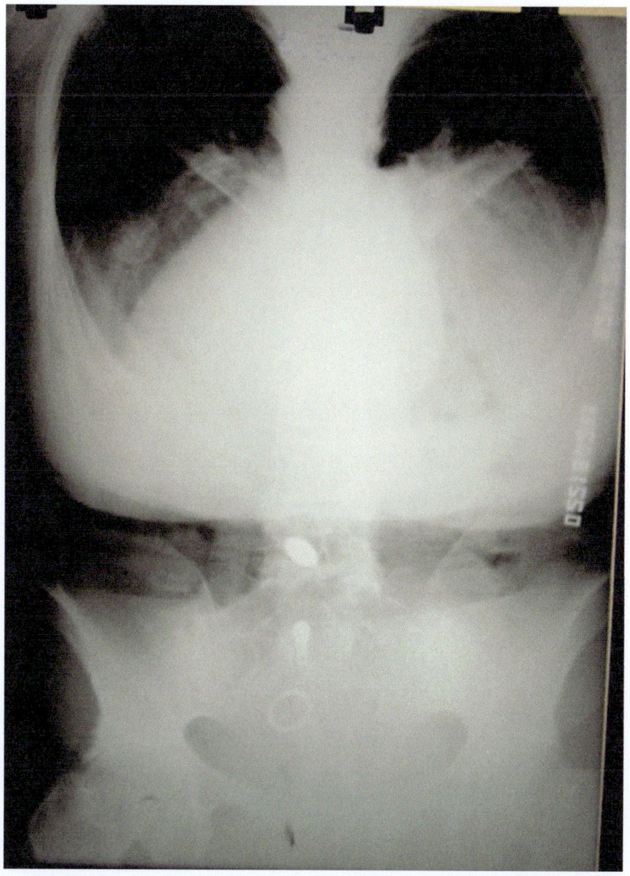

Fig. 6.40 Anteroposterior radiograph reveals segmented imaging

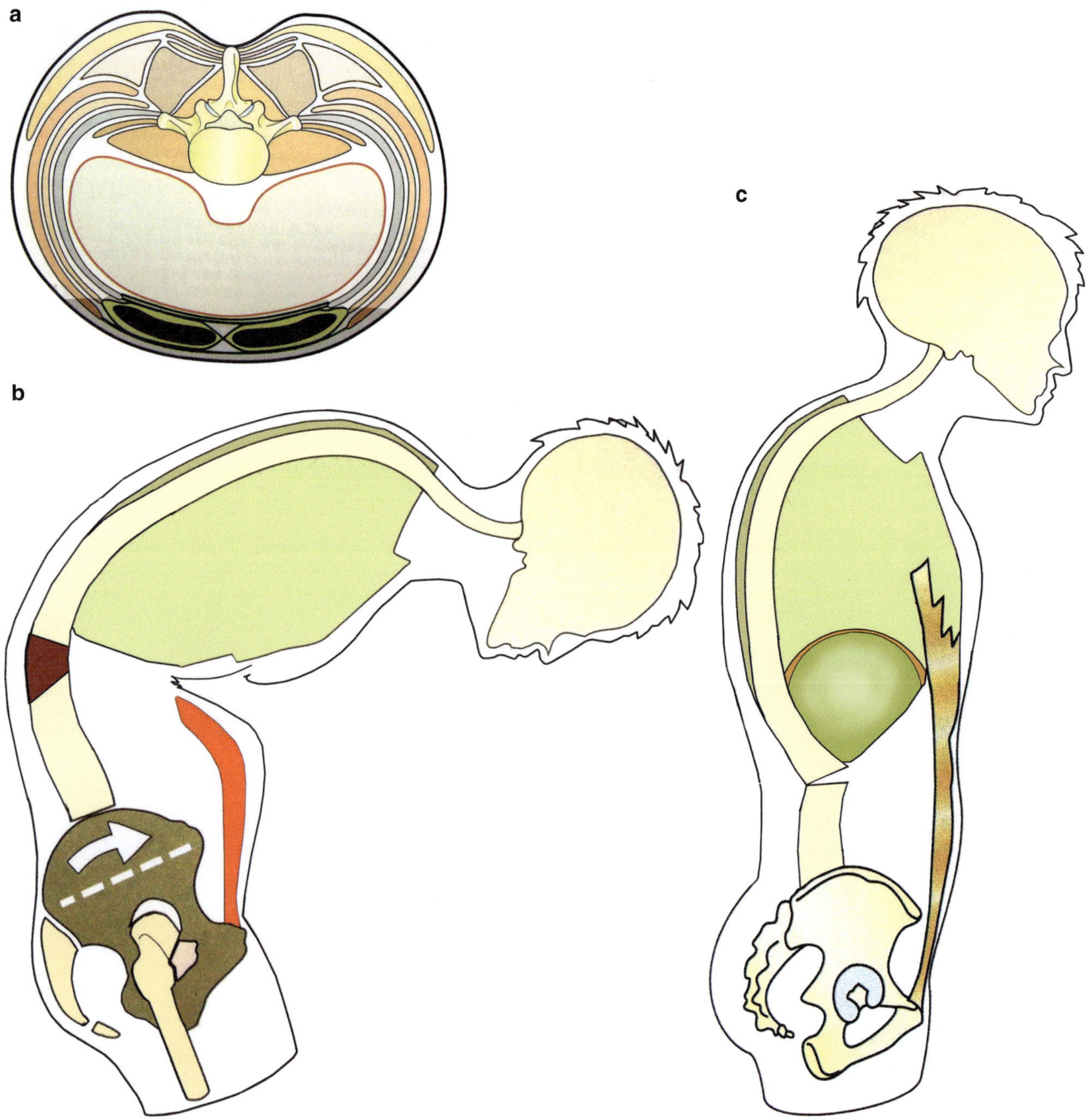

Fig. 6.41 Preoperative and postoperative diagram. (**a**) Severe contracture of rectus abdominis muscle. (**b**) The distance between xiphoid and symphysis pubis is reduced and abdominal bulging is seen. (**c**) After non-apical osteotomy, a large "C" spine is converted to spine improved respiratory movement with the restoration of the abdominal wall

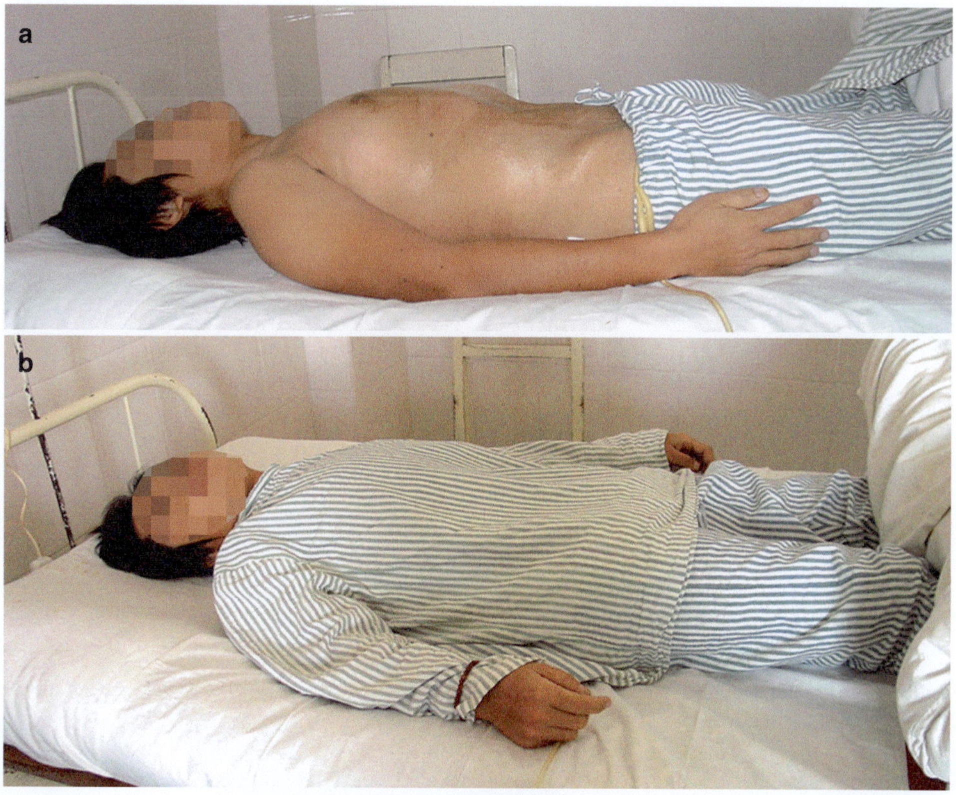

Fig. 6.42 The kyphosis had been completely corrected and the patient was able to sleep in the supine position.

Fig. 6.43 Fixed the trunk in hyperextended plaster vest, she can wear it to do some out-of-bed activity

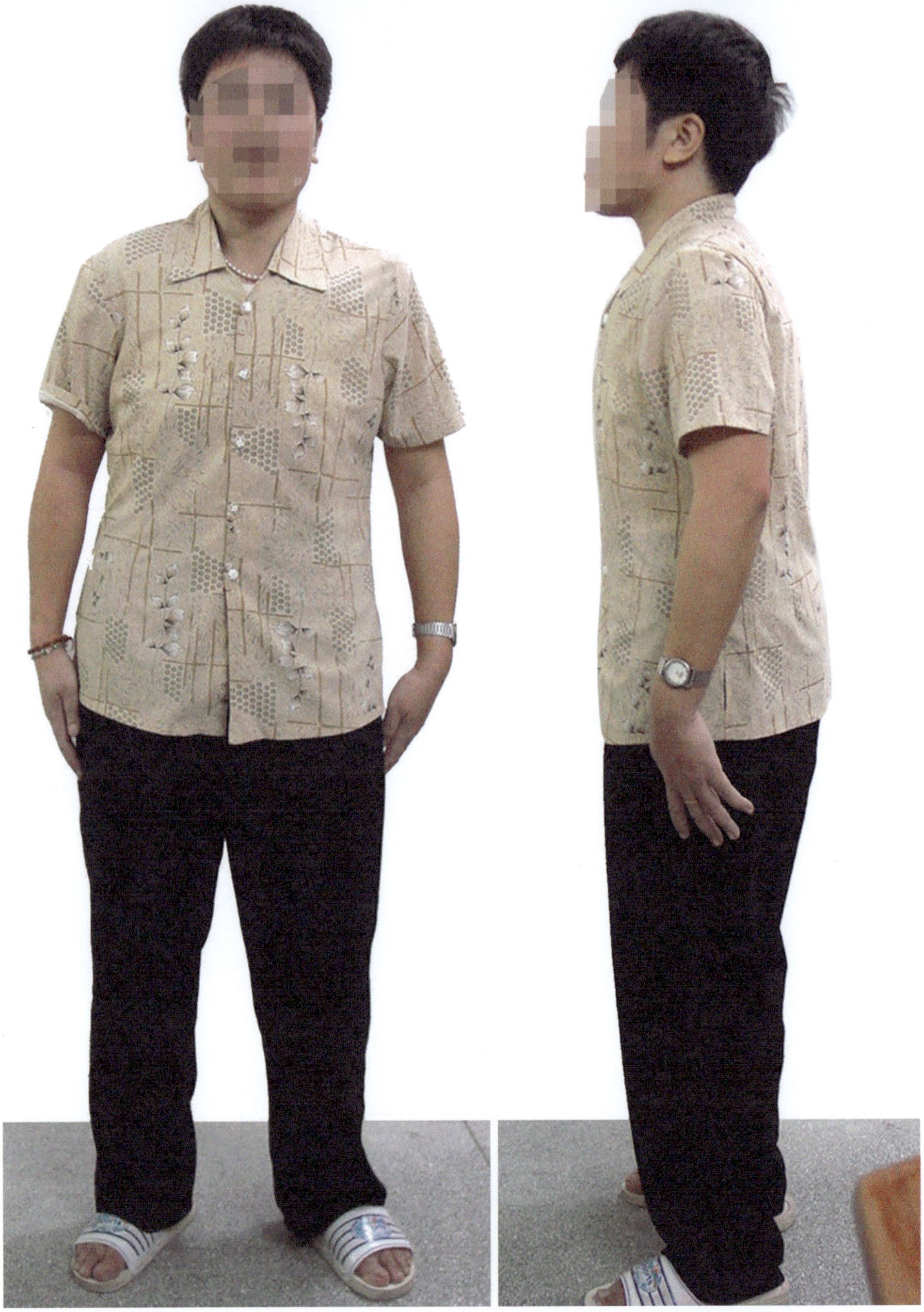

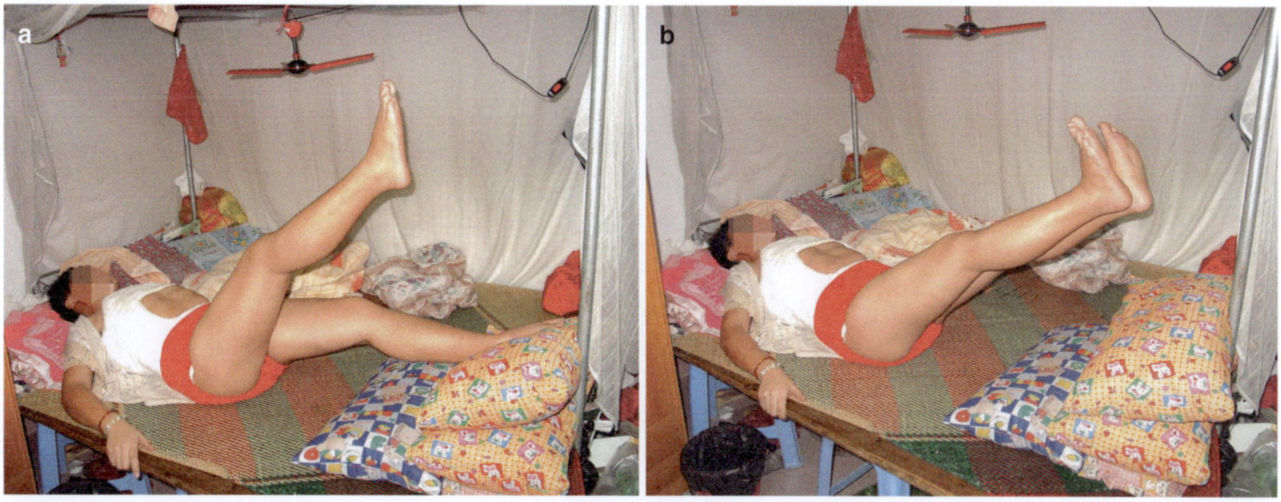

Fig. 6.44 She was lying on the bed wearing a plaster vest and doing straight leg raising exercise

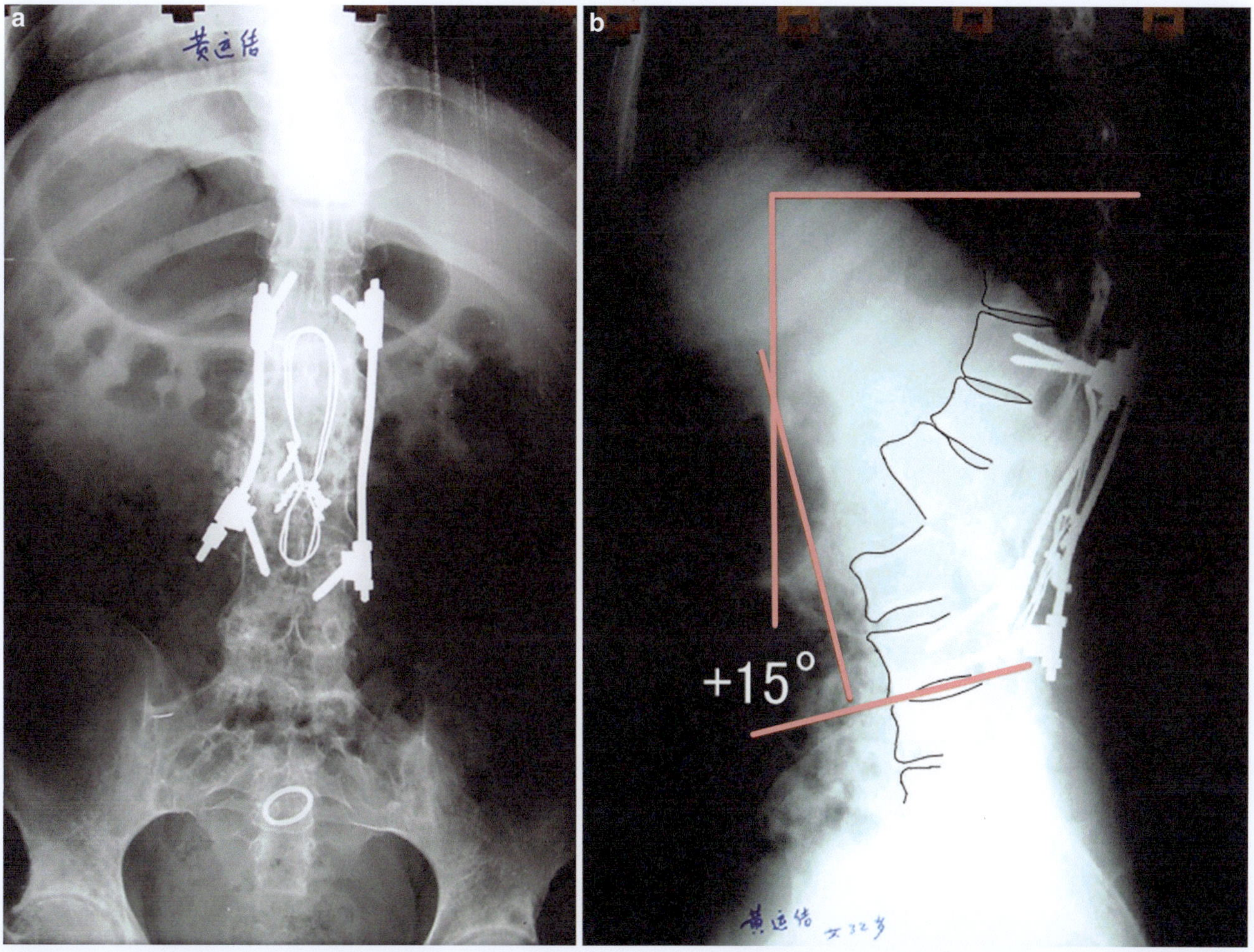

Fig. 6.45 The AP X-ray images after operation showed. (**a**) effective internal fixation. (**b**) The lateral image showed the kyphosis was corrected to lordosis

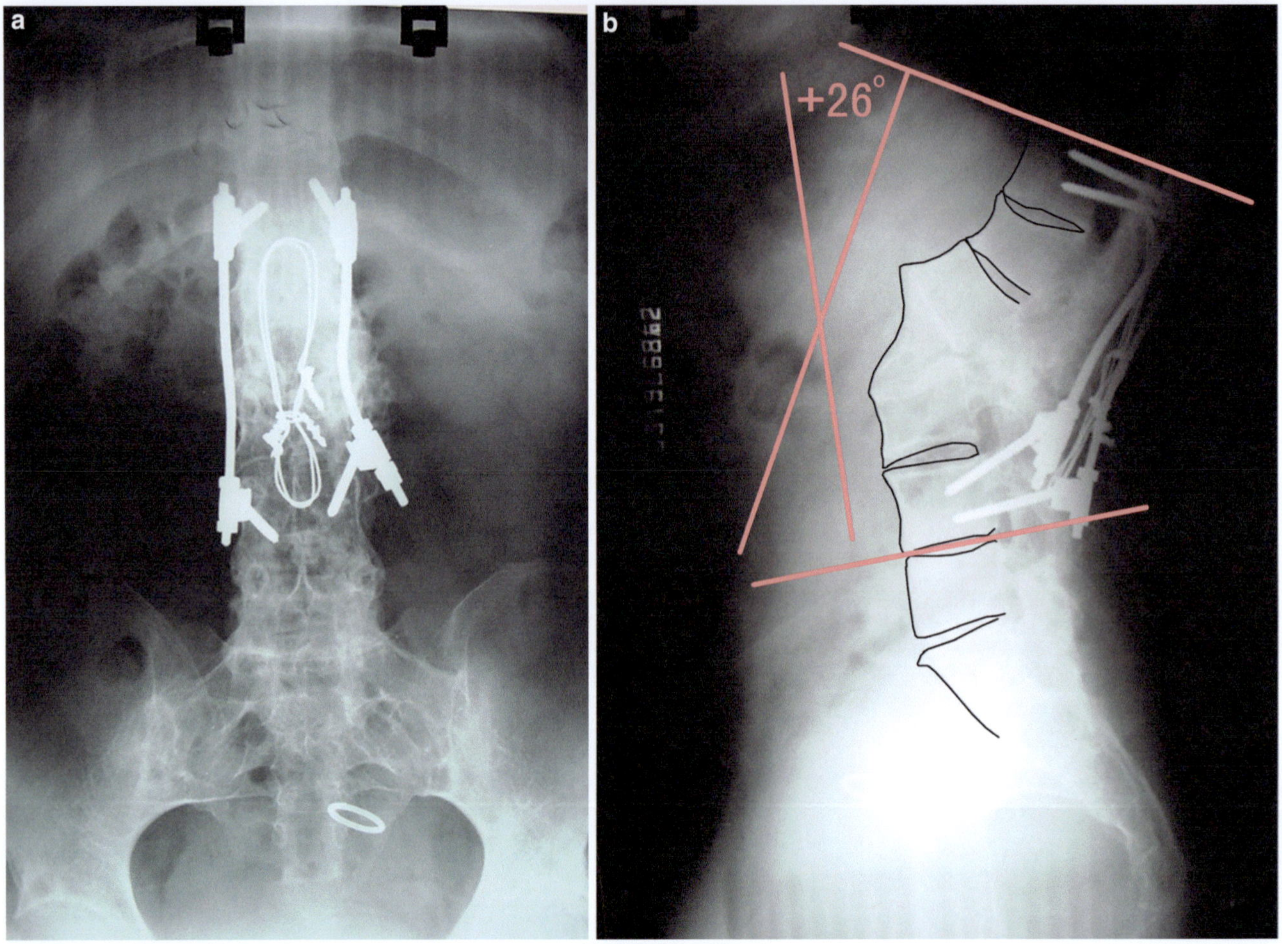

Fig. 6.46 X-ray film half a year after operation. (**a**) The postoperative AP X-ray showed the dynamic fixation was effective. (**b**) A gross correction of 124° was achieved. Bony fusion occurred in both interbody space and behind the lamina

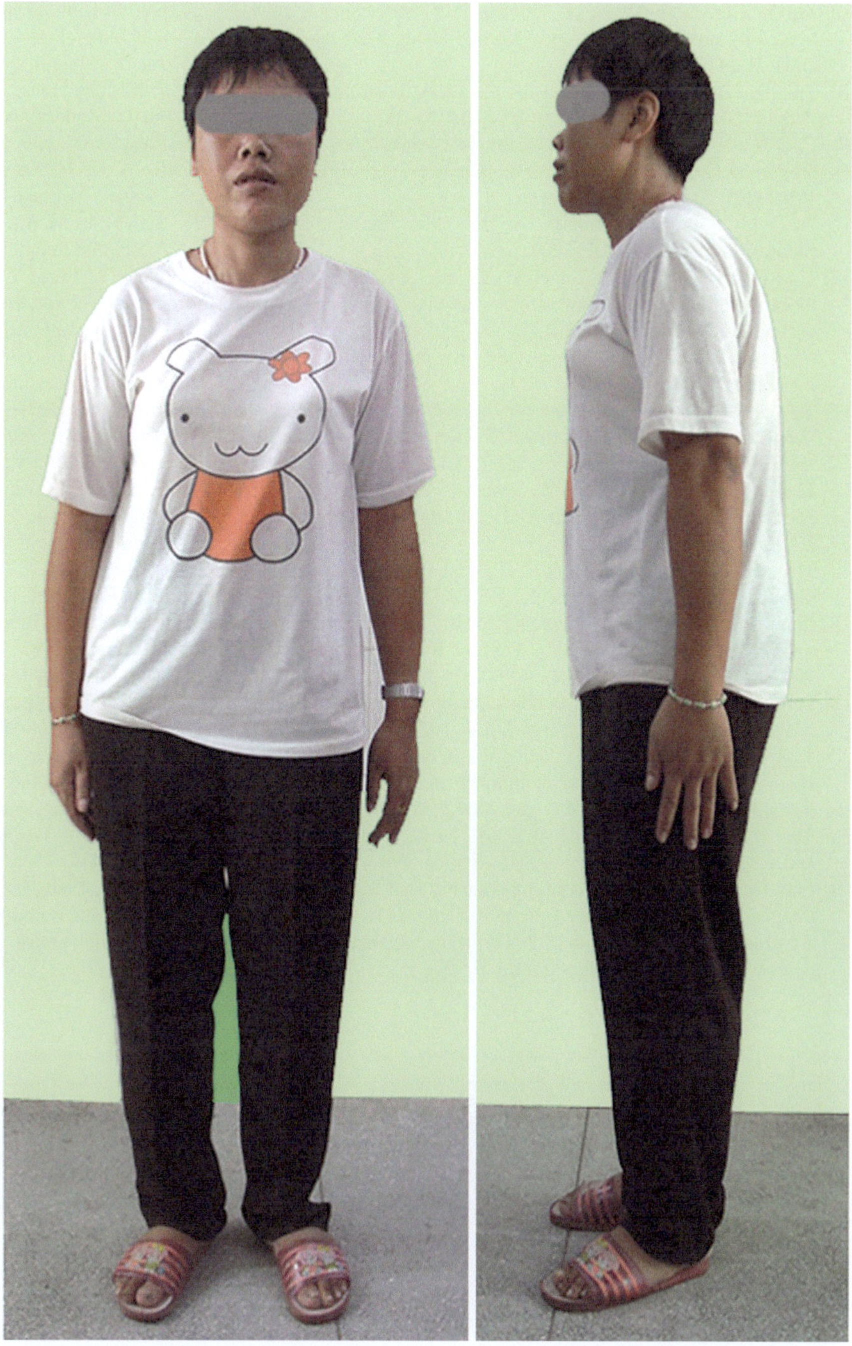

Fig. 6.47 Half-year appearance after operation

Suggested Reading

1. Tian H, Lin Q, Tan Y. Therapeutics of ankylosing spondylitis. Guangzhou: World Book Publishing Company; 2005. p. 165–95.
2. Tian H, Xiang Z. Spinal deformity surgery. Xinjiang: Science and Technology Medical Press; 1994. p. 314–24.
3. Tian H, Li F. Spinal deformity and osteotomy. Xi'an: World Book Publishing Company; 2001. p. 662–734.
4. Jiang M, Tian H. Clinical application of Tian's pedicle locator. Orthopedic Journal of China. 2003;11(7):448–50.
5. Tian H, Wang B, Lv X, et al. Correction and fixation of ankylosing kyphosis and osteotomy. Chinese Journal of Orthopaedics. 2005;13(7):509–12.
6. Tan J, Feng J. Orthopedic unpadded plaster technique. Shanghai: Second Military Medical University Press; 2000. p. 126–46.
7. Tian H. Application of the "Tian's spinal osteotomes" in orthopaedic surgery. Chinese Journal of Orthopaedics. 1994;14(4):236–40.
8. Chen Q. Programmed surgical treatment of ankylosing spondylitis deformity. U.S. Chinese Journal of Orthopaedics. 2001;7:85–7.

9. Ma Y. Clinical analysis of 200 cases of ankylosing kyphosis treated by posterior column resection. Xinjiang Medical Science. 2001;31(3):180–2.
10. Tian H, Liu S, Ma Y. Practical spine surgery illustration. Beijing: People's Military Medical Press; 2008. p. 316–21.
11. Chen L, Li F. Diagnosis and treatment of ankylosing spondylitis complicated with stress fracture. Chinese Journal of Surgery. 1994;32(8):512.
12. Dang G. Surgical techniques for the spine. Beijing: People's Medical Publishing House; 2004. p. 246–52.
13. Tian H, Lv X, Tian B. Correction of osteotomy of cervical and thoracic kyphosis with ankylosing spondylitis. Chinese Journal of Orthopaedics. 2006;14(7):522–3.
14. Chen A, Xu W. Spinal surgery atlas. Beijing: People's Medical Publishing House; 2001. p. 181–273.
15. Tian H. Total spinal osteotomy for the treatment of kyphosis and kyphoscoliosis. Japanese Scoliosis Society program of the 25th Annual Meeting, l991;25:23.
16. Tian H, Ma Y, Lv X. Minimally invasive V-shaped osteotomy for correction of ankylosing kyphosis. Chinese Journal of Orthopaedics. 2008;16(5):349–52.
17. Tian H, Liu S, Ma Y. Practical spine surgery. Guangzhou: Guangdong Science and Technology Press; 2008. p. 195–409.
18. Liang Z. Transpedicular osteotomy for the treatment of kyphosis caused by ankylosing spondylitis. Chinese Journal of Orthopaedics. 1997;17(6):351–2.
19. Leong JCY, Ma A, Yau A. Spinal osteotomy for fixed flexion deformity. Journal of Orthopaedic Translation. 1978;2:271.
20. Tian H , Lv X. Halo pelvic distraction in combination with total spine osteotomy and internal fixation for treatment of severe scoliosis. Orthopedic Journal of China. 2006;l(1):11–6.
21. Tian Huizhong, Yuan Tian, Zhengxing, Tian S. Posterior invasion and vertebral osteotomy. Spinal Deformation. 1992;7(1):4.
22. Tian H, Bai J, Liu S. Operative orthopaedics Gist & Atlas. Beijing: People's Medical Publishing House; 2009. p. 3–41.
23. Bradford DS, Zhang Y, Wang Y. The spine. Shenyang: Liaoning Science and Technology Press; 2003. p. 75–83.
24. Guo S. Clinical anatomy of orthopedics. Jinan: Shandong Science and Technology Press; 2000. p. 1–17.
25. Jin D. Modern spine surgery. Beijing: People's Military Medical Publishing House; 2001. p. 12.
26. Jia L. Modern spine surgery. Beijing: People's Military Medical Press; 2007. p. 9.
27. Xu S, Ge B, Xu Y. Practical orthopedics, vol. 2. 3rd ed. Beijing: People's Military Medical Press; 2011. p. 1776–7.
28. Tian H, Li M, Ma Y. Spinal deformity osteotomy orthopedics, vol. 5. Beijing: People's Medical Publishing House; 2011. p. 3–339.
29. Wang Y, Zhang Y, Zhang X, et al. Single posterior approach with multi-level vertebra column resection in severe kyphosis and scoliosis. Journal of Spine Surgery. 2007;2:65–7.
30. Xu S, Lu S Zhu B, et al. Prevention and treatment of complications of orthopedic surgery, vol. 4. Beijing: People's Military Medical Publishing House; 2002. p. 181–5.
31. Xu S, Ge B, Xu Y. Practice of orthopaedics. 2nd ed. Beijing: People's Military Medical Publishing House; 2003. p. 341–636.
32. Wang B. Spinal surgery. Beijing: Peking University Medical Press; 2009. p. 152–4.
33. Tian H. Surgical treatment of kyphosis kyphosis. Chinese Journal of Orthopaedics. 1992;12(3):162–5.
34. Tian H. Spinal surgeons should be good at using rongeurs and osteotome. Chinese Journal of Modern Operative Surgery. 2002;6(1):67–8.
35. Hou S. Spinal surgery. Beijing: People's Military Medical Publishing House; 2005. p. 444–610.
36. Tian H. Selection of internal fixation after osteotomy and correction of ankylosing kyphosis. Orthopedic Journal of China. 2011;19(9):784–6.
37. Tian H, Li M, Wang Z. Key points and diagrams of thoracolumbar surgery. Beijing: People's Medical Publishing House; 2012. p. 375–417.
38. Tian H, Liang Y. Ankylosing spondylitis spinal deformity osteotomy and orthopedic surgery skills. Beijing: People's Medical Publishing House; 2014. p. 1–328.

7 Non-apex Osteotomy for ASK

Yingsong Wang, Ying Zhang, and Huizhong Tian

7.1 Overview

The osteotomy technique for kyphosis correction is divided into two categories: non-apex osteotomy and apex osteotomy. These two techniques have different indications: non-apex osteotomy is suitable for the round kyphosis of ankylosing spondylitis. It means the osteotomy site is not at the apex of the thoracic segment, but rather below the kyphotic apex. In this way, a large C-curve is corrected into a figure of "3" after osteotomy and correction (Fig. 7.1), which enlarges the lumbar lordosis and compensates for the kyphosis, so that the patient will straighten the trunk, move the gravity line more posterior, have eyes look forward, extend the distance between the xiphoid and the pubic symphysis, and resolve abdominal compression. Therefore, ankylosing kyphosis is the absolute indication for non-apex osteotomy while apex osteotomy is the absolute indication for congenital or tuberculous angular kyphosis, although sometimes the latter is also used for ankylosing kyphosis, e.g., when the apex of round kyphosis is below T10. In particular, PSO or VCR is commonly performed at the apex level to treat kyphosis due to ankylosing spondylitis.

7.1.1 Rationale of Non-apex Osteotomy

Back in 1945, Smith Petersen began applying this method to treat ankylosing spine. Non-apex osteotomy is simpler and time-saving than apex osteotomy, with safe and reliable treatment outcomes. When it is not to achieve the complete straightening of the spine (just to convert the large C-curve to a figure of "3"), it restores the normal appearance of the ankylosing spine. Resolves pathological impact on visceral organs while making the life of AS patients much easier. In particular, the improvement of the respiratory and circulation system refreshes patient condition. Relief of pressure on the abdomen greatly improves the appetite and the nutritional status of the patients. Patients thus embrace the restoration of normal life.

7.1.2 Selection of Osteotomy Site

Non-apex osteotomy position is usually performed in L2–3 levels as transverse lamina or V-shape osteotomy. Most cases can be treated with single-level osteotomy. In some cases, lamina osteotomy for 2–3 levels followed by manual correction and dynamic compress to close the gap of three levels and

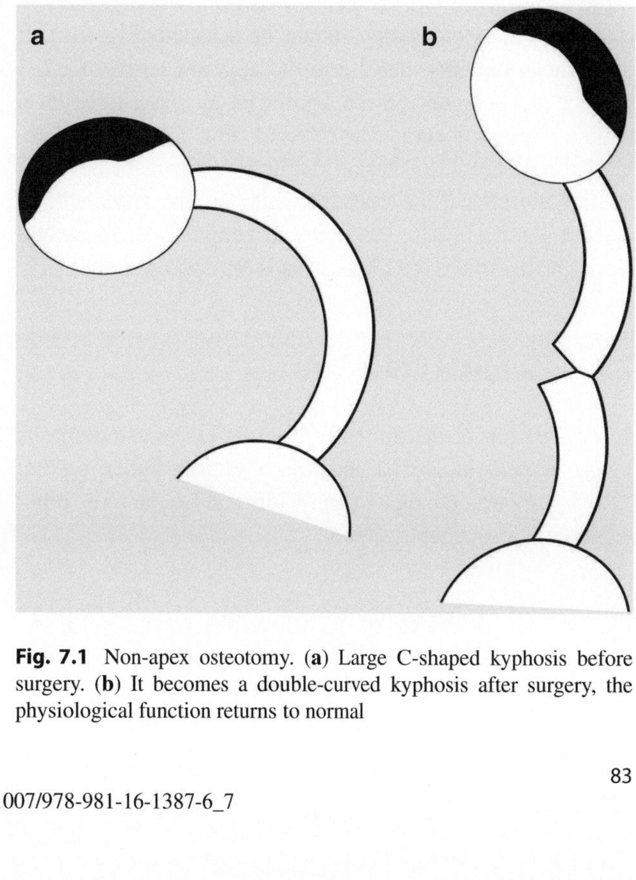

Fig. 7.1 Non-apex osteotomy. (**a**) Large C-shaped kyphosis before surgery. (**b**) It becomes a double-curved kyphosis after surgery, the physiological function returns to normal

Y. Wang (✉) · Y. Zhang
Department of Orthopedics, The 2nd Affiliated Hospital of Kunming Medical University, Kunming, China

H. Tian
The Sixth Affiliated Hospital of Xinjiang Medical University, Urumqi, China

H. Tian et al. (eds.), *Spinal Osteotomy Orthopaedics*, https://doi.org/10.1007/978-981-16-1387-6_7

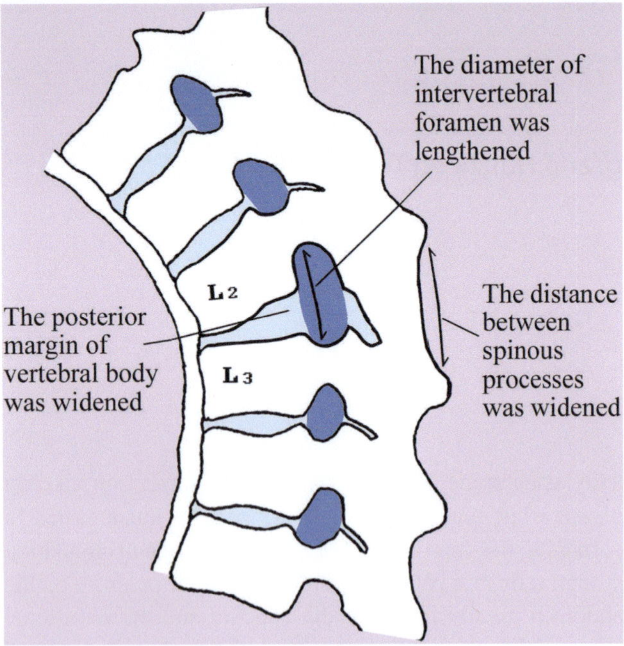

Fig. 7.2 Suitable for non-apex L2–3 single level osteotomy

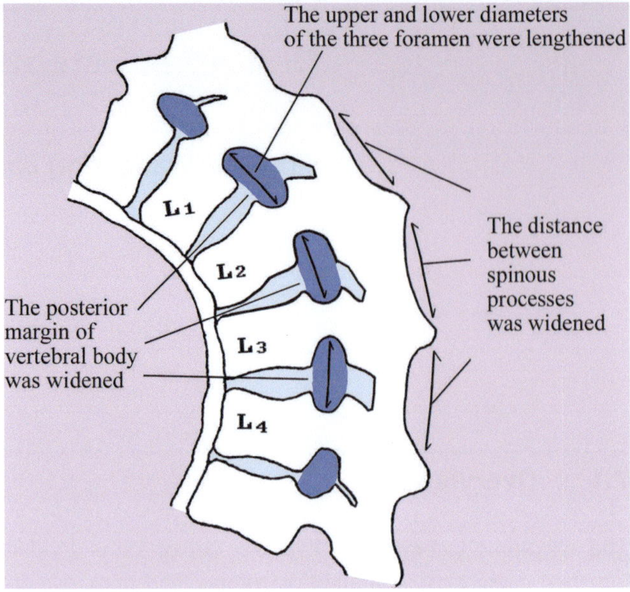

Fig. 7.3 Suitable for non-apex multilevel osteotomy

correct severe kyphosis to a great extent. However, the problem often encountered is that the anterior longitudinal ligament tear and anterior opening caused by corrective maneuver which is often limited to one intervertebral space. If the case is selected properly, the anterior opening can also occur in three levels. Lateral X-rays should be carefully reviewed before surgery. If L2–3 interspinous process space and the superior-inferior dimension of intervertebral foramen (IVF) is the widest while these measurements do not increase in the adjacent levels, single-level osteotomy should be selected (Fig. 7.2). If these measurements increase in the adjacent levels of L2–3 while L2–3 does not have a significant increase, three-level lamina osteotomy should be selected (Fig. 7.3). After three-level osteotomy, the anterior longitudinal ligament covering the three levels will be extended while the disc space will be opened anteriorly as correction and compression force will work on all of the three levels. This is the optimal result.

7.2 Surgical Procedure

1. Preparation of instruments: A set of Tian's osteotome, a set of pedicle screws and rod, a pedicle finder, several 0.8–1.2 mm diameter Luque wires and Luque rods; other general instruments.
2. Anesthesia: General anesthesia with tracheal intubation or bronchoscopic intubation, local infiltration anesthesia.
3. Position: The patient takes a prone position. The operation table is set to an inverted V shape, with the lumbar bridge raised and pads applied (Fig. 7.4). The headrest and shoulder rest should be installed. The feet should be fixed to the end of the bed (Fig. 7.5). A traction reduction band should be under the armpits (Fig. 7.6).
4. Surgical procedure:

   The first step, incision, and exposure: Make an incision over skin and subcutaneous tissue along the spinous process and expose the spinous processes and the posterior layer of the lumbar dorsal fascia. Dissect along the spinous processes with an electric cutter, expose the spinous process under the periosteum, and expose the bilateral lamina to the transverse process of the spine.

   The second step, selection of the osteotomy site: Pinpoint the osteotomy site under the C-arm. Non-apex osteotomy is generally performed between L2–3, as this site is below the conus where cauda equina lies (Fig. 7.7). Since it is relatedly safe for neurological structure, L2–3 space is the preferable level. If the anterior side of L2–3 has bony fusion, the level above or below should be selected as the level for non-apical vertebral osteotomy (Fig. 7.8).

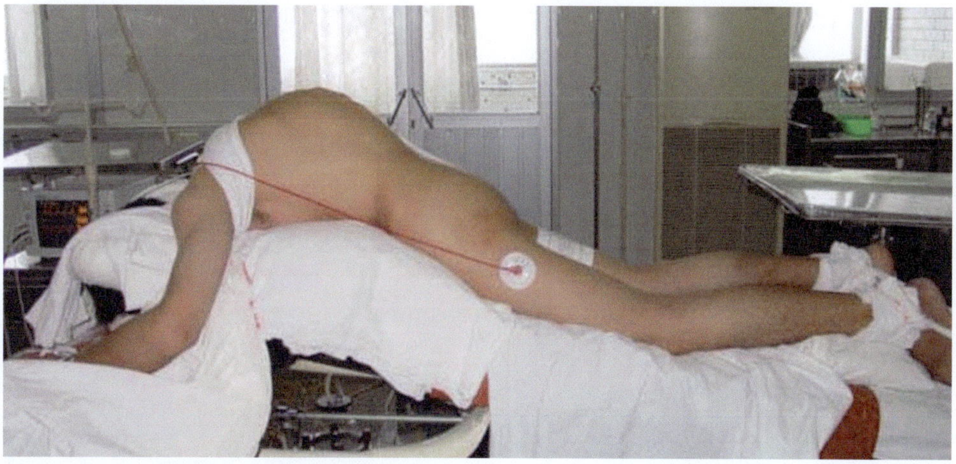

Fig. 7.4 Positioning of surgery for ankylosing kyphosis

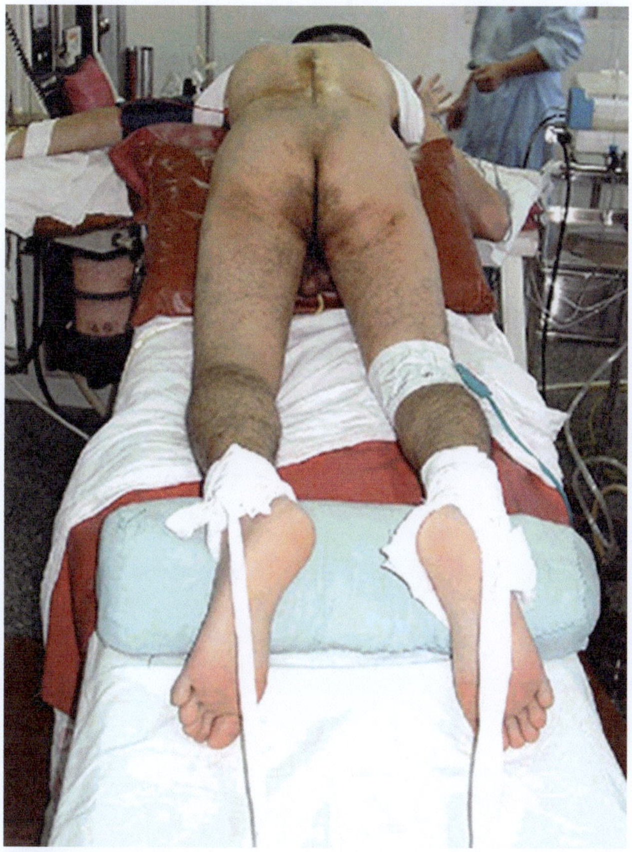

Fig. 7.5 Surgical position: both legs are fixed at the end of the bed to prevent the patient from sliding forward and to facilitate traction reduction

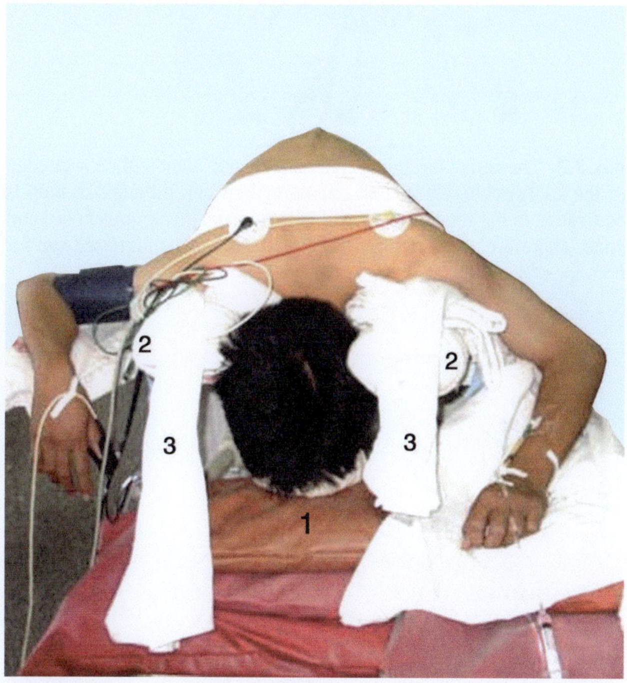

Fig. 7.6 Surgical position: 1. Headrest (round stool that can be raised and lowered automatically); 2. shoulder support; 3. traction band

Third step non-apex osteotomy:

1. Simple lamina osteotomy: If there is no bony connection anterior to the disc space, especially in the lateral view where the disc space is narrow anteriorly and wide posteriorly, transverse laminar osteotomy (Fig. 7.9) or laminar V-shape osteotomy (Fig. 7.10) should be selected. With a complete laminectomy, the gap will spontaneously close. So after the lamina is resected on one side, a wooden spacer should be inserted to distract the space (Fig. 7.11), before resecting the lamina on the other side. This technique prevents spontaneous closing of the gap with laminectomy on both sides, which is causing difficulty in clearing up the deeper space.
2. PSO: This technique is suitable for those who have a bony connection anterior to the vertebra and the kyphotic curve is not too large (Fig. 7.12). Only the arch and the two pedicles of one level are removed (Fig. 7.13). The tip of

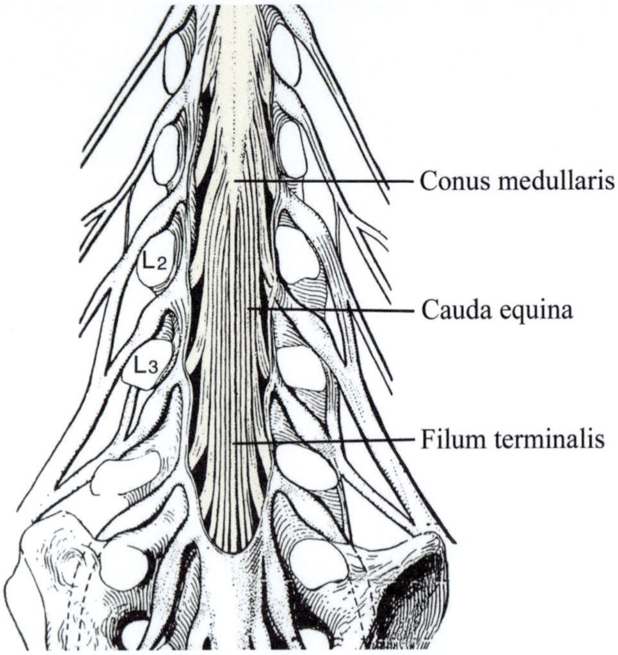

Fig. 7.7 The end of the spinal cord cone is equivalent to the lower edge of the L1 vertebra. Choose an osteotomy between L2 and 3, which is equivalent to the cauda equina, and will not damage the spinal cord and cone. Therefore, the vertebra between L2 and 3 is the preferred site for non-apex osteotomy

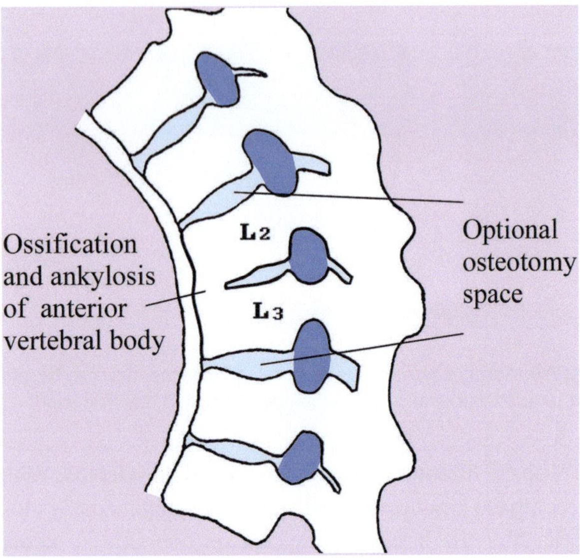

Fig. 7.8 Non-apex osteotomy if the anterior edge of the vertebral body has been ossified and ankylosed, the gap above or below is selected

the wedge-shaped resection does not go beyond the anterior 1/4 of the vertebral body (Fig. 7.14). The wedge is closed by breaking the anterior 1/4 of the vertebral body (Fig. 7.15), followed by internal fixation to achieve the correction of kyphosis.

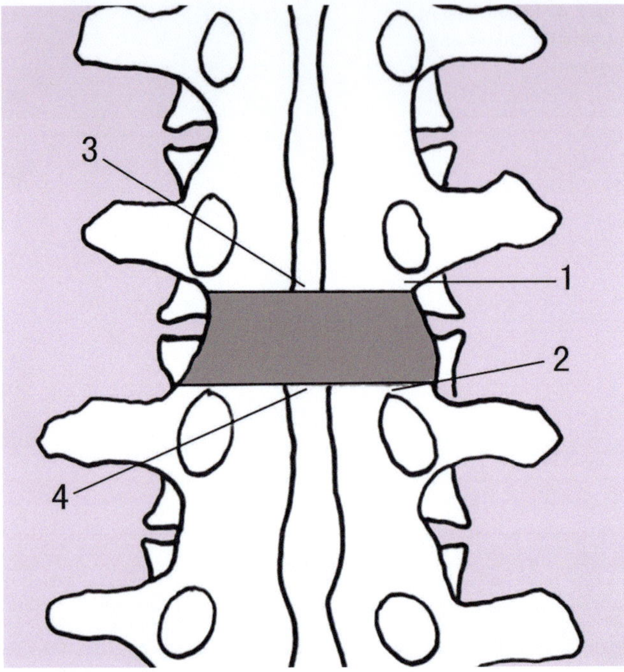

Fig. 7.9 Laminar transverse osteotomy. 1. 2 mm below the lower edge of the pedicle. 2. 2 mm above the upper edge of the pedicle. 3. Spinous process upper edge. 4. Spinous process lower edge. Osteotomy width: 8 ~ 12 mm. Single-gap osteotomy

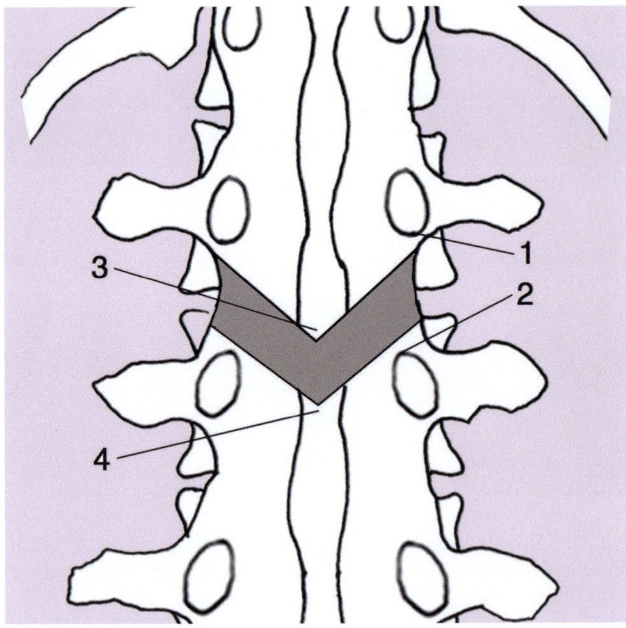

Fig. 7.10 Laminar V-shaped osteotomy. 1. The lower edge of the pedicle; 2. The upper edge of the pedicle; 3. The lower edge of the spinous process; 4. The upper edge of the spinous process; The width of the osteotomy is 8–12 mm. Osteotomy gap: single gap or multiple gaps

3. VCR: VCR is suitable for those with extensive bony fusion between the vertebral arches and vertebral bodies and severe kyphotic curves (Fig. 7.16). According to the

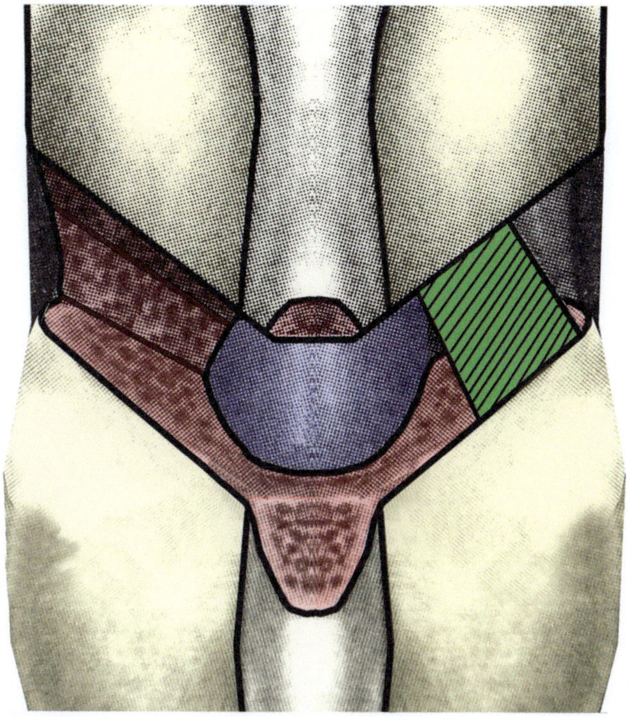

Fig. 7.11 After the right side is done, use a wooden plug to open the osteotomy space, and then use the same method to perform the left osteotomy

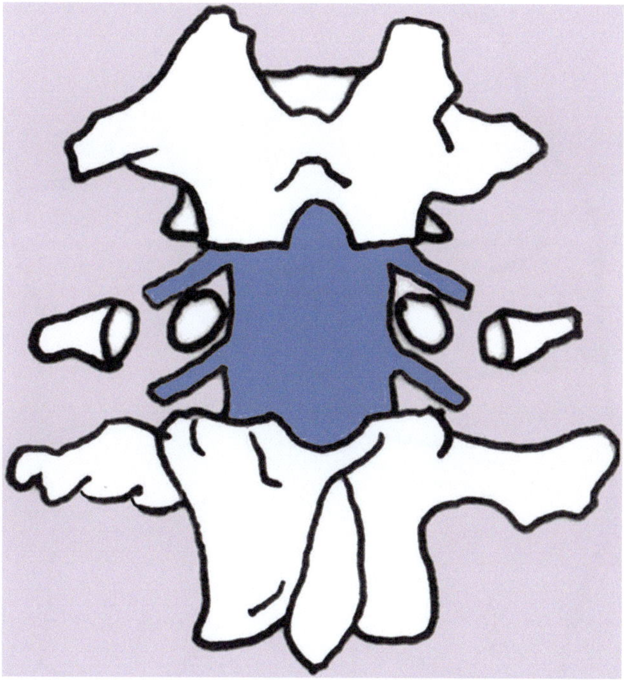

Fig. 7.13 Subtotal osteotomy of vertebral body, one section of vertebral arch and two pedicles are removed posteriorly, exposing the dura mater and spinal nerve root

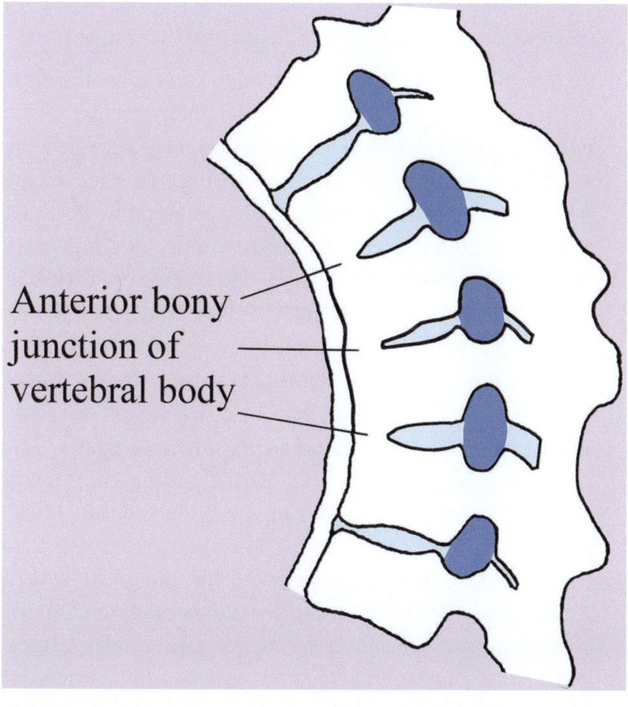

Fig. 7.12 Bone connection of the anterior margin of the three intervertebral vertebrae, which is an indication for subtotal osteotomy of the vertebral arch

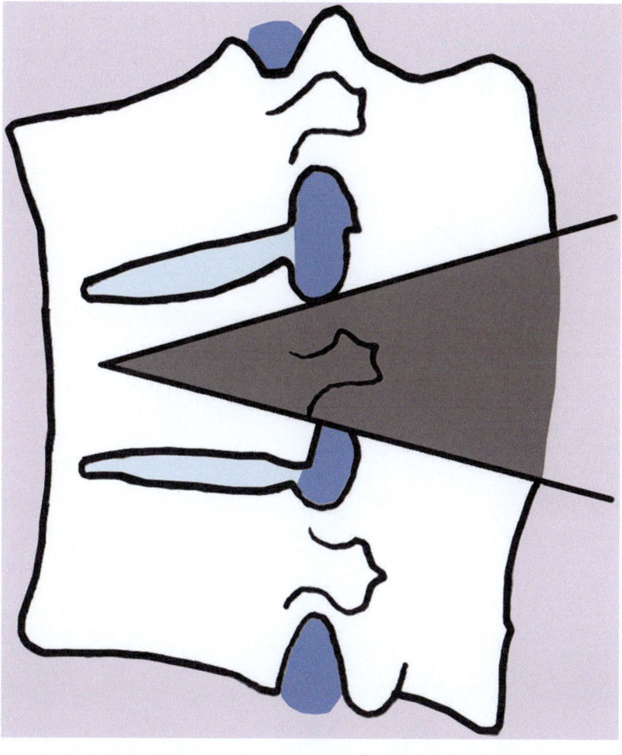

Fig. 7.14 Subtotal osteotomy of the vertebral arch. The tip of the wedge resection reaches the front 1/4 of the vertebra, and its base is backward

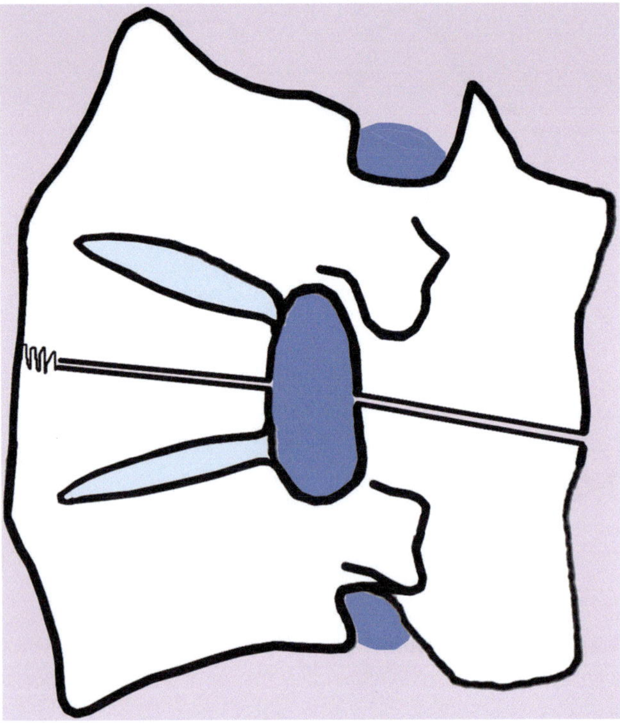

Fig. 7.15 Manual reduction of the anterior margin of the vertebral body to close the osteotomy space, correcting the kyphosis deformity changes, and make the two foraminal vertebrae become one

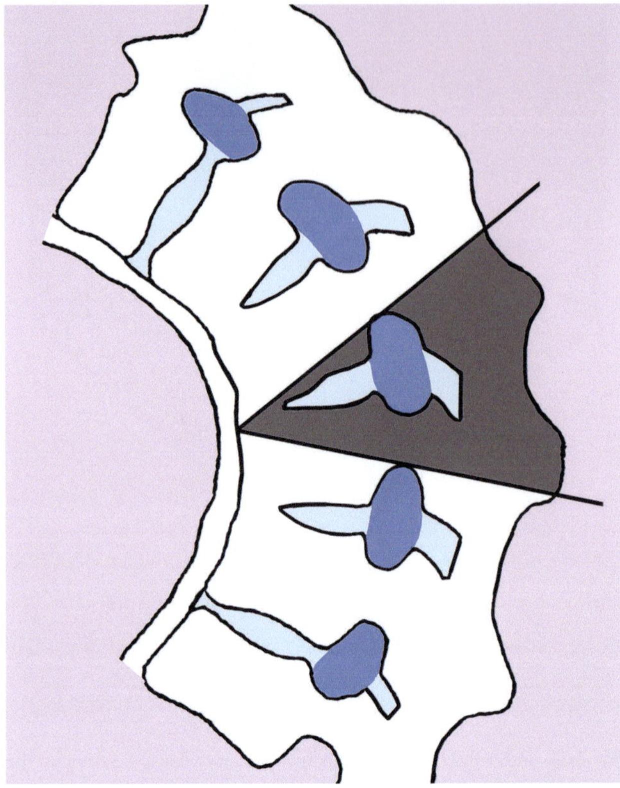

Fig. 7.17 The wedge-shaped tip of a full spine osteotomy reaches the front edge of the vertebral body and completely truncates the spine. The width of the wedge-shaped base can include 1–2 intervertebral spaces

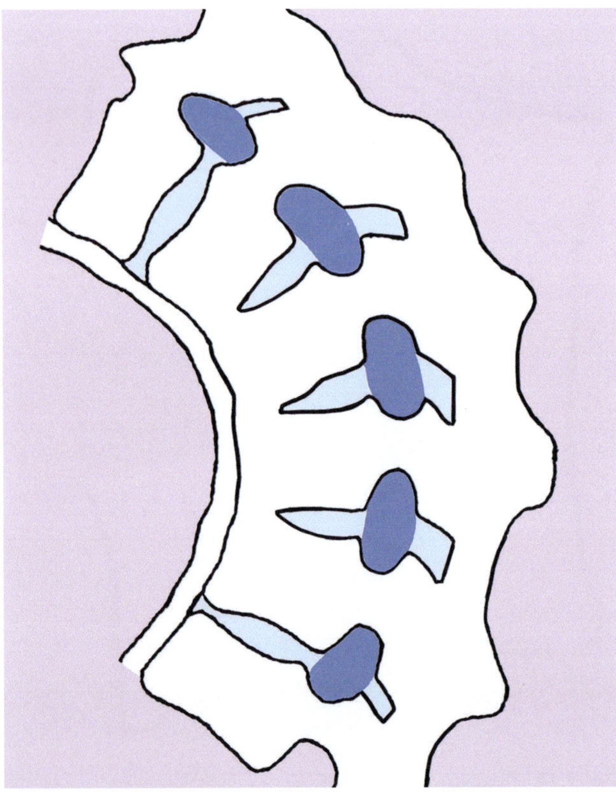

Fig. 7.16 Severe kyphosis, vertebral vertebrae with osseous fusion; a 3-column osteotomy should be performed

degree of kyphotic angle, the wedge should be designed to make the wedge tip reaching the anterior edge of the vertebra (Fig. 7.17). The reduction is performed by anterior opening and posterior closing. This technique provides powerful correction, so it is suitable for ASK with 80 ~ 90°kyphosis. If the osteotomy is completely intra-body (waist osteotomy), the anterior vertebral space does not need to be grafted (Fig. 7.18a, b). Closing posteriorly to make it bone-on-bone between lamina and bone grafting behind the lamina is sufficient. For extensive resection involving one disc space or two disc spaces, a strut graft should in the anterior space. The posterior edge of the lamina should not be completely closed to avoid over-shortening the spine and dura buckling (Fig. 7.19).

4. Spinal Shortening: It is suitable for the most severe ASK (Fig. 7.20). In order to reduce the tension of abdominal wall muscles, the superior mesenteric artery, and visceral organs and major vessels, spinal shortening is needed during operation on those patients (Fig. 7.21). Operation in stages is required for selected cases in order to extend the spine. This is a challenge in the treatment of ASK.

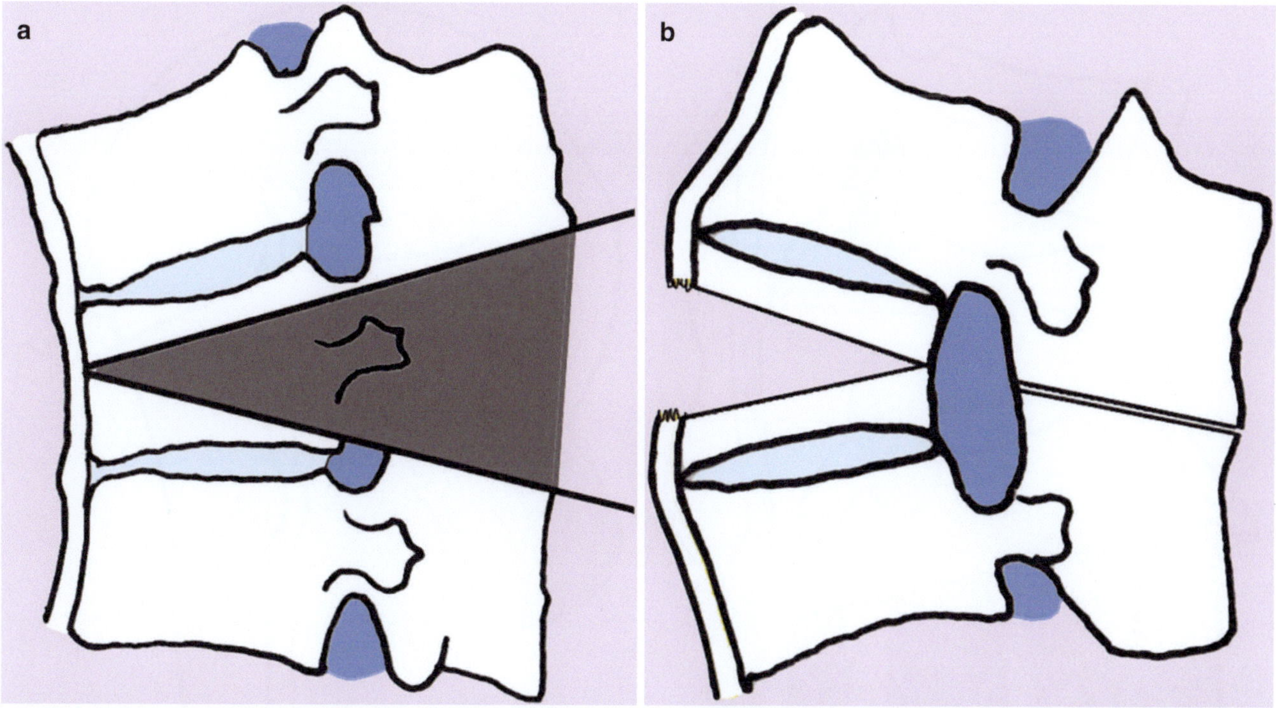

Fig. 7.18 Osteotomy of the whole spine of the vertebral body, which can open the front of the spine. No bone graft is needed in the gap between the vertebral bodies. Spontaneous bone fusion will occur at the leading edge of the vertebra in patients with ASK. (**a**) The width of the vertebral lumbar osteotomy. (**b**) Schematic diagram of opening before closing

The fourth step: reduction and internal fixation:

1. Reduction technique: After the osteotomy is completed, perform a corrective procedure with head and foot traction, making the lumbar bridge of the operating table flat, adjust the inverted V-shaped bed to a V-shape, and perform compression force on the spinous processes between the upper and lower sides of the osteotomy site, so that the spine is extended to close the osteotomy space, and then perform bilateral pedicle screw insertion and rod fixation. After the internal fixation is completed, irrigate the wound, and hemostasis by electrocoagulation. The bone chip is grafted on the lamina. A drainage tube is left and the wound is closed by layers to finish the operation.
2. Stable internal fixation: Suitable for cases of severe kyphosis after large wedge resection or spinal shortening. A stable strong screw–rod system is required for internal fixation. Some patients even need combined anterior and posterior internal fixation (see Figs. 7.19 and 7.21).
3. Elastic internal fixation: Suitable for kyphosis deformity within 90°, such as wire internal fixation (Fig. 7.22), elastic compression rod fixation, Luque rod fixation (Fig. 7.23). This fixation technique allows further self-correction by best rest, or maneuver reduction in multiple stages after operation. It is a safe and reliable method.
4. External fixation without internal fixation: For ankylosing spondylitis with mild kyphosis, internal fixation is generally not required. After V-shape lamina osteotomy, the patient may experience further correction by bed rest or maneuver reduction in multiple stages. Upon X-ray confirmation of correction of kyphosis and closure of osteotomy gap, a hyperextensive plaster vest is applied as an immobilization tool (Fig. 7.24a, b) for 8–10 months.
5. Postoperative management:

(a) When moving the patient to a flatbed in the ward, keep the patient straight. (b) Use suitable pillows and cotton pads to support the patient. Connect the negative pressure drainage tubes on both sides of the bed. After recovery from anesthesia, use pillows to support either side of the body alternatively once every 2–3 h to prevent pressure ulcers. (c) Remove the drainage tube in 24 or 48 h, and take an X-ray bedside. (d) After stitches are removed on Day 10, the plaster vest should be applied for 8–10 months. Patients should come back periodically for follow-up.

7.3 Essentials and Notes

1. The non-apex osteotomy is supposed to be performed on L2–3 level. After the osteotomy, the large C-shaped kyphosis of ASK is converted to a figure of "3" shape, which improves the physiological function, and reduces the cardiopulmonary dysfunction and digestive dysfunction caused by cardiopulmonary compression and poor

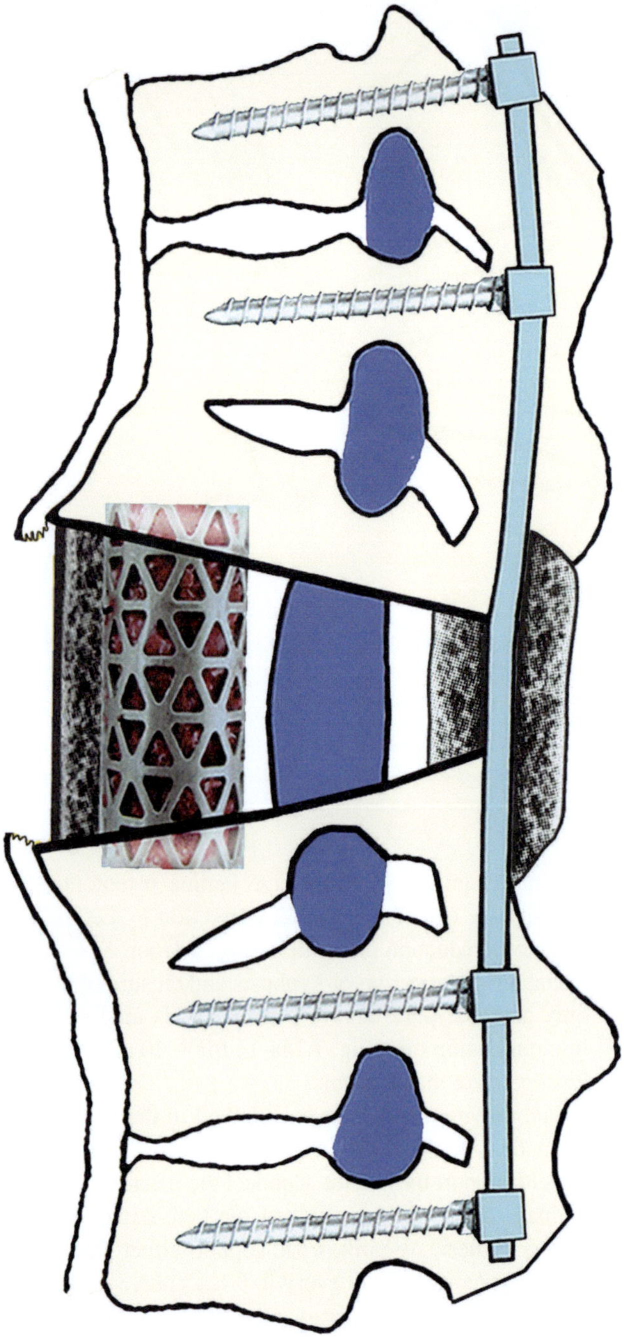

Fig. 7.19 After an extensive VCR, interbody strut grafting and post-lamina grafting should be applied with stable fixation by pedicle screw system

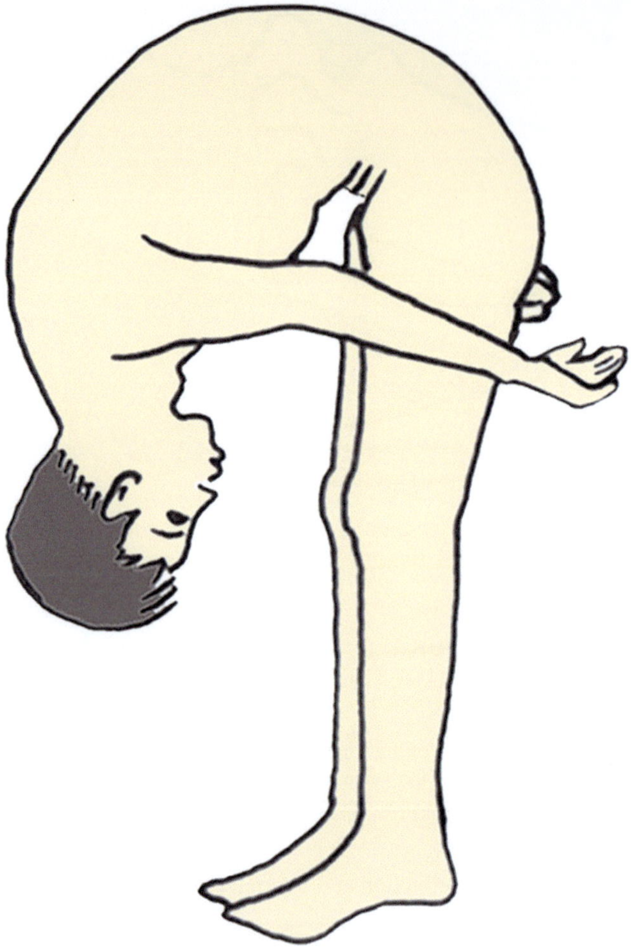

Fig. 7.20 Correction for severe ASK requires shortening of the spine

appetite. The physical and nutritional conditions of ASK patients are also improved significantly after surgery. This is the biggest advantage of non-apex osteotomy.

2. ASK osteotomy between L2 and L3 reconstructs the relationship between lower ribs and lower outlet of thorax cage and abdominal cavity by setting them apart from each other. It restores the vertical movement of the diaphragm, and increases the abdominal respiration function. Due to the rigidity of coastal joints of ASK patients, chest respiration is impaired. Abdominal aspiration is the only way left to maintain carbon and oxygen exchange. Non-apical osteotomy improves the respiration function of the diaphragm as an important way to prolong the patient's life.
3. L2–L3 space is at the level of cauda equina, which is more resistant to traction and dissection during the operation than the spinal cord. Therefore, it is safer to perform osteotomy at this level to reduce the possibility of spinal cord injury.
4. If bony fusion forms at the anterior edge of the L2–L3 vertebral space, L3–L4 or L1–L2 level should be selected for osteotomy.

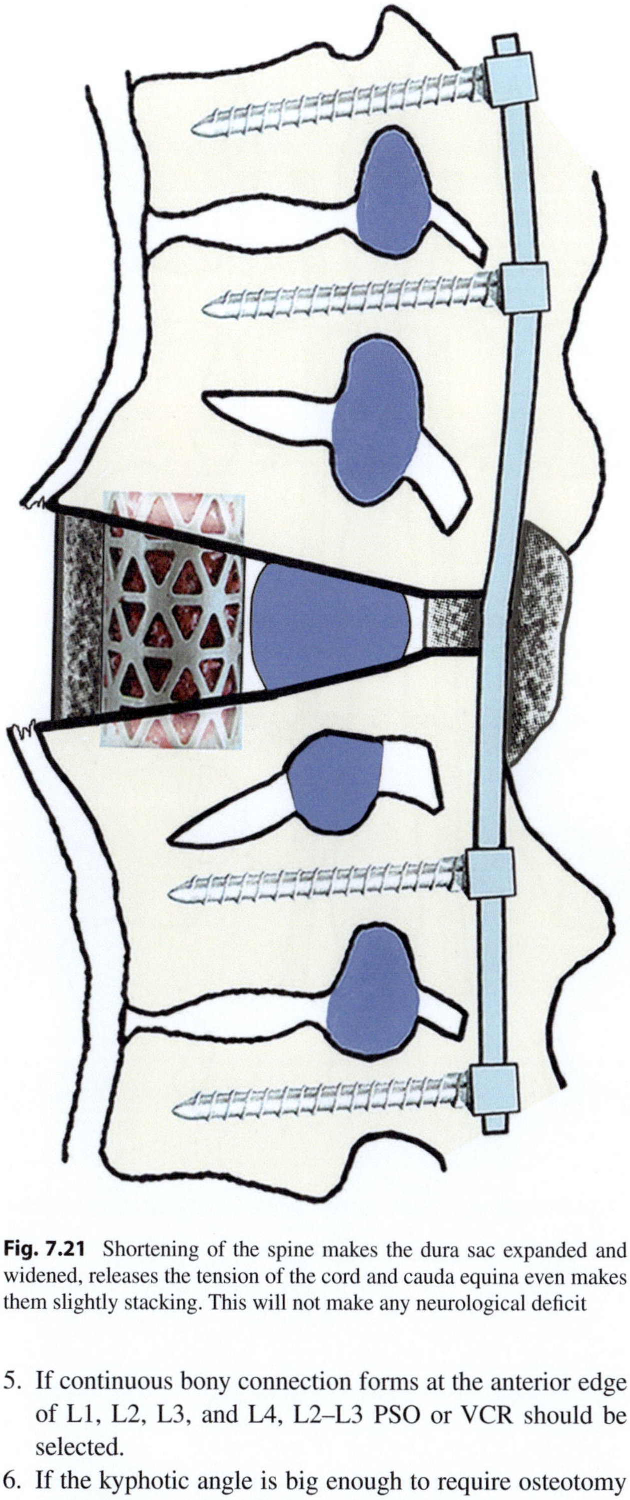

Fig. 7.21 Shortening of the spine makes the dura sac expanded and widened, releases the tension of the cord and cauda equina even makes them slightly stacking. This will not make any neurological deficit

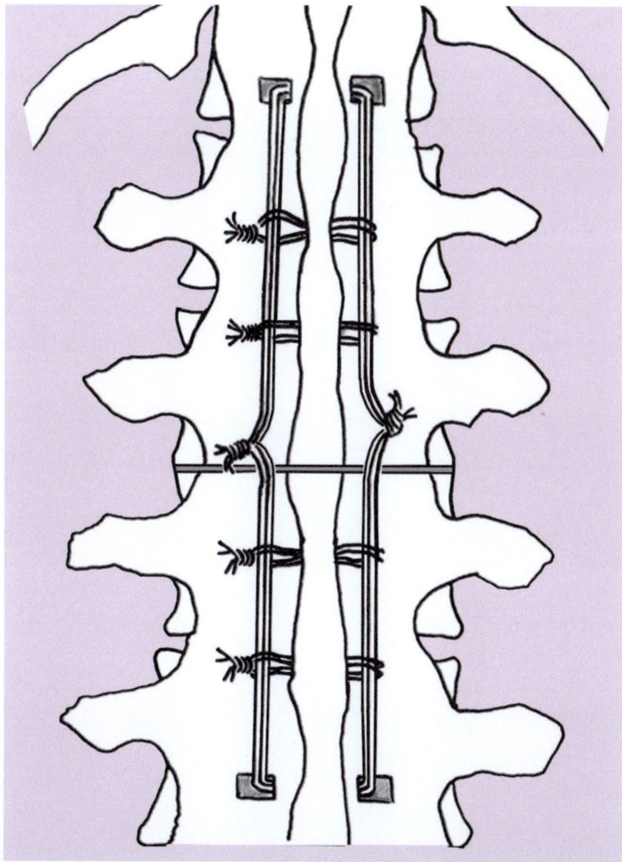

Fig. 7.22 Internal fixation by spinous process wiring is a dynamic internal fixation, allowing self-correction by bed rest after the operation. The method is simple and reliable, but plaster vest immobilization is needed

5. If continuous bony connection forms at the anterior edge of L1, L2, L3, and L4, L2–L3 PSO or VCR should be selected.
6. If the kyphotic angle is big enough to require osteotomy involving two disc spaces or shortening osteotomy, strut grafting in the anterior space and incomplete wedge closing and grafting posterior to the lamina should be considered.
7. Internal fixation could be spared for mild ASK correction. Once self-correction is achieved by bed rest, a hyperextensive plaster vest should be applied.
8. If three disc spaces, that is, L1–L2, L2–L3, L3–L4 are all narrow anteriorly and wide posteriorly, without bony connection, one may consider three-level transverse lamina osteotomy to correct kyphotic deformity, if the kyphotic angle is relatively big. Manual correction and plaster vest immobilization should be applied after operation.
9. Non-apex osteotomy has wide application. Non-apex osteotomy between L2–L3 is suitable to treat thoracic kyphosis and lumbar kyphosis. Except for cervical and thoracic kyphosis, most of the kyphotic curves can be solved by non-apex osteotomy.

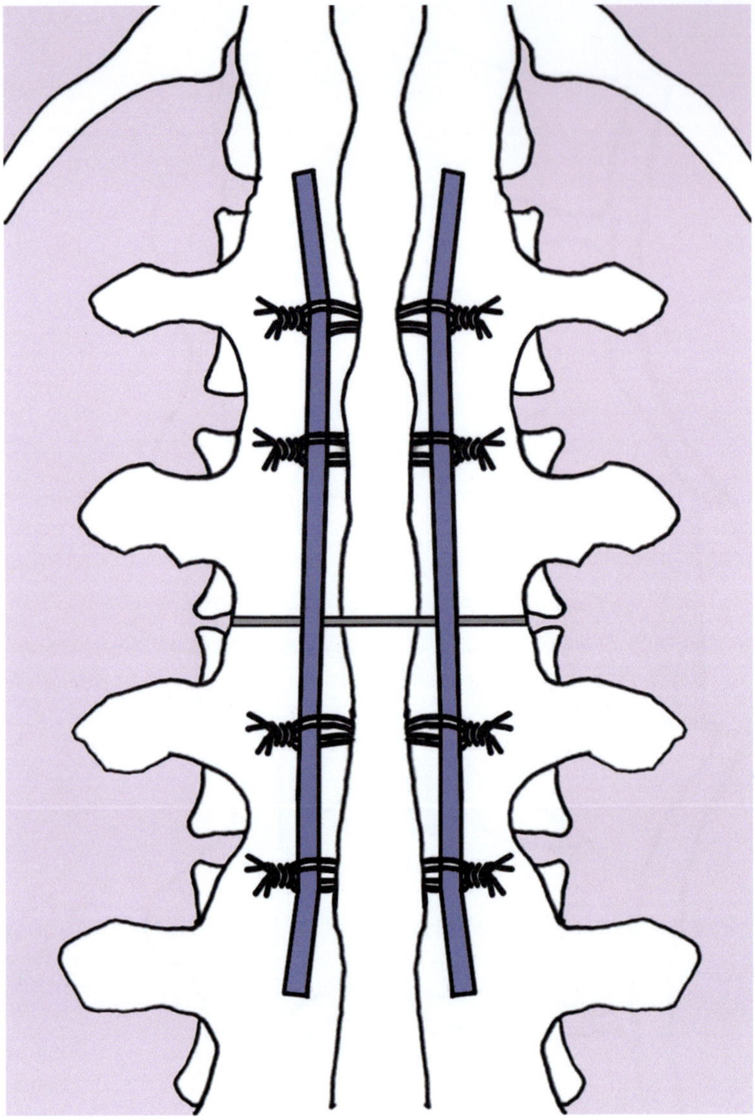

Fig. 7.23 Luque rod application and interspinous process wiring allows gliding between the rod and wiring and self-correction with bed rest after the operation

Fig. 7.24 For mild ASK, internal fixation after osteotomy could be spared by self-correction on flatbed or maneuver correction. When satisfactory correction is achieved, hyperextensive plaster vest immobilization is applied for 8–10 months. (**a**) Preoperative, (**b**) Postoperative

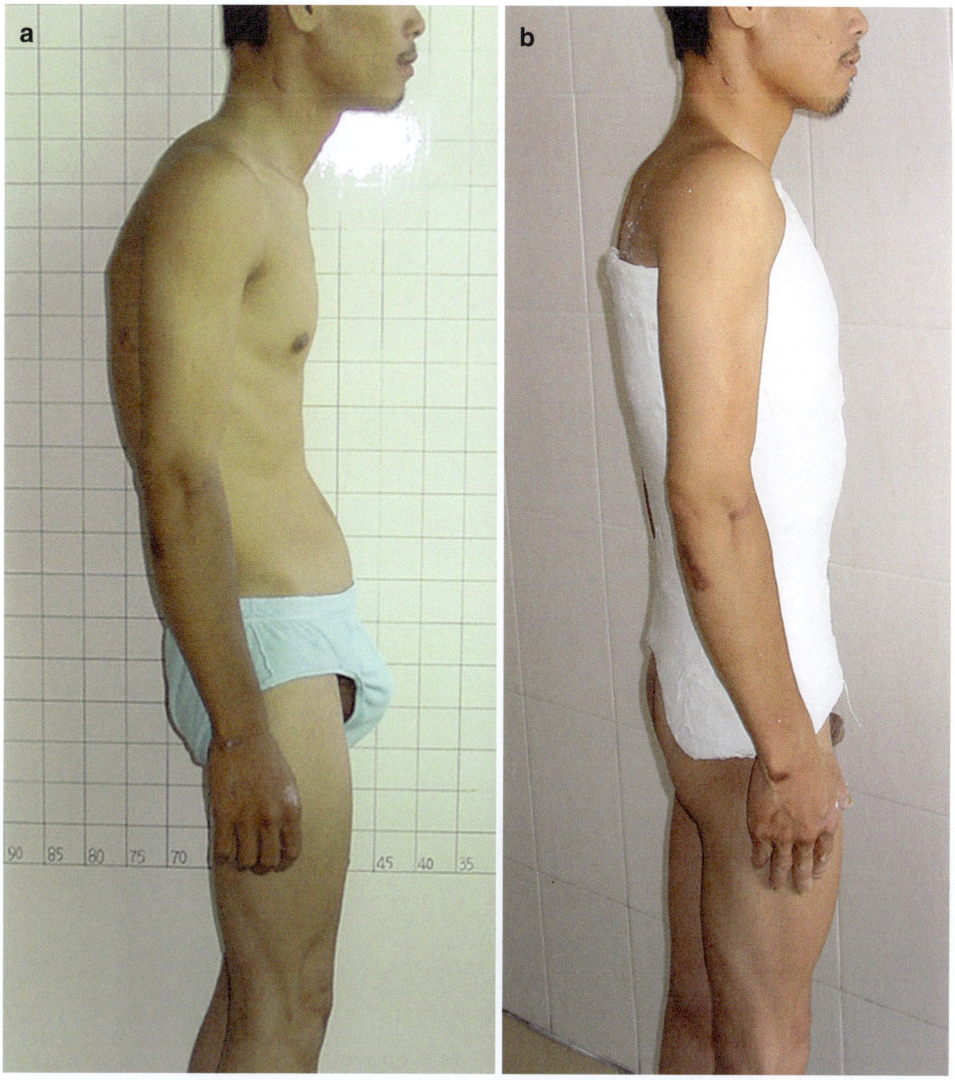

Suggested Reading

1. Tian H, Lin Q, Tan Y. Therapeutics of ankylosing spondylitis. Guangzhou: World Book Publishing Company; 2005. p. 165–95.
2. Tian H, Li F. Spinal deformity and osteotomy. Xi'an: World Book Publishing Company; 2001. p. 662–734.
3. Tian H, Wang B, Lv X, et al. Correction and fixation of ankylosing kyphosis and osteotomy. Chinese Journal of Orthopaedics. 2005;13(7):509–12.
4. Tian H. Application of the "Tian's spinal osteotomes" in orthopaedic surgery. Chinese Journal of Orthopaedics. 1994;14(4):236–40.
5. Tian H. Selection of internal fixation after osteotomy and correction of ankylosing kyphosis. Orthopedic Journal of China. 2011;19(9):784–6.
6. Tian H, Liu S, Ma Y. Practical spine surgery illustration. Beijing: People's Military Medical Press; 2008. p. 316–21.
7. Dang G. Surgical techniques for the spine. Beijing: People's Medical Publishing House; 2004. p. 246–52.
8. Chen A, Xu W. Spinal surgery atlas. Beijing: People's Medical Publishing House; 2001. p. 181–273.
9. Tian H, Ma Y, Lv X. Minimally invasive V-shaped osteotomy for correction of ankylosing kyphosis. Chinese Journal of Orthopaedics. 2008;16(5):349–52.
10. Tian H, Liu S, Ma Y. Practical spine surgery. Guangzhou: Guangdong Science and Technology Press; 2008. p. 195–409.
11. Liang Z. Transpedicular osteotomy for the treatment of kyphosis caused by ankylosing spondylitis. Chinese Journal of Orthopaedics. 1997;17(6):351–2.
12. Leong JCY, Ma A, Yau A. Spinal Osteotomy for fixed flexion deformity. Journal of Orthopaedic Translation. 1978;2:271.
13. Bradford DS, Zhang Y, Wang Y. The spine. Shenyang: Liaoning Science and Technology Press; 2003. p. 75–83.
14. Tian H, Li M, Ma Y. Spinal deformity osteotomy orthopedics, vol. 5. Beijing: People's Medical Publishing House; 2011. p. 101–279.
15. Wang B. Spinal surgery. Beijing: Peking University Medical Press; 2009. p. 152–4.
16. Tian H, Liang Y. Ankylosing spondylitis spinal deformity osteotomy and orthopedic surgery skills. Beijing: People's Medical Publishing House; 2014. p. 1–328.

8 Apex Osteotomy for AS Kyphosis

Yijian Liang, Shaoyu Liu, Huizhong Tian, and Junyi Ma

8.1 Overview

Most thoracolumbar ASK patients are treated with apex osteotomy. For patients with apex on T10–L4, apex osteotomy is also a favorable technique to achieve a sound outcome. As the spinal canal between T10 and L4 is relatively wide, it is not easy to lead to spinal stenosis after osteotomy and correction. As this segment is not constrained by the chest cage and ribs, it is easier to close the osteotomy gap of the lamina during hyperextension reduction. The osteotomy correction is performed on the apex; it is very effective to extend and lengthen the spine, and thus increase the body height. Therefore, thoracolumbar apex osteotomy is also an optional surgical technique.

The spinal canal of T3–T9 segment is narrower, with nourish blood supplying and exiting the spinal cord. The spine is supported by the ribs and chest cage on both sides, forming a "birdcage-shaped" elastic fixation. The osteotomy gap on those levels will be difficult to be closed. Therefore, it is not an ideal location to perform ASK apex osteotomy, considering complication prevention. The spinal canal of T10–L4 is wider and is not affected by chest cage support. Anatomically, it is the preferred site for apex osteotomy.

The vast majority of ASK patients can be corrected with apex or non-apex osteotomy of T10–L4. As ASK most frequently occurs in T10–L4, nearly 79% of ASK osteotomy and correction are performed in this segment, regardless of apex or non-apex osteotomy. Therefore, T10–L4 is the preferred segment for ASK osteotomy (Fig. 8.1).

When selecting an osteotomy site, lateral X-ray should be evaluated to observe how the spinous process gap widens at the apex level, how the superior-inferior dimension of the intervertebral foramen is lengthened, and anterior closing and posterior opening of disc space. If the apex is located at T12–L1, osteotomy should be performed between T12 and L1. Thus, osteotomy is not necessarily performed between L2 and L3. Instead, it should be performed on the apex level. This is called apex osteotomy. However, the osteotomy site should be within T10–L4. As the spinal canal of T10–L4 is wide, it is not easy to produce secondary spinal stenosis after osteotomy, and it is not restricted by the chest cage and ribs.

Ankylosing Spondylitis Kyphosis: Ankylosing spondylitis often forms a typical round kyphotic deformity in the late stage of the disease. With the patient's age and disease progression, the spine and surrounding tissue experience bone remodeling. A three-dimension reconstructive and print model may be helpful for preoperative plan and guidance of osteotome during operation.

Selection of surgical segments: At present, posterior osteotomy is one of the most effective techniques for correction for severe ankylosing spondylitis. The surgical site is mostly selected at the apical level of the spinal deformity. However, instrumentation applied in osteoporotic areas bears a potential of failure. ALL ossification tissue should also be noted preoperatively. Simulation examples and experience of ankylosing spondylitis correction, 1 is a single-segment VCR case (Figs. 8.2a–d and 8.3a,b); 2 is a case of laminectomy combined with VCR (Figs. 8.4a–g and 8.5a,b).

8.2 Surgical Procedure

1. Preoperative preparation
   (a) Guide the patient through physical preparation:
      I Routine preoperative laboratory work-up and imaging examinations, organ functional performance, and tolerance to anesthesia and surgery should be evaluated. Patients planned for spinal osteotomy

Y. Liang
Spinal Surgery, Affiliated Hospital of Southwest Jiaotong University, Chengdu, China

S. Liu
Spinal Surgery, The Seventh Affiliated Hospital, Sun Yat-sen University, Shenzhen, China

H. Tian (✉) · J. Ma
Spinal Surgery, The Sixth Affiliated Hospital of Xinjiang Medical University, Urumqi, China

H. Tian et al. (eds.), *Spinal Osteotomy Orthopaedics*, https://doi.org/10.1007/978-981-16-1387-6_8

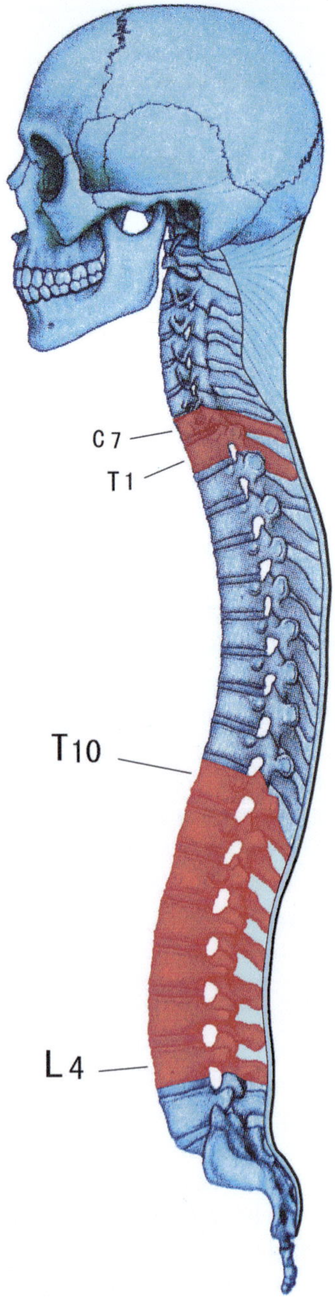

Fig. 8.1 C7–T1 is the osteotomy site of the cervical thoracic segment. T10–L4 are the preferred sites for parietal and non-parietal vertebral osteotomy. Seventy-nine percent of ASK patients undergo spine osteotomy at this segment

and correction should receive lung function measurement, which includes pulmonary volume and aspiration functions such as vital capacity, functional residual capacity, total lung volume, minute ventilation, FEV1, forced expiratory vital capacity, and mid-expiratory flow rate. It is also necessary to calculate the corresponding value according to the estimated formula of vital capacity and maximum ventilation according to age, gender, height, weight, etc., and then calculate the percentage by comparing the actual measured value against the predicted value to determine the degree and grade of pulmonary impairment.

II Adaptive exercise for postoperative changes: Eating in bed. bowel movement and urination in bed, limb exercise in bed, long-term bed rest, correct cough and sputum production, pulmonary improvement exercise (deep breathing, balloon blowing, hand-assisted breathing), abdominal massage training, etc.

III Surgical posture training for patients scheduled for spinal osteotomy and correction: The positioning for ASK osteotomy and correction is the key to success. Sometimes it takes 1 h to set the surgical position, which osteotomy and internal fixation take 2–3 h. Before the surgery, the patient should be trained for taking a prone position (Fig. 8.6). The duration should be gradually extended until the patient is able to maintain the position for more than 2 h. The nurse should check the acceptance of the patient and any potential respiratory failure.

(b) Preparation of instruments: A set of Tian's spine osteotome, a complete set of pedicle screw and rod system, a set of Tian's pedicle finders, some 0.8–1.2 mm Luque wires, Luque rods as well as other general instruments.

2. Anesthesia: Tracheal intubation anesthesia or bronchoscopy intubation anesthesia.
3. Position: The patient should be put into a prone position. The operating table should be set to an inverted V shape. The waist bridge should be elevated, with cushion, headrest, and shoulder support applied. The patient's feet should be fixed to the bed end. The traction reduction band should be placed under the armpits. The incision line should be marked, followed by sterilization and draping (see the positioning of non-apex osteotomy).
4. Operation procedures:

   The first step, incision and exposure. Make an incision on the skin and subcutaneous tissue along the spinous process, expose the spinous process and the posterior layer of the back fascia, dissect with an electric cutter along the spinous process. The spinous process should be exposed by subperiosteal elevation. Lamina is then exposed bilaterally until the transverse process (Fig. 8.7).

   The second step, select the osteotomy level. According to preoperative X-ray, osteotomy site should be selected where the proudest spinous process of the kyphotic curve, with the widest gap between the spinous processes, the biggest intervertebral foramen superior-inferior dimension on the lateral X-ray, the anterior narrow

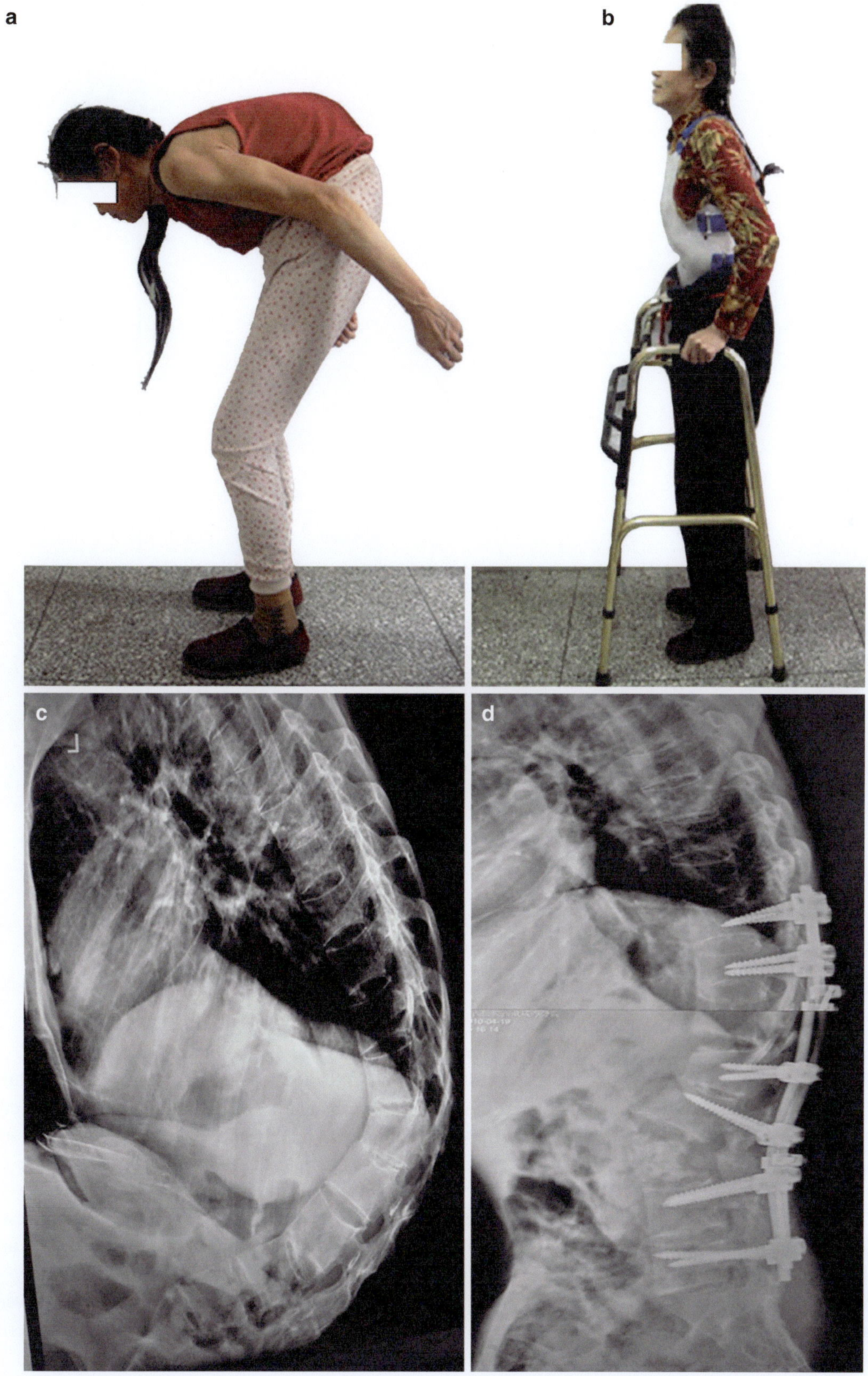

Fig. 8.2 Female, 45 years old, ankylosing spondylitis with severe kyphosis, Comparison before and after apex osteotomy. The Cobb angle decreased from 110° before to –28° (lumbar lordosis restored) after. (**a**) Preoperative appearance; (**b**) postoperative appearance; (**c**) preoperative lateral X-ray ; (**d**) postoperative lateral X-ray

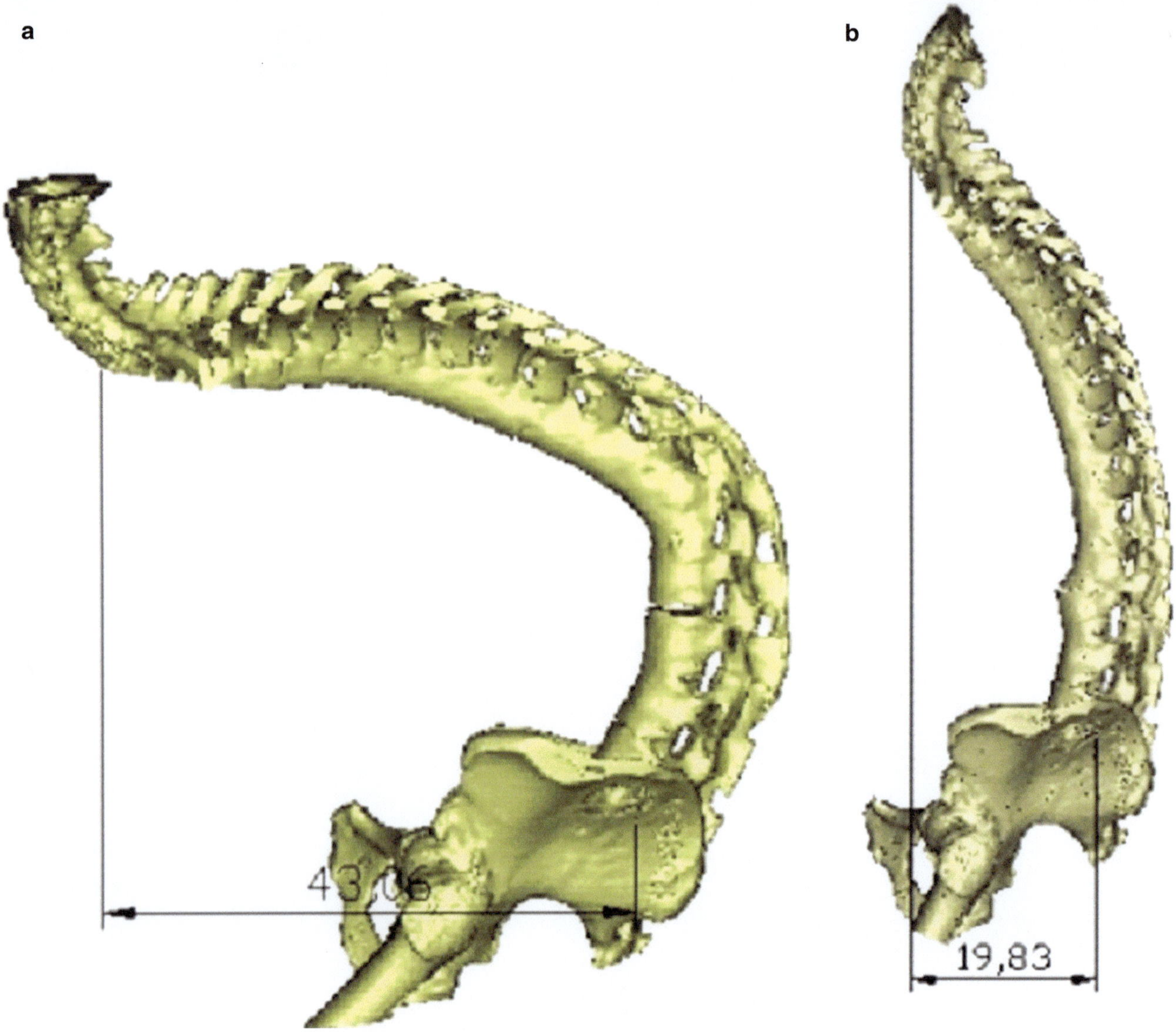

Fig. 8.3 Simulation of VCR procedure of L3 and comparison. (**a**) Preoperative, (**b**) postoperative

and posterior widen intervertebral space and free of bony fusion anterior to the vertebral body (Fig. 8.8). Apex osteotomy is not limited to L2–L3. Any intervertebral space between T10 and L4 may be the potential site of apex osteotomy. Thus, the indications for apex osteotomy are more extensive.

The third step: osteotomy. Simple transverse laminar osteotomy, laminar V-shape osteotomy, pedicle subtraction osteotomy (PSO), and vertebral column resection (VCR) are all possible options for apex osteotomy.

(a) Transverse laminar osteotomy (Fig. 8.9): It is intended for ASK patients with Cobb angle <80°. A thin blade straight osteotome is be used to make a transverse osteotomy wedge resection from the spinous process toward the posterior edge of the vertebral body. The width of the wedge resection is 8–12 mm between the lamina. After resection, head and foot traction and manual correction are applied to achieve the closure of the osteotomy gap, which means opening the anterior side of the vertebral body and extension of the spine. Static internal fixation,

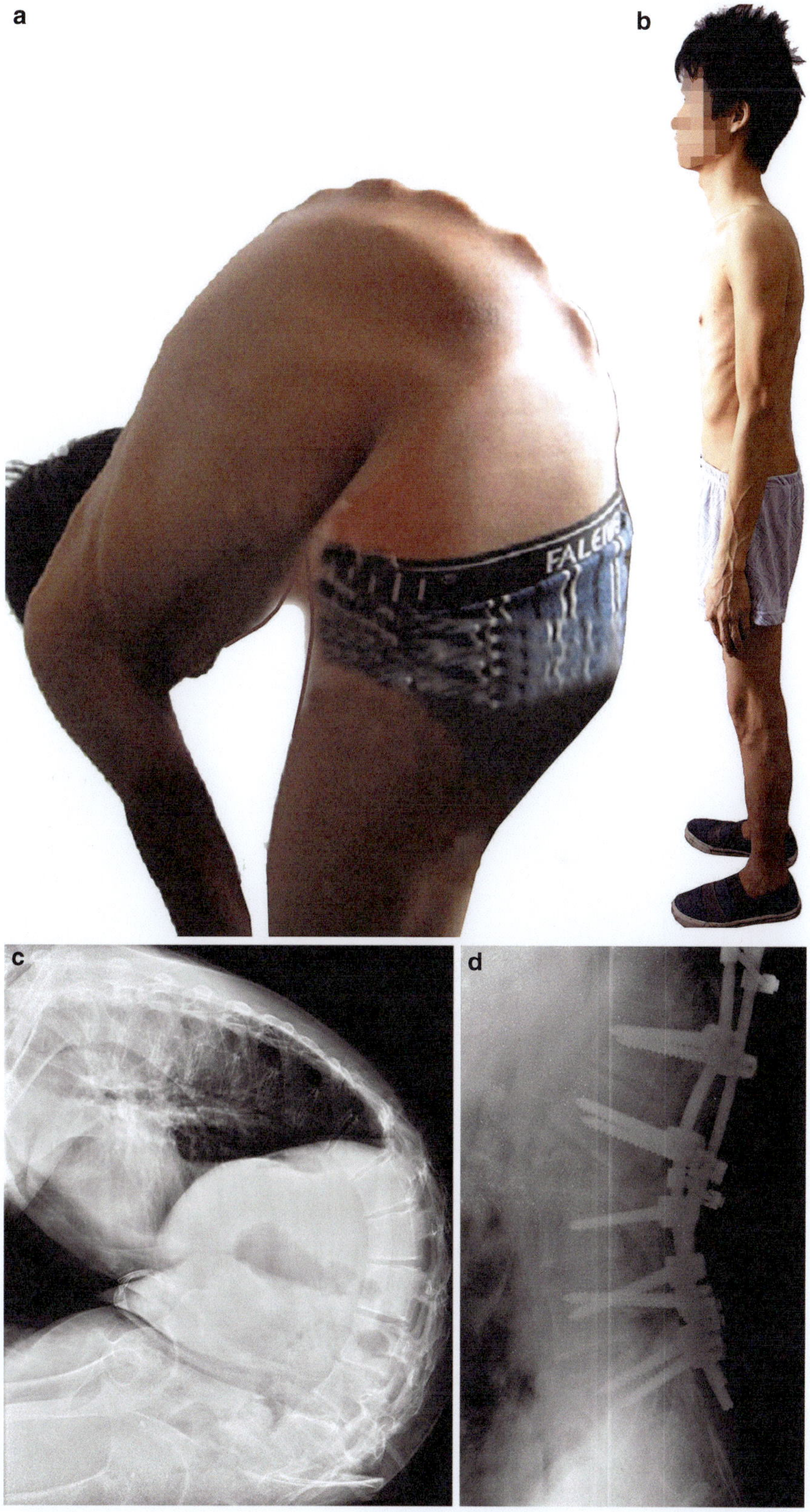

Fig. 8.4 Patient Liu XX with severe ankylosing kyphosis deformity. After two operations, the patient's appearance was significantly improved. He was able to lie flat without a pillow. The abdominal skin folds completely disappeared, and his height increased from 122 to 170 cm. The sagittal Cobb angle was 151° before apex osteotomy and –20° after operation (lumbar lordosis restored). (**a**) Appearance before operation, (**b**) appearance after operation, (**c**) preoperative lateral X-ray, (**d**) postoperative lateral X-ray

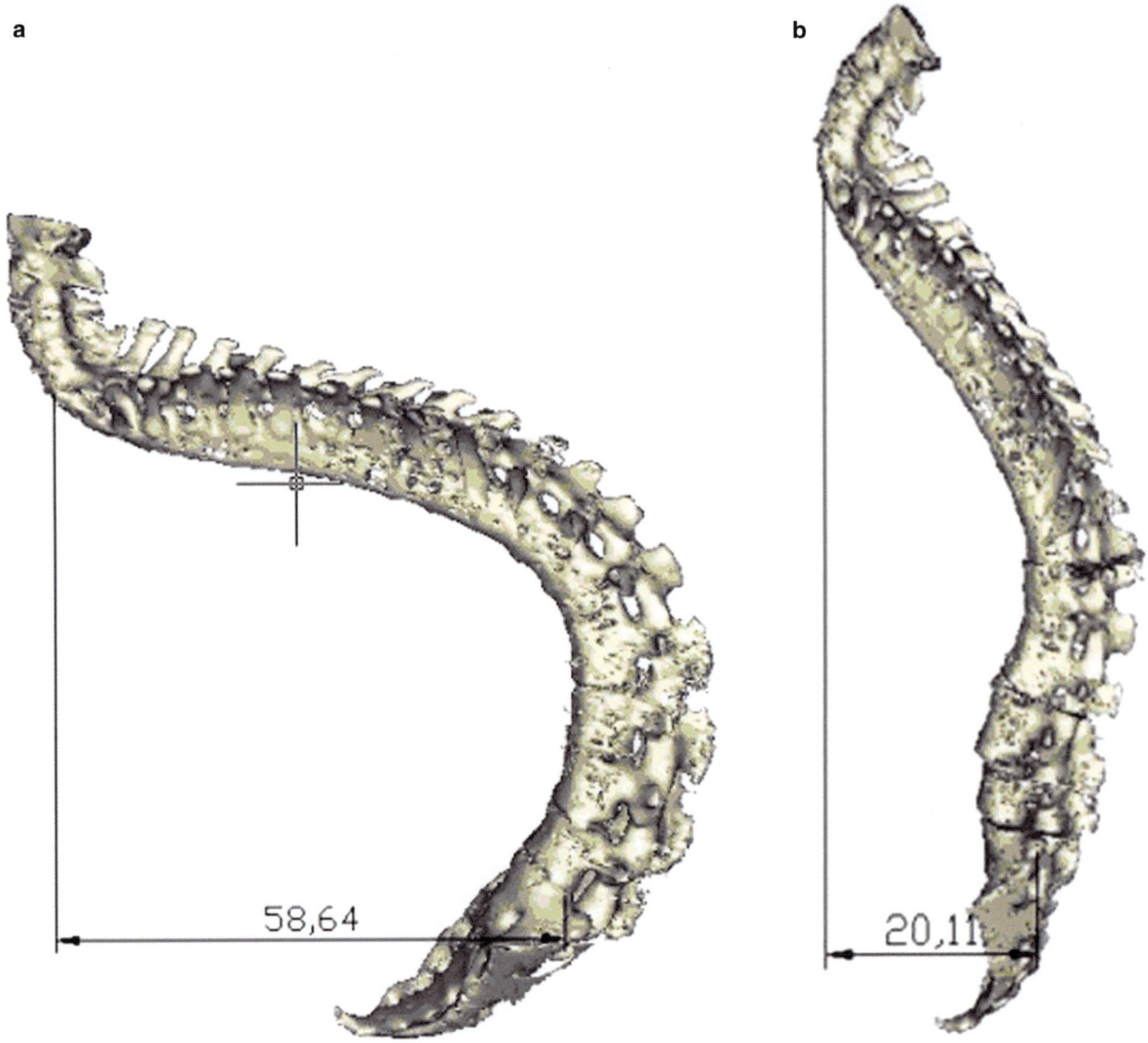

Fig. 8.5 Simulated surgery of L2 VCR and lumbar 4/5 laminectomy. (a) Before operation, (**b**) after operation

that is, the pedicle screw system, is to be used to have primary correction of kyphosis with bracing postoperatively. This will allow for early ambulation. D Dynamic fixation is to be used combined with postoperative plaster vest immobilization for 6–8 months, given the correction is achieved by intraoperative manipulation and self-correction of kyphosis by bed rest. X-ray evaluation should be performed once the plaster is removed to check up graft healing.

(b) Lamina V-shape osteotomy (Fig. 8.10): The direction of the laminar V-shape osteotomy is slightly inclined to the cranial side. After closing the gap of V-shape osteotomy, the osteotomy surfaces are tightly overlapped to prevent lateral and longitudinal displacement. The surgical technique of V-shape osteotomy is more complicated than transverse osteotomy. It requires special surgical skills and tools, namely "thin blade osteotome with different curves." This set of osteotomes make laminar V-shape osteotomy fast and convenient. The osteotomy surface remains smooth. After reduction, the V-shaped ends are seamlessly impacted into each other to facilitate bony fusion. Therefore, this technique is more commonly used in single- or multiple-level apex osteotomy.

(c) PSO (Fig. 8.11): When the apex of ankylosing spondylitis kyphosis is located in T10–L4 and the anterior edge of the vertebral body and the anterior longitudinal ligament present ossification, it is predicted that simple lamina osteotomy is difficult to open the anterior edge of the vertebral body. PSO at the apex is a

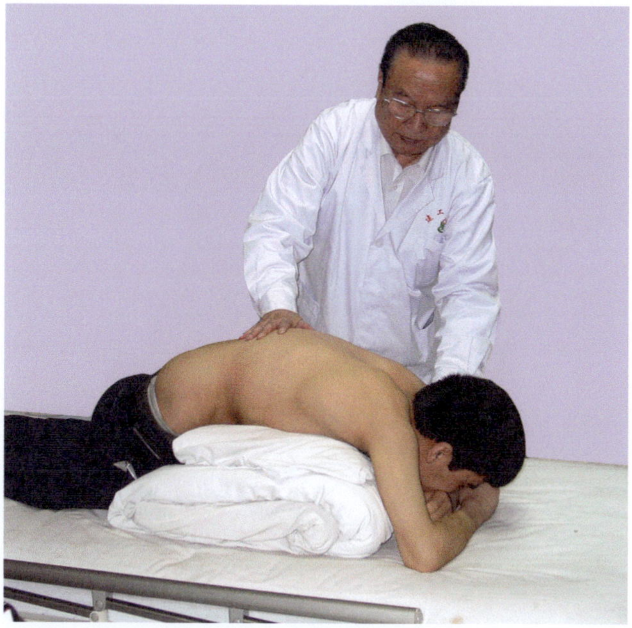

Fig. 8.6 ASK patients undergoing training in the prone position before surgery

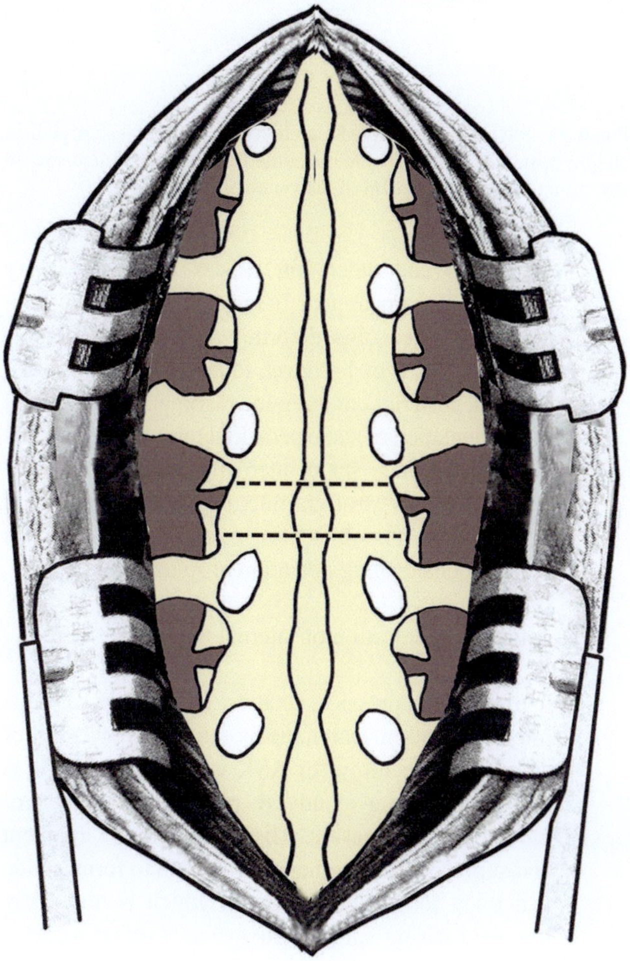

Fig. 8.7 Incision and exposure

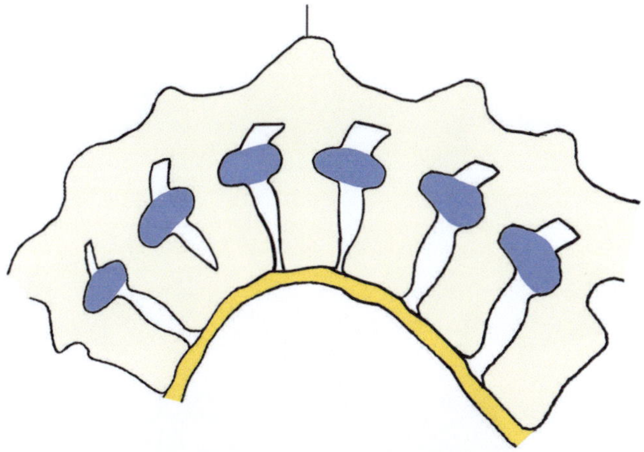

Fig. 8.8 Selecting the parietal vertebral part as the osteotomy gap

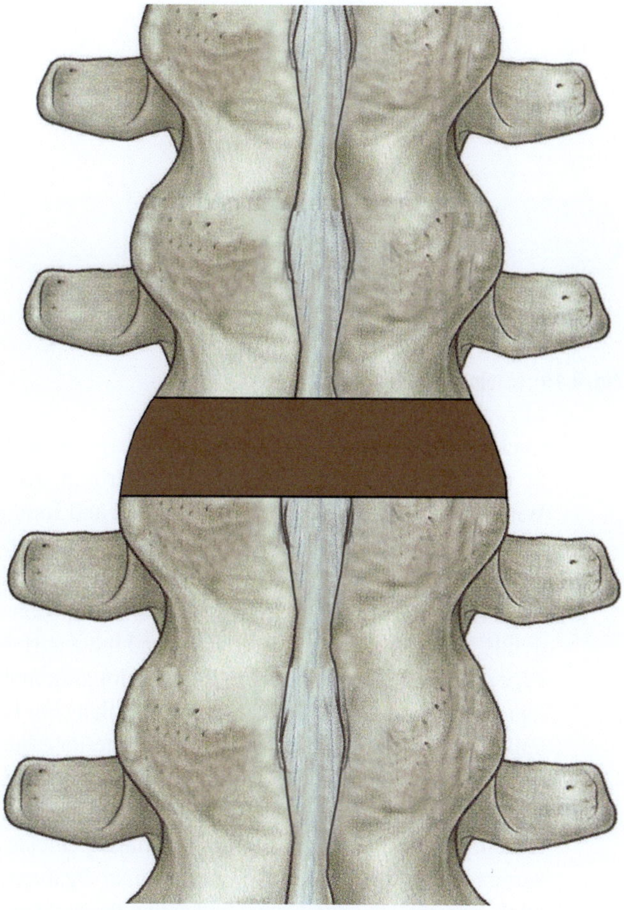

Fig. 8.9 Laminar transverse osteotomy

good option in this case. PSO includes wedged resection of the vertebral arch, pedicle, and the posterior 3/4 of the vertebral body. The tip of the wedge-shaped resection reaches the front 1/4 of the vertebral body. With hyperextension manipulation, the front 1/4 of the vertebral body experiences compression fracture

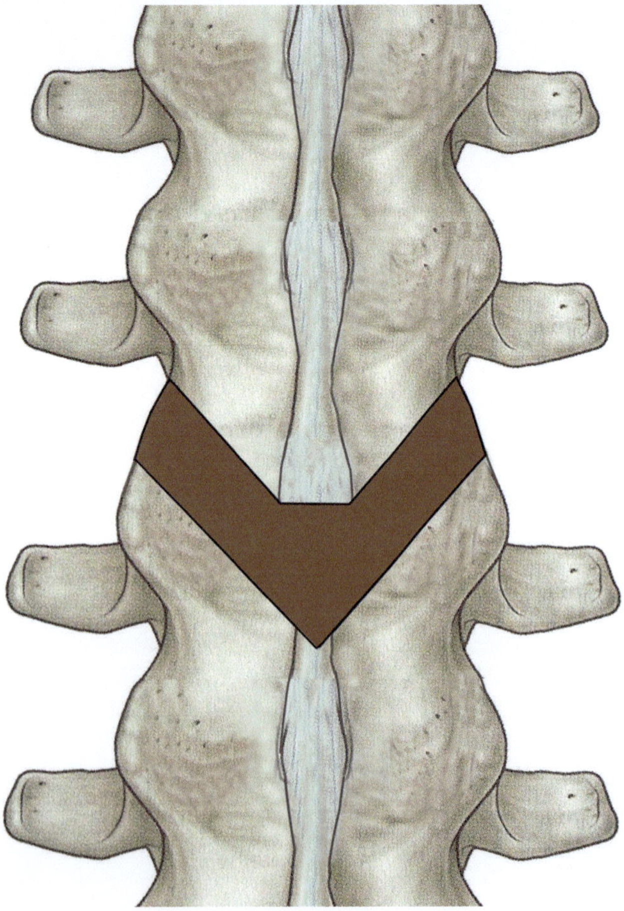

Fig. 8.10 Lamina V-shaped osteotomy

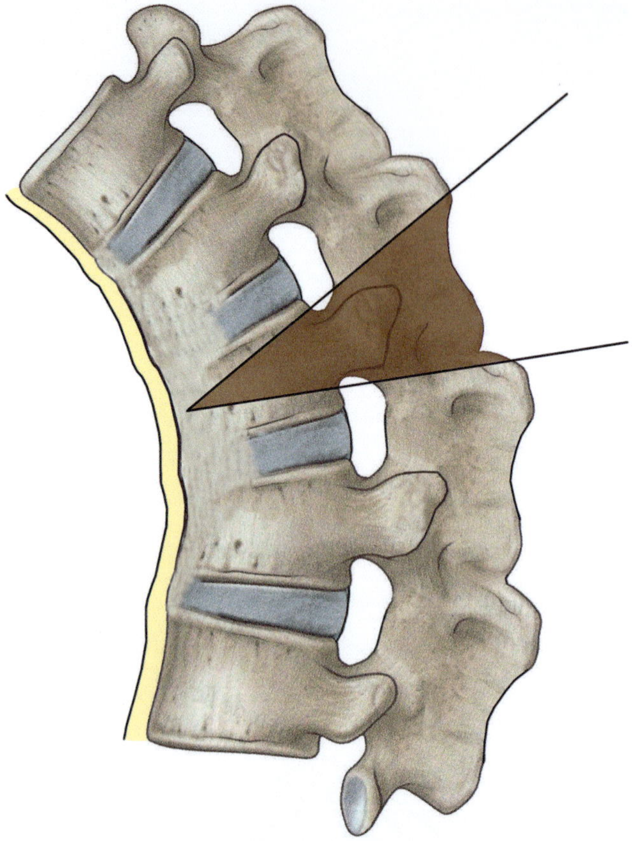

Fig. 8.11 PSO includes wedged resection of the vertebral arch, pedicle and the posterior 3/4 of the vertebral body. The tip of the wedge-shaped resection reaches the front 1/4 of the vertebral body.

to close the osteotomy gap. The osteotomy surfaces in this surgical technique are well approximated. With compression posterior to the lamina and internal fixation, the bone-on-bone interface is stable and reliable.

(d) VCR (Fig. 8.12): When the apex of ankylosing spondylitis kyphosis is located in T10–L4 and the anterior edge of the vertebral body and the anterior longitudinal ligament present ossification, it is predicted that simple lamina osteotomy is difficult to open the anterior edge of the vertebral body. VCR at the apex is another good option in this case. VCR means the complete wedge resection from the spinous process, lamina, pedicles, vertebral body to the anterior longitudinal ligament while retaining the dural canal and spinal nerve roots. To achieve this, Tian's osteotome set is the essential tool. It works around the dura canal to get circular resection which means resecting the anterior structure through the posterior approach in one stage. Bone grafting is needed. Static fixation with pedicle screw system is only suitable for severe ASK cases with Cobb angle above 90°, because these patients have developed severe kyphosis, high contracture of rectus abdominis and other soft tissues while mesentery artery and neurovascular tissues are also in high tension. To correct this deformity, spine shortening is needed by VCR of 1–2 level, followed by anterior distraction, posterior compression manipulation, and long instrumentation of static pedicle screw system. For this class of patients, static internal fixation is essential while interbody strut grafting, posterior grafting, and postoperative immobilization are all important. VCR is the most challenging operation in spinal surgery.

The fourth step, selection of internal fixation:

(a) Dynamic compression fixation (Fig. 8.13a,b): This internal fixation technique is suitable for cases of simple laminectomy for ASK whose Cobb angle is <80°. Ankylosing spondylitis patients have hypertrophic spinous processes. Their interspinous ligament and supraspinous ligament are ossified to form a wide and thick longitudinal septum, which is not easily removed during surgery. However, it offers a favorable condition for dynamic compression fixation. The interspinous process wiring plus Luque rods provide

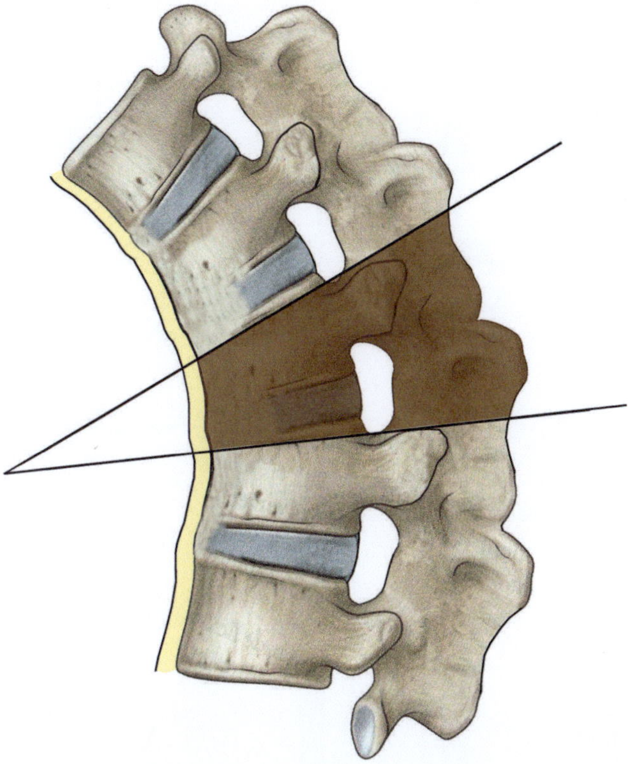

Fig. 8.12 The scope of VCR depends on the degree of kyphosis, including waist osteotomy through the vertebral body retaining the endplates, osteotomy involving one disc space, and osteotomy involving two disc spaces

dynamic compression which allows the kyphosis to be further corrected and extended by bed rest in supine position after returning to the ward. It is not limited by the fixation device and is more effective than static internal fixation by the pedicle screw system. In the process of correcting ASK deformity, any internal fixation is not able to replace the role of external immobilization with hyperextensive plaster vest with a good fit. The latter is the truly effective way to prevent the recurrence of kyphosis deformity and promote solid bone fusion.

(b) Static pedicle screw system fixation (Fig. 8.14a,b): Applicable to severe ASK cases with Cobb angle above 90°. These patients have developed severe kyphosis, high contracture of rectus abdominis and other soft tissues while mesentery and neurovascular tissues are also in high tension. To correct this deformity, spine shortening is needed by VCR of 1–2 level, followed by anterior distraction, posterior compression manipulation, and long instrumentation of static pedicle screw system (Fig. 8.15). For this class of patients, static internal fixation is essential while interbody strut grafting, posterior grafting, and postoperative immobilization are all important.

5. Postoperative treatment:

   After the operation, the patient with dynamic fixation should be placed in a supine position. According to the extent of kyphosis correction, a pillow or cotton pad should be properly used. Pillows could be used alternatively on each side to prevent pressure ulcers. The suction tubes on both sides are connected to the suction bottle. The patency of the drainage tube should be absolutely maintained. During the ward round on the next day, 200–400 mL of blood in the suction bottle indicates free of blood collection in the wound. The drainage tube can be removed on day 2 or day 3 after surgery. Upon suture removal on Day 10, the hyperextensive plaster vest will be applied for external immobilization. Patients are allowed to ambulate with the protection of a plaster vest which lasts for 6–8 months.

8.3 Key Aspects and Cautions

1. Apex osteotomy is the most widely used technique, covering a wide range of indications from round kyphosis to angular kyphosis. However non-apex osteotomy is limited to ASK correction.
2. The way to correct the curvature of the spine is to resect a wedge shape from the apex of the deformity. After resection of a wedge specific to the degree of curve, the spinal deformity is corrected on any planes. It is applicable to either kyphosis, scoliosis, or kyphoscoliosis.
3. The principle of apex osteotomy to correct spinal deformity is the same as that for limb deformity. However, it is not as simple and easy as long bone osteotomy. Due to the existence of neurovascular tissue of and around the spine, outstanding surgical skills are required to ensure the safety of neurovascular tissues and sufficient correction of spinal deformities. This is a highly challenging surgical operation that requires special surgical tools and solid basic skills.
4. The apical vertebrae of ASK are protruding to the back and are located under the skin on the back of the body. A posterior approach is thus more convenient. The anterior side is the concave side of the spine. It is difficult to expose as it forms a deep recess covered by lower ribs and iliac crest. Therefore, it is more convenient to expose the vertebral arch and vertebral body from the posterior; thus, the role of anterior and posterior two-stage surgery is limited.
5. The apical vertebra is the most prominent part that bulges backward, and it is most convenient to do a wedge osteotomy from the posterior. The more the kyphosis angle is, the more suitable it is for the posterior approach. Exposure of the vertebral arch and vertebral

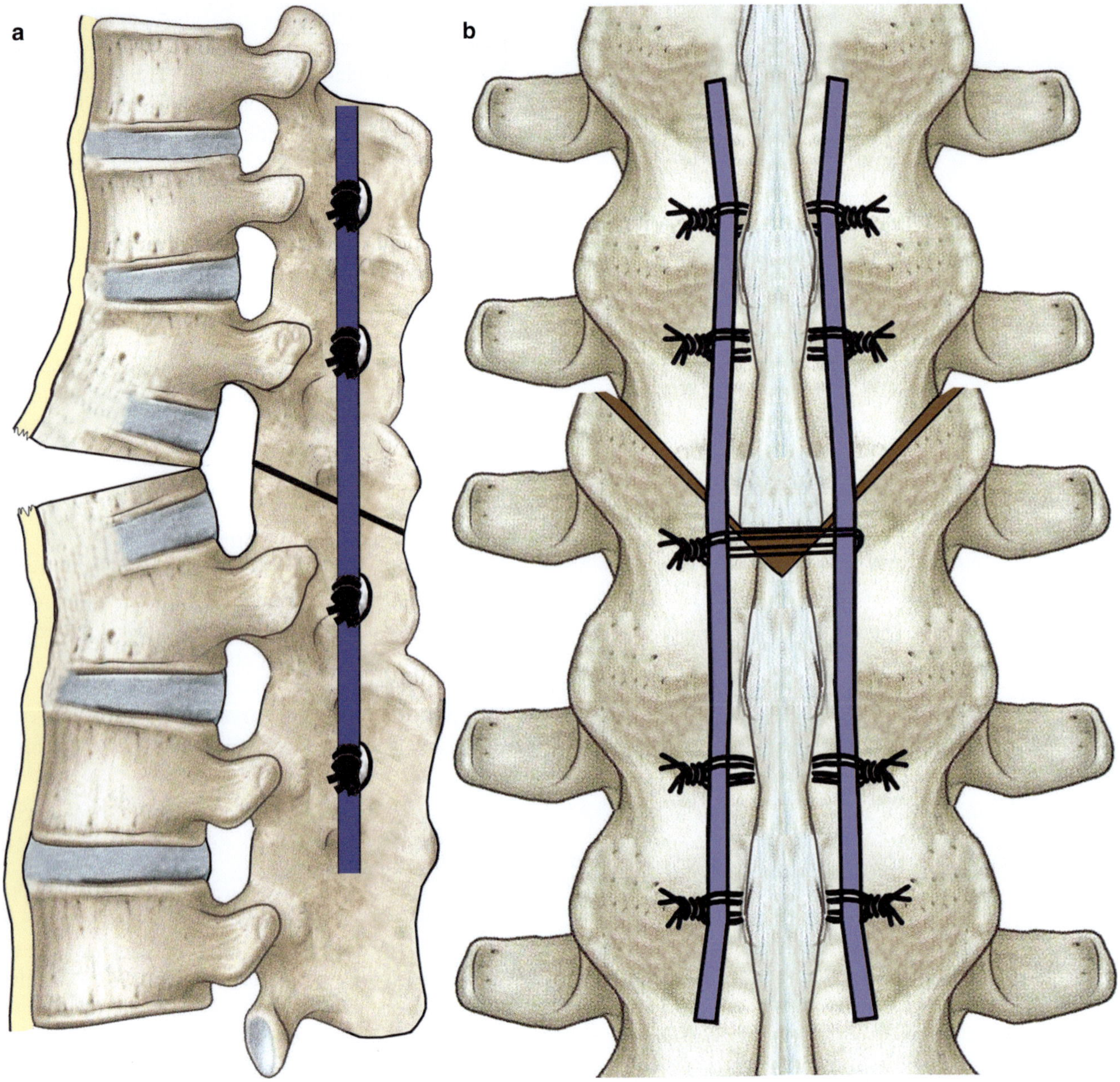

Fig. 8.13 Dynamic compression fixation with Luque rods and interspinous process wiring. The technique is simple and practical and allows self-correction after surgery. (**a**) Lateral view, (**b**) posterior view

body is not a problem by extending the incision and more dissection to both sides.

6. As long as the principle of subperiosteal elevation is strictly followed, there is no need to ligate the segmental vessels. By using the retractor osteotome, a clear surgical field is completely guaranteed. Losing a clear surgical field is losing the way toward a successful osteotomy.
7. Osteotomy should be performed in a step-by-step manner, starting from pedicle and lateral osteotomy and then moving to the central part of the vertebral body while retaining a posterior sheet of the vertebral body which is reserved for final push down and resection. This is the way to reduce bleeding and save surgery time.
8. In case of cancellous sinus bleeding, a thin blade straight osteotome is used to make a smooth cut, and then apply bone wax for hemostasis.
9. Bleeding of epidural venous plexus can be stopped by quickly removing and pushing down the thin sheet of bone on the posterior edge of the vertebral body and quickly closing the osteotomy space.

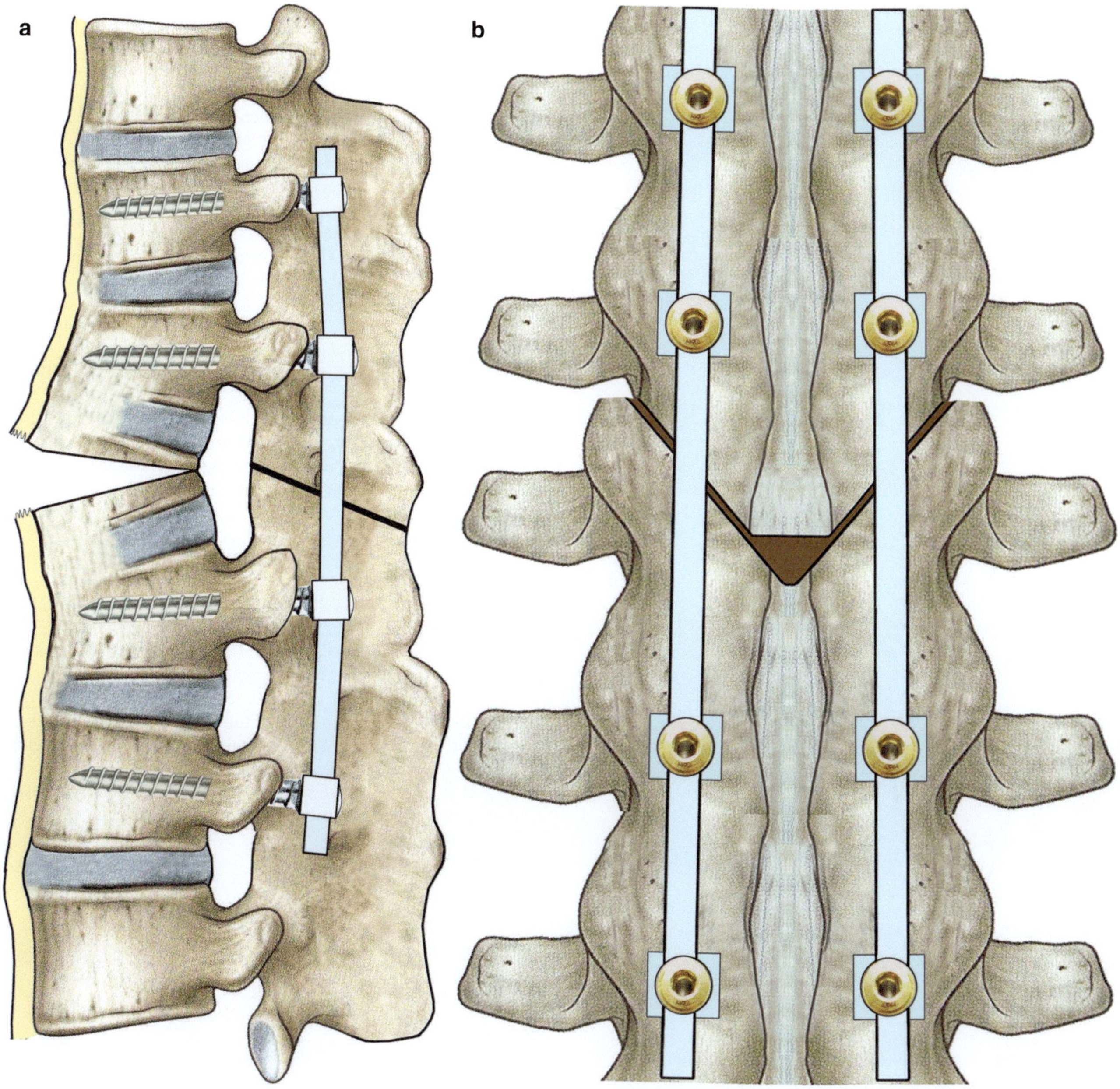

Fig. 8.14 Static pedicle screw system fixation, suitable for severe ASK cases with Cobb angle above 90°. After VCR, a static pedicle screw and rod system is used for internal fixation. Postoperatively plaster vest or brace will allow early ambulation. (**a**) Lateral view, (**b**) posterior view

10. After the osteotomy space is closed, the dura mater should be slightly shortened and widened, so that the dura mater expands and presses the epidural venous plexus, and the bleeding naturally stops.
11. After reducing the osteotomy gap, the dural sac should not be stretched to avoid nerve injury and epidural venous plexus bleeding.
12. Choose appropriate internal fixation according to the needs of osteotomy, such as dynamic internal fixation or static internal fixation.
13. The role of postoperative external immobilization with plaster vest should not be underestimated as it outperforms internal fixation in ASK patients.

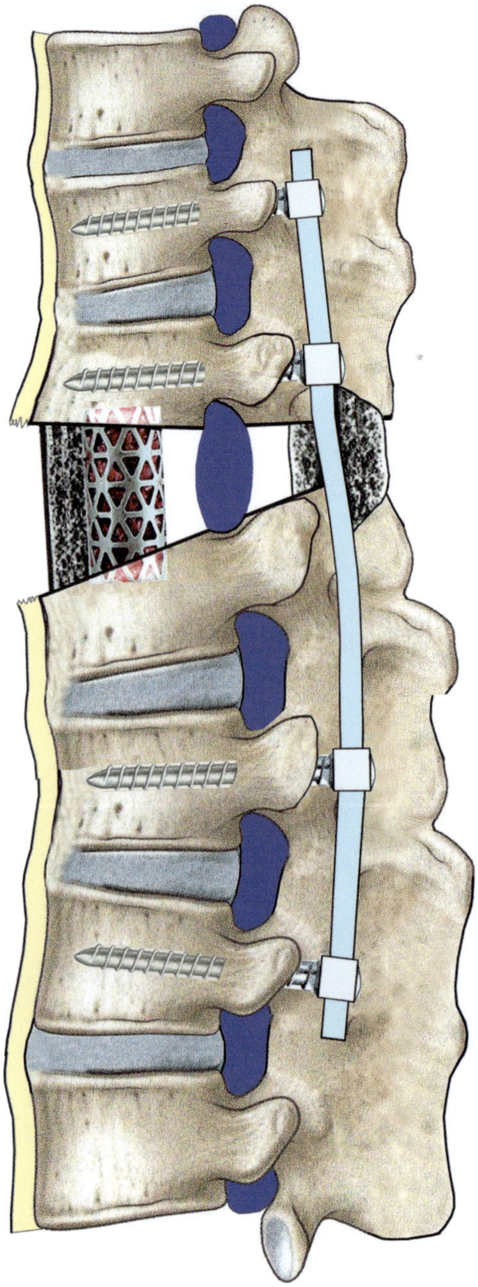

Fig. 8.15 If spinal shortening is required, osteotomy is performed with strut grafting anteriorly. The posterior edge of the lamina should not be completely closed to avoid buckling of the dura sac

Suggested Reading

1. Standring S. Gray's anatomy. Beijing: Peking University Medical Press; 2006. p. 14–98.
2. Zhong S, Fu Z, Liang M. Introduction to digital medicine. 1st ed. Beijing: People's Medical Publishing House; 2009. p. 1–3.
3. Pei G, Xiang D. Current development and prospects of computer assisted orthopedic surgery. Chin J Orthop Trauma. 2003;5:85–8.
4. Canale S , et al. Campbell's operative orthopaedics, 10th ed., vol. 12, issue 38. Philadelphia, PA : Mosby/Elsevier; 2007. p. 2792–6.
5. Norio K, Sun G, Tian H. One-stage posterior closed-open combined wedge osteotomy to correct kyphosis. Orthop J Chin. 2007;15(17):1307–12.
6. Tian H, Lin Q, Tan Y. Therapeutics of ankylosing spondylitis. Guangzhou: World Book; 2005. p. 165–95.
7. Tian H, Li F. Spinal deformity and osteotomy. Xi'an: World Book; 2001. p. 662–734.
8. Tian H, Wang B, Lv X, et al. Correction and fixation of ankylosing kyphosis and osteotomy. Chin J Orthop. 2005;13(7):509–12.
9. Tian H, Liu S, Ma Y. Practical spine surgery illustration. Beijing: People's Military Medical Press; 2008. p. 316–21.
10. Dang G. Surgical techniques for the spine. Beijing: People's Medical Publishing House; 2004. p. 246–52.
11. Tian H, Ma Y, Lv X. Minimally invasive V-shaped osteotomy for correction of ankylosing kyphosis. Chin J Orthop. 2008;16(5):349–52.
12. Chen A, Xu W. Spinal surgery atlas. Beijing: People's Medical Publishing House; 2001. p. 181–273.
13. Tian H, Liu S, Ma Y. Practical spine surgery. Guangzhou: Guangdong Science and Technology Press; 2008. p. 195–409.
14. Liang Z. Transpedicular osteotomy for the treatment of kyphosis caused by ankylosing spondylitis. Chin J Orthop. 1997;17(6):351–2.
15. Leong JCY, Ma A, Yau A. Spinal osteotomy for fixed flexion deformity. Orthop Trans. 1978;2:271.
16. Tian H, Liang Y. Ankylosing spondylitis spinal deformity osteotomy and orthopedic surgery skills. Beijing: People's Medical Publishing House; 2014. p. 1–328.
17. Tian H, Zhang H, Liang Y. Surgical treatment of spinal deformity. Guangzhou: Guangdong Science and Technology Press; 2012. p. 1–483.

9 Spinal Osteotomy for Congenital Angular Kyphosis

Huizhong Tian, Weibin Sheng, Yilihamu Tuoheti, Li Li, and Junyi Ma

9.1 Overview

Two common types of kyphosis are round kyphosis and angular kyphosis. The main causes of angular kyphosis include: (1) congenital posterior hemivertebra, anterior malsegmentation, wedge vertebra or absence of vertebra caused by congenital dysplasia of anterior vertebra; (2) vertebral dysplasia due to damage of vertebral body and disc secondary to spinal tuberculosis while the growth of vertebral arch and lamina is not impacted. Traumatic angular kyphosis with spinal cord compression are commonly seen as well.

On the basis of osteotomy for ankylosing kyphosis, Tian Huizhong in China has carried out VCR for angular kyphosis. He believes that posterior VCR is an effective way of treating this. He has accumulated extensive surgical experiences from a large number of cases and considered that congenital angular kyphosis has the following features: (1) Angular kyphosis in short segment which is in favor of posterior wedge osteotomy to resect the vertebral arch and body. (2) In congenital kyphosis, it is easier to dissect the epidural level sac with less bleeding due to less adhesion. (3) The spine is shortened to prevent spinal cord distraction when closing the osteotomy gap. It is safer and more reliable than correction by anterior distraction and cord lengthening.

Kyphosis secondary to spinal tuberculosis is more difficult to be treated: (1) the kyphotic angle is typically large, e.g., more than 90°; (2) epidural adhesion creates trouble for dissection which is technically demanding. Ideally, the patient should be operated during the early stage of development.

H. Tian (✉) · L. Li · J. Ma
Spinal Surgery, The Sixth Affiliated Hospital of Xinjiang Medical University, Urumqi, China

W. Sheng
Spinal Surgery, The First Affiliated Hospital of Xinjiang Medical University, Urumqi, China

Y. Tuoheti
Department of Orthopedics, The Seventh Affiliated Hospital of Xinjiang Medical University, Urumqi, China

Causes of congenital angular kyphosis include congenital posterior hemivertebra as well as congenital anterior malsegmentation or semi-fused disc space (Figs. 9.1 and 9.2). Posterior correction and instrumentation will not work for congenital angular kyphosis. Anterior disc space distraction and bone grafting will not help to correct the deformity satisfactorily due to the deep anterior recess where grafting is the only thing to do. The surgical trauma of combined ante-

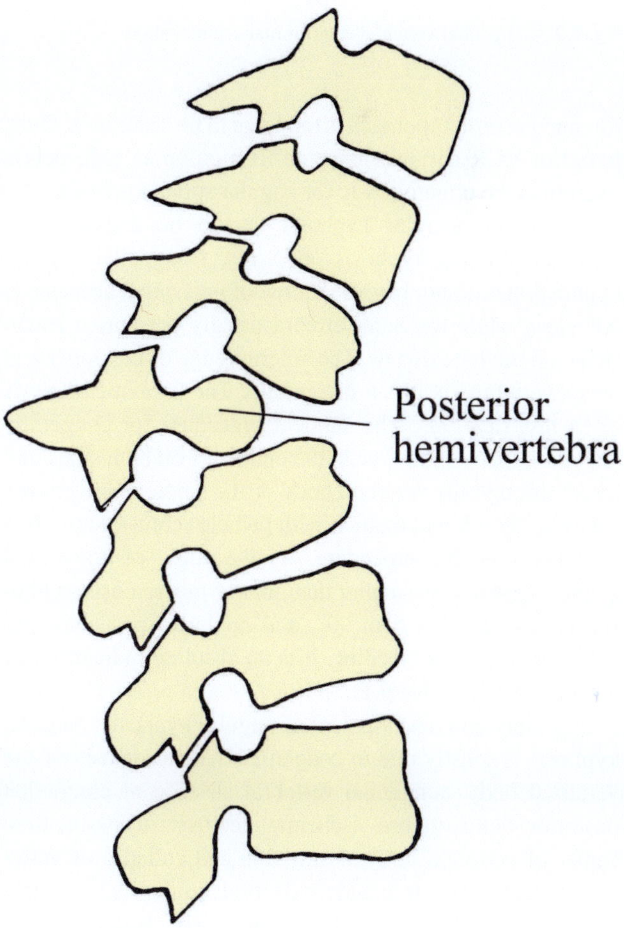

Fig. 9.1 Congenital posterior hemivertebra

H. Tian et al. (eds.), *Spinal Osteotomy Orthopaedics*, https://doi.org/10.1007/978-981-16-1387-6_9

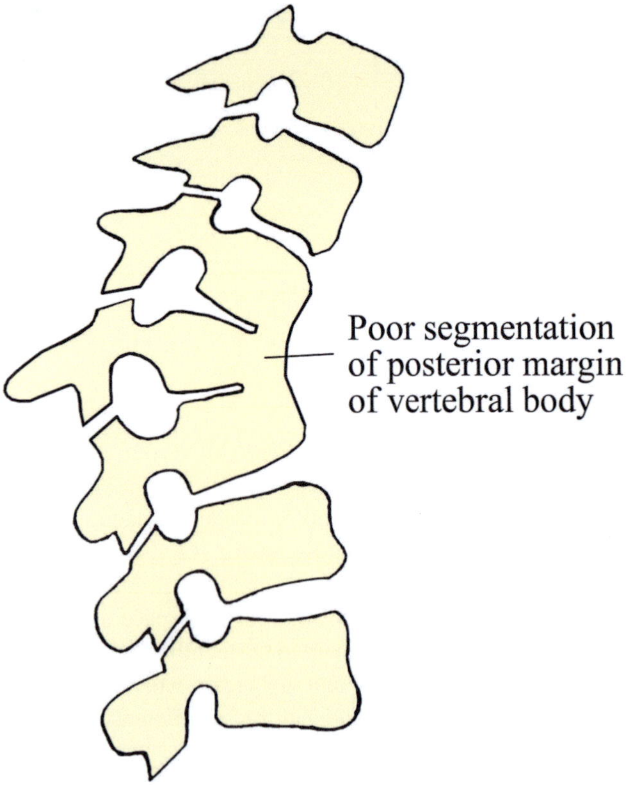

Fig. 9.2 Congenital vertebral anterior mal-segmentation

Table 9.1 Differential diagnosis for congenital angular kyphosis and tuberculosis angular kyphosis

No.	Congenital spinal kyphosis	Tuberculosis spinal kyphosis
1	Kyphotic angle less than 90° and involved only 1 vertebra usually	Kyphotic angle more than 90° and involved 2–4 vertebrae usually
2	Rare adhesions in epidural space	Wide adhesion in epidural space
3	No osseous connection between involved vertebrae	Bony fusion between involved vertebrae
4	Kyphotic angle <90° without curled deformity	Kyphotic angle >90° with curled deformity
5	Absolute indication of correction by VCR	Correction by VCR an option

rior and posterior approach is too large to be necessary. Thus, posterior VCR and instrumented fixation under halo-pelvic traction is the effective way for angular spinal kyphosis.

Congenital angular kyphosis should be distinguished from tuberculous kyphosis on X-ray. Congenital angular kyphosis should not have a shadow of paraspinal abscess on AP view, while the hemivertebra usually presents a round shape on the lateral view. The anterior edge of the upper and lower vertebrae is like a fish mouth. The kyphotic angle is often less than 90°. The surgical procedure for congenital angular kyphosis may retain the endplates on both sides and resect through the vertebral body or the whole hemivertebra followed by internal fixation with pedicle screw system. It is a highly effective procedure. As the angle of congenital angular kyphosis is smaller than that of tuberculosis kyphosis, e.g., often less than 90°, and epidural space has less adhesion with less bleeding, it is an absolute indication for posterior VCR (Table 9.1).

Anatomy and development of angular kyphosis: Angular kyphosis is mostly due to congenital achondroplasia of the vertebral body, congenital vertebral absence or congenital posterior hemivertebra, ischemic necrosis of ossification center of vertebral body, destruction and collapse of vertebral tuberculosis, traumatic vertebral compression, iatrogenic vertebral body defect, and early fusion. These incentives lead to asymmetric growth between the vertebral body and vertebral arch so that angular deformity progressed with increasing age (Fig. 9.3a–c). When bony fusion forms between adjacent vertebrae, the kyphosis becomes stabilized. The spinal canal forms a narrow U-shaped loop while neurological function is generally normal (Fig. 9.4).

Understanding of angular kyphosis: Multilevel laminar osteotomy and compression fixation has been widely used to treat adolescent kyphosis. Non-apical lamina osteotomy has been widely used to treat ankylosing kyphosis. However, angular kyphosis, such as congenital and tuberculosis kyphosis, still lacks effective surgical techniques. Although some surgeons demonstrated that anterior and posterior staging surgery with anterior column bone grafting could correct the kyphosis, this technique is not adequate to eliminate deformity. We believe that this kind of surgery performed in children and adolescents may face the risk of kyphotic recurrence due to uncertain spinal growth potential. The author believes that posterior wedge osteotomy plus closing osteotomy gap with instrumentation and fixation is the ultimate solution (including one or two vertebral arch and vertebral body, the wedge tip extends to the anterior edge of the vertebral body).

The formation and development of angular kyphosis: The common causes of angular kyphosis include congenital factors and tuberculous infection. In disturbance of cartilage formation in the center of primary vertebral ossification (posterior hemivertebra or vertebral absence), the vertebral arch grows faster to make the anterior edge of lower and upper adjacent vertebral gradually approximated, with three vertebrae involved usually (Fig. 9.5). Spinal tuberculosis often invades two adjacent vertebral bodies and the disk in between while posterior accessories are reserved. The destruction and collapse of these structures make the anterior edge of lower and upper adjacent vertebral gradually approximated, with more than four vertebrae involved usually so that kyphosis tends to be more severe than congenital kyphosis (Fig. 9.6). Cobb angle of congenital kyphosis is usually less than 90°, while Cobb angle of tuberculosis kyphosis may be more than 90°. In

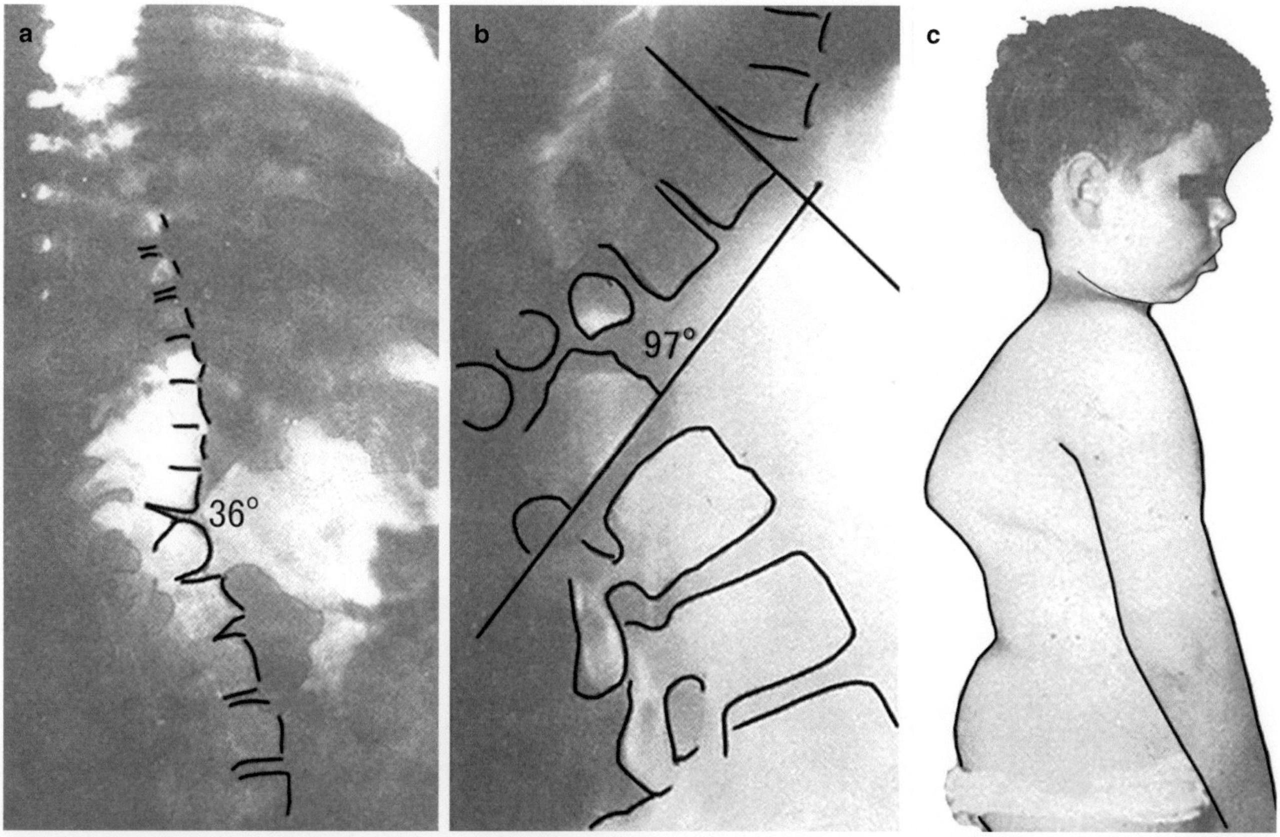

Fig. 9.3 Congenital angular kyphosis. (**a**) Male, 1 year old, congenital posterior hemivertebra, kyphotic angle 36°, untreated. (**b**) The same case, 7 years old, kyphotic angle 97°. (**c**) Appearance at 7 year old

angular kyphosis, the pedicles curled close to the residual vertebral body and spontaneous bone fusion finally forms which will arrest the growth of other vertebrae to stabilize the spine. In severe tuberculosis kyphosis, the Cobb angle is more than 135° to form a V-shape curve (Fig. 9.7). Compensatory lordosis forms in the upper thoracic and lower lumbar segments. This type of deformity is a challenge to any surgical technique and remains a contraindication for VCR.

Biomechanical perspectives for correcting angular kyphosis. Posterior compression, anterior distraction, and horizontal translation-based VCR forms the synergy of correction mechanically. Permitting hinged reduction by a wedge osteotomy at the curve apex of kyphosis firstly, and then using three mechanical forces above to keep the truncated spine in a stable state to complete the correction procedure. This biomechanical principle of posterior compression and anterior distraction is suitable not only for spinal osteotomy but also for the treatment of unstable spinal fractures to avoid spinal cord distraction injury in the process of reduction while alignment cannot be restored. The spine is like a rope. If you cut the rope without connecting its broken end and pull it only by the distal end, the rope will not be straightened. Only by ligating and connecting the broken end of the rope can it be straightened. Posterior compression without anterior distraction will make the instrumentation prone to fail, due to lack of counterforce and loss of correction. The horizontal translation prevents the lateral displacement of the spine and ensures the alignment of the bony spinal canal and the dural canal. To stabilize the spine, these three mechanical effects are indispensable.

The necessity of early osteotomy and compression correction for angular kyphosis during growth and development: Some authors suggest early bone graft fusion for congenital scoliosis to prevent the progressive aggravation of the curvature. However, we consider the issue is not that easy. Whether simple posterior fusion prevents the curve progression is not definitively known. From the 1950s to 1960s, the author widely used posterior bone grafting to fuse tuberculosis kyphosis during development and growth ages, but kyphosis still aggravated year by year, which proved that posterior fusion only could not effectively prevent the aggravation of kyphosis. Through the summary of follow-up experience in recent years, the author proposed that the procedure of osteotomy, followed by compression, bone grafting, and fixation can prevent the transition from mild kyphosis to severe kyphosis in children during the early development stage (3–12 years old). The effect may be associated with direct resection of posterior structures having growth potential like lamina, pedicle, and posterior edge of the vertebral body by

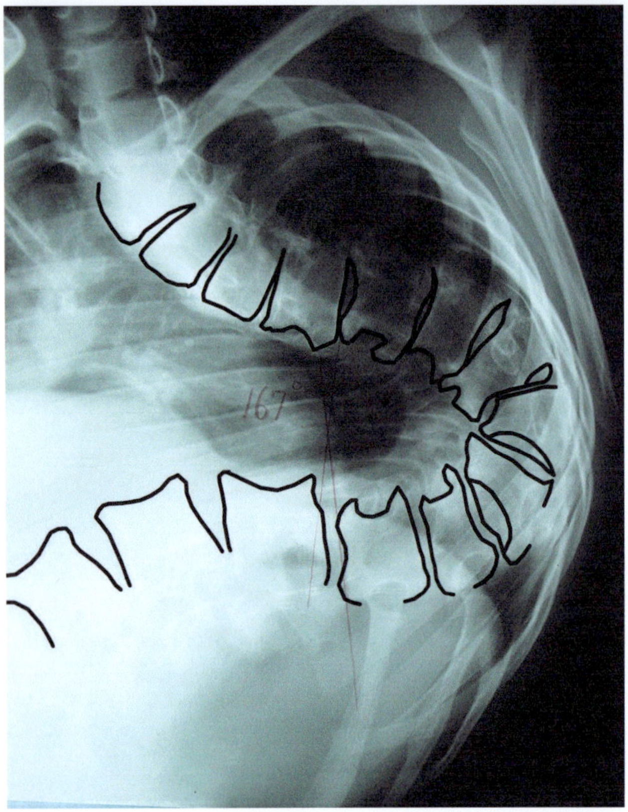

Fig. 9.4 Congenital kyphosis untreated in early stage, with age increased a U-shaped loop formed, unacceptable appearance, no neurological deficits

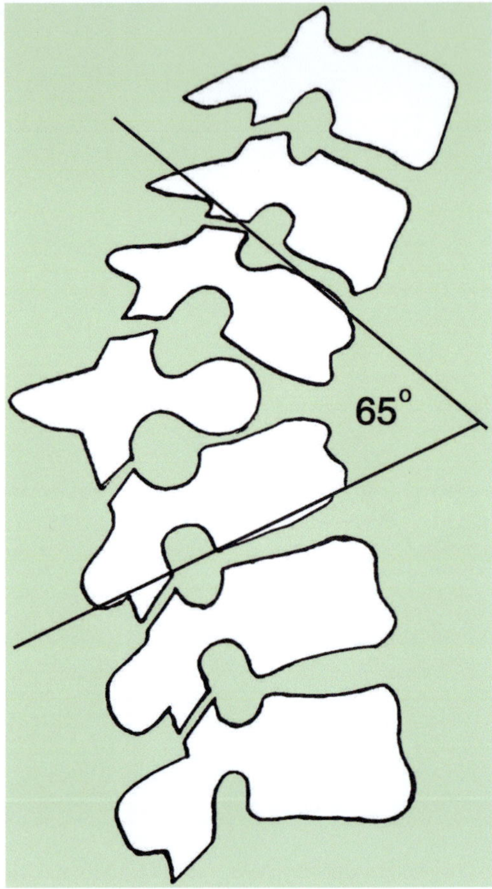

Fig. 9.5 Congenital kyphosis usually one vertebra diseased and three involved, kyphotic angle <90°

wedge osteotomy and epiphyseal arrest effect of compression fixation. After long-term follow-up, there are cases confirming that compression force does limit the aggravation of kyphosis. We suggest that osteotomy with bone grafting plus compression and fixation should be performed as early as possible for congenital or tuberculosis kyphosis during development (for TB, the timing should be beyond 1 year after TB lesion clearance, stable lesion under X-ray).

9.2 Surgical Indication

No matter what causes angular kyphosis, the best timing for osteotomy correction is 8–20 years old. For children with potential aggravation of kyphosis, early osteotomy and compression fixation can also be done in advance at the age of 3–7 years old, without the need for Halo-Pelvic traction. Over 20 years old, the correction effect attenuates as age grows.

Apex and osteotomy site: Apex is the only site where the author performs VCR. T10-L3 is the most favorable area. Angular kyphosis above T10 is often complicated with chest deformation, so it is not the indication of this procedure. Kyphosis below L3 is compensated by physiological lumbar lordosis, usually without significant appearance change. Thus, for this segment, there is no role for VCR, and fusing by bone grafting only is enough.

The most favorable condition for VCR is when the Cobb angle of angular kyphosis is less than 90°. The patients whose kyphosis is less than 90° with good flexibility can be treated directly without Halo-Pelvic traction. For the cases with a Cobb angle of more than 90°, Halo-Pelvic traction should be applied first. The decision of go or no-go with VCR depends on the traction outcome. In the case of higher age, bigger kyphosis, or poor response to traction, VCR should be carefully considered.

9.3 Total Spinal Osteotomy in Congenital Angular Kyphosis

It is difficult to obtain a corrective effect on the angular kyphosis with a posterior instrument only. In the anterior, a deep depression is formed in the front of the spine due to the curled kyphosis. Except for bone grafting on the concave

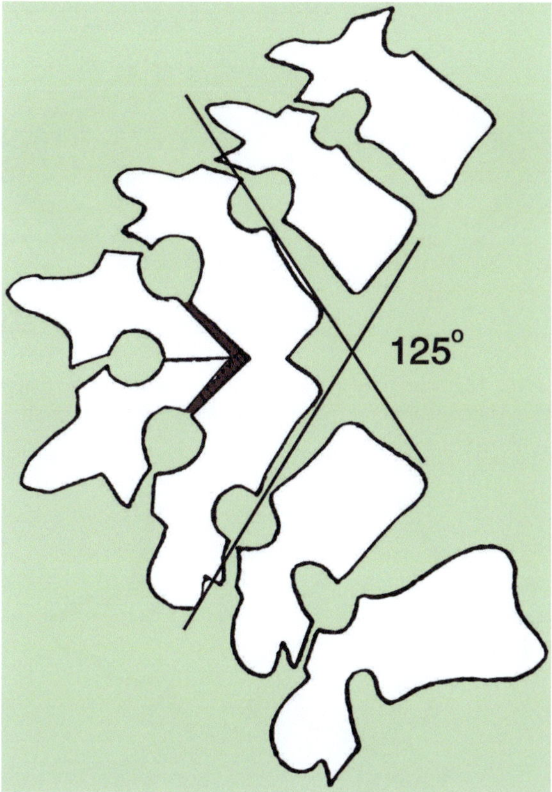

Fig. 9.6 Tuberculosis kyphosis usually two vertebrae diseased and 4 involved, kyphotic angle >90°

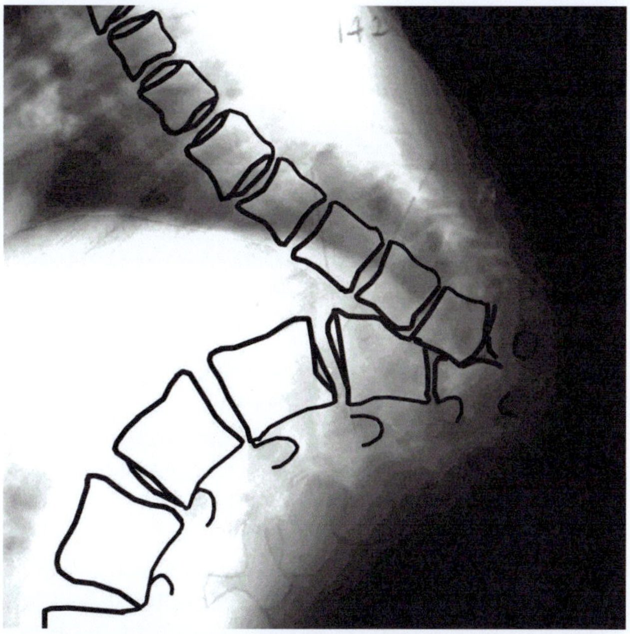

Fig. 9.7 Tuberculosis angular kyphosis, upper thoracic and lower lumbar vertebrae form compensatory lordosis, like V-shaped loop, it is contraindication for total spinal osteotomy

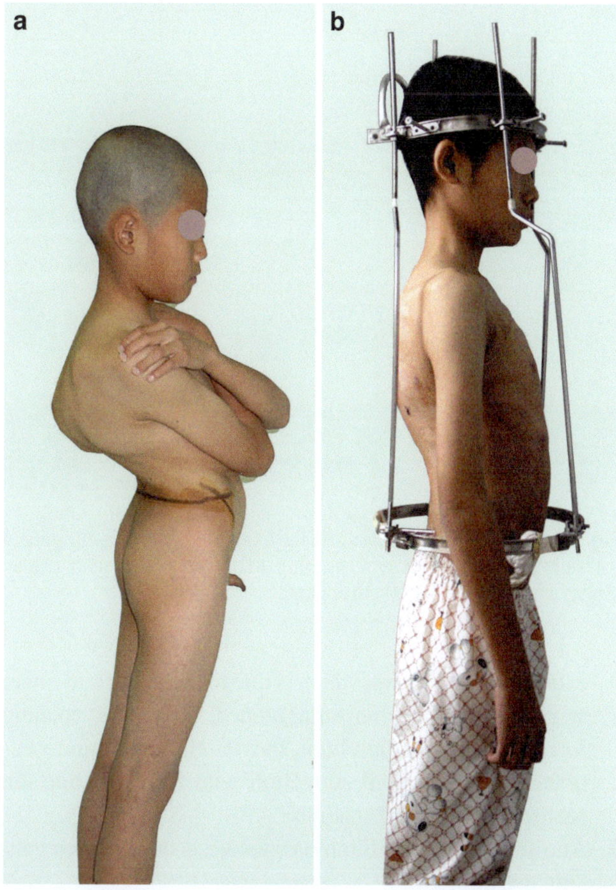

Fig. 9.8 Congenital angular kyphosis, 4-week after preoperative halo-pelvic traction, the height was increased by 6 cm, and the patient was planned to be operated by vertebral column resection under traction. (**a**) Before traction; (**b**) after traction

side, it is incapable of doing anything else to correct the deformity. The staged anterior plus posterior surgery makes a severe trauma to the patient, although it is more effective. The only effective method to correct the angular kyphosis is posterior vertebral column resection and instrumented correction with the halo-pelvic traction. Surgical indications for congenital angular kyphosis include: (1) congenital posterior hemivertebra; (2) congenital vertebral anterior malsegmentation (semi-fused vertebra).

1. Halo-pelvic traction for preoperative preparation: For the cases with larger kyphosis, the duration of preoperative halo-pelvic traction is 3–6 weeks (Fig. 9.8a, b). During traction, X-ray evaluation is periodically performed to observe the changes of spinal deformity. Whether there are changes in the angle of several vertebrae to determine whether there is bone fusion, even if there is bony fusion at the curve apex, and the halo-pelvic traction can still be

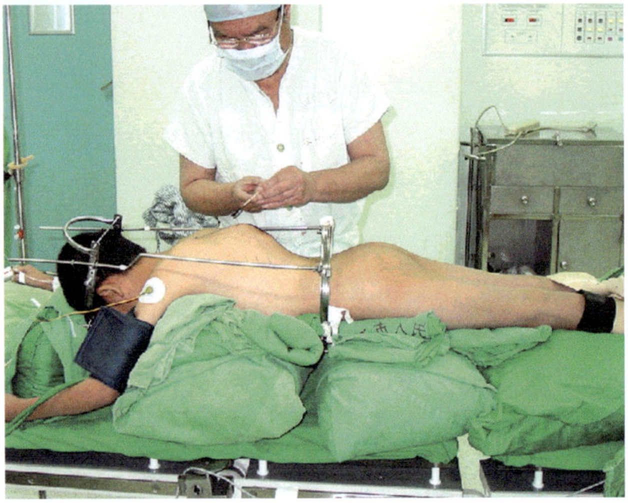

Fig. 9.9 At the prone position with the halo-pelvic traction, the patient was well padded. Always avoid hanging. Mark the incision with gentian violet, which was about 20–30 cm long

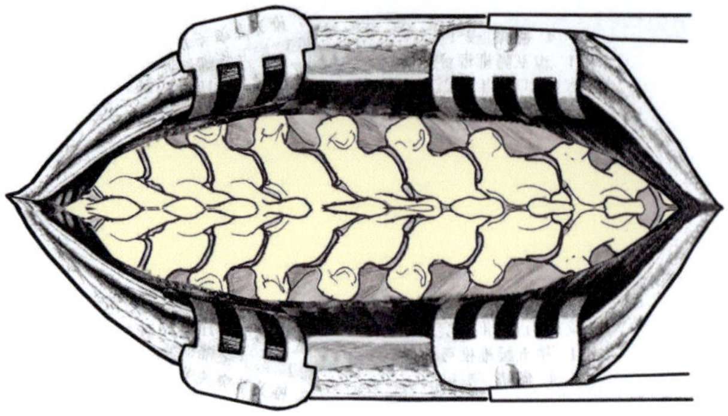

Fig. 9.10 The osteotomy site is exposed to the tip of the transverse process. At two ends of the incision, only the lamina is exposed

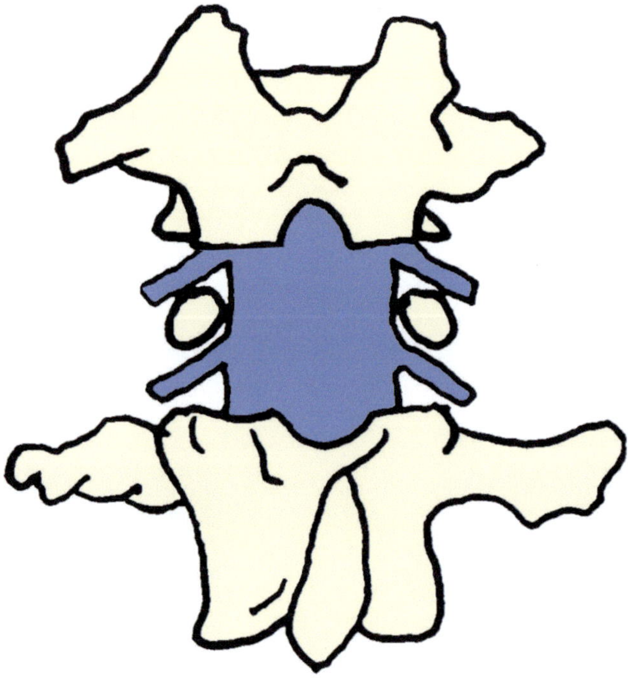

Fig. 9.11 The dural sac, the bilateral spinal nerve roots, and pedicles are exposed by resecting the arch

extended by 6–10 cm, which is due to the upper and lower spine segments being straightened. After the opening force reaches a certain limit, the vertebral column resection and instrumental correction with bone grafting are performed under the traction.

2. Anesthesia: Local infiltration anesthesia or intubated general anesthesia.
3. Intraoperative position: During the operation under the halo-pelvic traction, the patient is placed on the table with sufficient support of pads (Fig. 9.9). The four rods on the skull ring are loosened 5 cm upward and downward and the two rods on the backside should be adjusted, or, one of them should be removed to avoid affecting the following operation.
4. Surgical procedures (for example: congenital posterior vertebral body (see Fig. 9.1), Congenital vertebral progenitor dysplasia (see Fig. 9.2):

The first step is to make an incision. The incision is on top of the spinous processes, 20–30 cm in length, covering the apex of the kyphosis. The osteotomy site is expected to be elevated toward the tips of the transverse processes. On the two ends of the incision, only lamina is exposed (Fig. 9.10).

The second step is transpedicular osteotomy: The extent of lamina resection is determined according to the kyphosis angle. Generally, lamina of 1–2 levels need to be resected. The dural sac and bilateral pedicles are exposed (Fig. 9.11) while carefully exploring the existence of diastematomyelia. Then the transverse process is cut off from the plane of the outer edge of the pedicle, and along the lateral edge of the pedicle, to strip from the subperiosteum to the anterior lateral edge of the vertebral body with the vertebral body stripper. Push the periosteum and anterior longitudinal ligament, put the tarsal plate to expose the lateral side of the vertebral body, and prepare for the following vertebral osteotomy.

The third step is vertebral osteotomy: To put two sacral plates on each side of the vertebral body under the periosteum and anterior longitudinal ligament, and to open the anterior longitudinal ligament to expose the vertebral body. On the lateral side of the vertebral body, with an osteotome to make a predetermined wedge-shaped line for following osteotomy process (Figs. 9.12 and 9.13): the wedge-shaped tip to the anterior edge of the vertebral body, and the size of the angle is determined by the upper and lower width of the laminectomy. The vertebral circular osteotomy around the spinal canal through the bilateral posterior approaches is a key step in this procedure. The bleeding of the anterior soft tissue of the vertebral body is

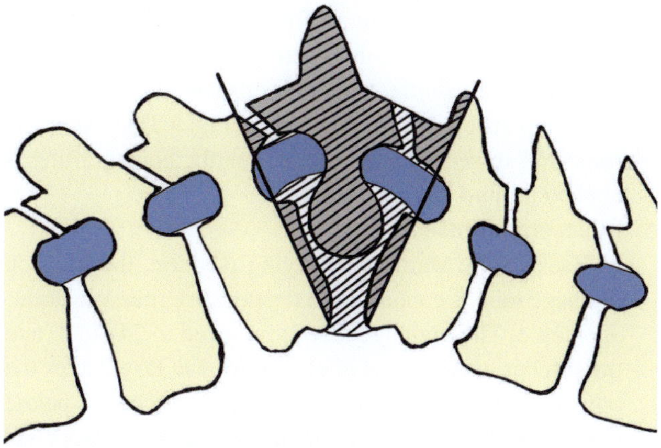

Fig. 9.12 Osteotomy for congenital posterior hemivertebra

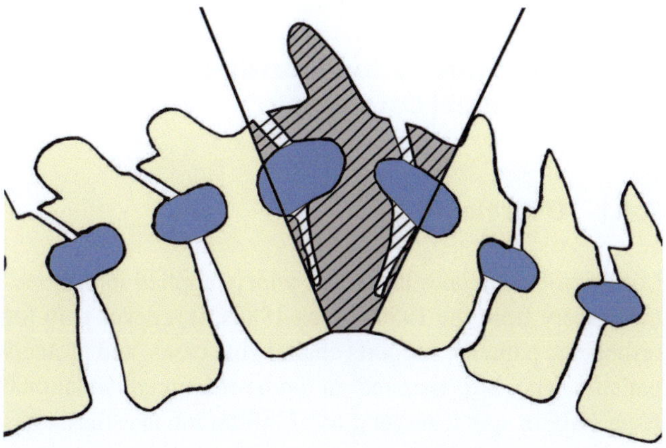

Fig. 9.13 The extent of congenital cone dysfunction syndrome

stopped by the compression of the tarsal plate (Fig. 9.14), and there is no need to ligate the intercostal artery or the lumbar artery and vein. The spinal nerve roots exiting the superior and inferior intervertebral foramen are retracted with a special nerve root retractor (Fig. 9.15). After the clear exposure being performed, the vertebral body osteotomy is started. Before starting osteotomy, the upper and lower separation hooks are placed (Fig. 9.16, 9.17, and 9.18), pedicle screw and Luque wire are inserted (Figs. 9.19 and 9.20), etc. Firstly, to resect the pedicle and the outer part of the vertebral body (Figs. 9.21 and 9.22), then the central part of the vertebral body is removed (Figs. 9.23, 9.24, and 9.25). A thin cortical bone of the posterior margin of the vertebral body is preserved to avoid bleeding of the epidural venous plexus. To use a special posterior vertebral instrument to remove the medial edge of the pedicle (Fig. 9.26) and the posterior edge of the vertebral body (Fig. 9.27) as fast as possible. At this time, the epidural venous plexus will have active bleeding. After finger palpation to ensure no residual bony fragments in the osteotomy space (Fig. 9.28), the

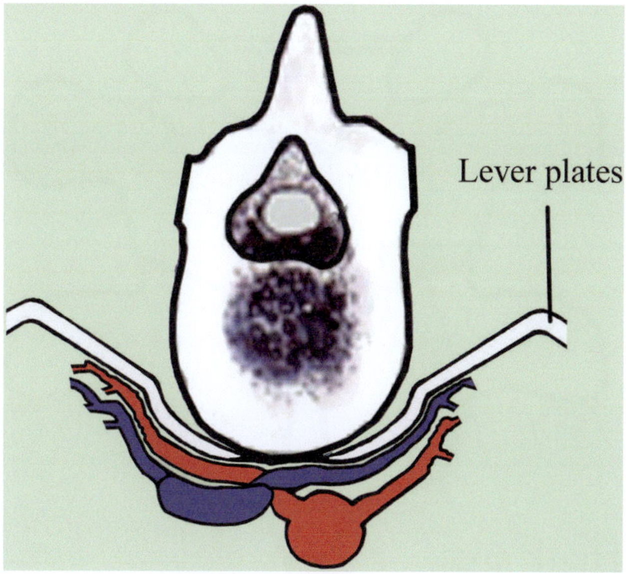

Fig. 9.14 Insert the tarsal plate to expose the vertebral body, compress the anterior segmental arteries and veins to stop bleeding. Segmental arteries and veins ligation is not necessary

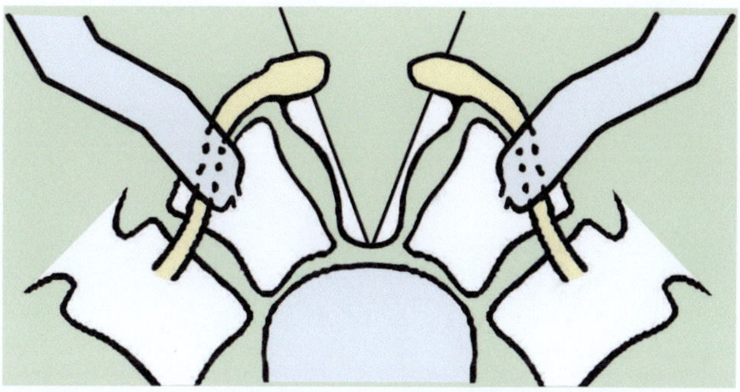

Fig. 9.15 The spinal nerve roots exiting the upper and lower intervertebral foramen are protected by the nerve root retractor outside the field to avoid damage during vertebral osteotomy

osteotomy gap is immediately closed to correct the deformity. Wire is used to drag the screws that have been inserted into the pedicles (Fig. 9.29a, b) closer. Tension is applied to close the osteotomy gap. After the dura sac is loosened and expanded, the epidural venous plexus is more compressed and bleeding will stop. After the gap is completely closed, bleeding deep in the wound can be completely stopped.

The range of vertebral wedge osteotomy: (1) the endplates at both ends of the vertebra are preserved, only to perform wedge-shaped osteotomy through the lumbar body, so that the cancellous bony surfaces are touched to without grafting; (2) wedge osteotomy including one intervertebral disc; (3) vertebral column resection including two adjacent intervertebral discs and two endplates resections. Longitudinal bone grafting or strut bone graft

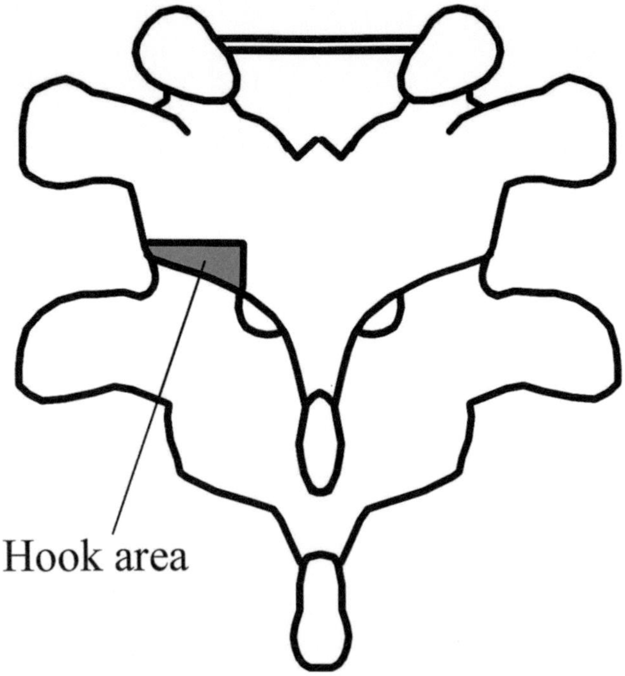

Fig. 9.16 L-shaped osteotomy to prepare the inferior articular process for hook

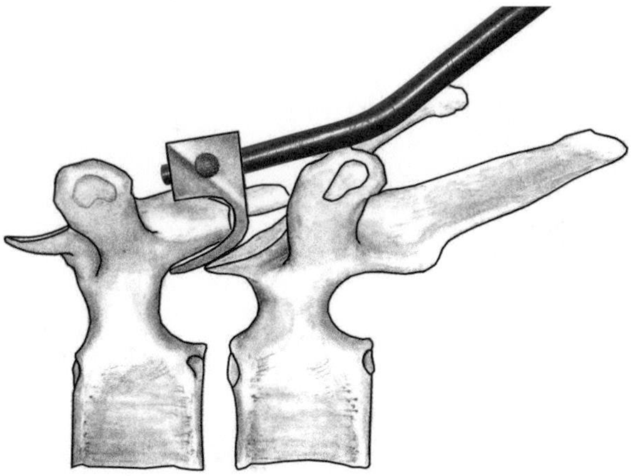

Fig. 9.17 Cranial hook is attached to the thoracic facet joint, to insert the hook into the facet joint space, preferably sitting on the pedicle

is filled between the upper and lower ends of the anterior space (Fig. 9.30). After the posterior edge of the vertebral body is closed, the anterior strut graft plays a supporting role.

The fourth step is internal fixation: Sublamina wiring or bilateral pedicle screw plus wire tightening techniques can be used to close the osteotomy gap to produce proximal compression; then at the upper and lower ends of the osteotomy site, the separation rod is used to open and maintain the straightening of the spine, and the inserted Luque wire is fixed on the separation rod, thus producing three mechanical effects includes proximal compression, distal expansion and lateral tension (Fig. 9.31) to keep the truncated spine in a stable state. Finally, bone grafting is applied around the lamina.

5. Postoperative management:

   Back to the ward with a lying position, the incision drainage tube is connected to the negative pressure drainage bottle. The drainage tube is removed in 24–48 h, and the stitches are removed after 10 days. On Day 2 after the operation, the patient may try to walk with the halo-pelvic rings protection. After the stitches are removed, the pelvic ring is be removed, and the halo ring is suspended on the vertical traction frame to be fixed in the plaster vest. The immobilization period is 8–10 months.

9.4 Local Infiltration Anesthesia for Spinal Osteotomy

9.4.1 Overview

Local infiltration anesthesia was widely applied in orthopedic surgery from the 1950s to the 1980s. It relieves pain for orthopedic patients, supports challenging cases, and protects patients who are operated in under-resourced situations. Especially in spinal surgery, local infiltration anesthesia has its advantages when decompression near dura or nerve roots and correcting spinal deformity. Being awake, the patient is able to respond to the surgeons' questions and tell the surgeon the feelings at any time. Due to tension and stimulation of spinal cord or nerve root by instruments, displacement like circumference resection, and shortening caused by opening and closing of the osteotomy gap, there will be a series of early neurological symptoms such as bilateral leg numbness. Surgeons will notice the onset of these symptoms in time. This is the greatest advantage of local infiltration anesthesia, which is not comparable with any monitoring equipment and wake-up test under general anesthesia. By the means of close cooperation with anesthesiologists and timely reporting feeling by patients, Tian Huizhong the author has completed vertebral column resection for 855 spinal deformity cases under local infiltration anesthesia.

General anesthesia with endotracheal intubation is not always feasible when the patient undergoes an operation with Halo-Pelvic traction perioperatively. Therefore, the author used posterior long segmental local infiltration anesthesia for most of these patients and achieved remarkable results. It guarantees painless operation. In particular, when osteotomy is performed near the dura mater and nerve

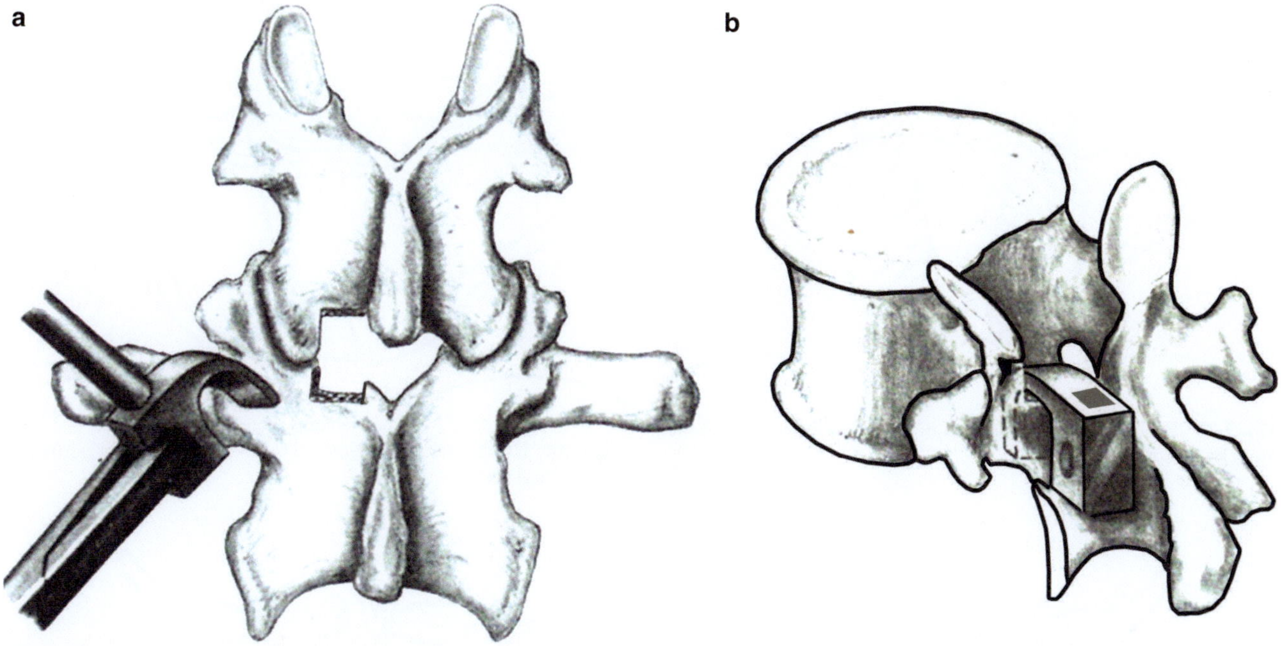

Fig. 9.18 Insert the caudal hook. (**a**) Make a U-shaped opening on the superior margin of the lumbar lamina and prepare to hang the caudal hook in the opening. (**b**) The square hole hook is hung on the lamina

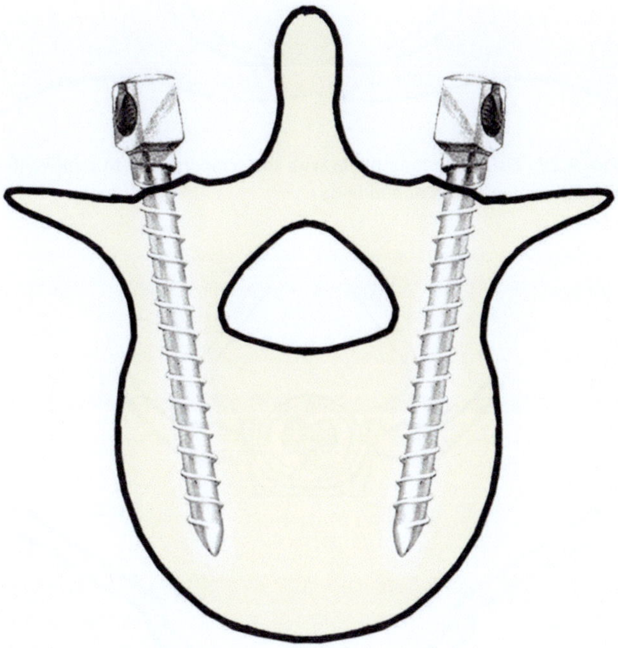

Fig. 9.19 Pedicle screws were inserted into the bilateral pedicles above and below the osteotomy gap for proximal compression

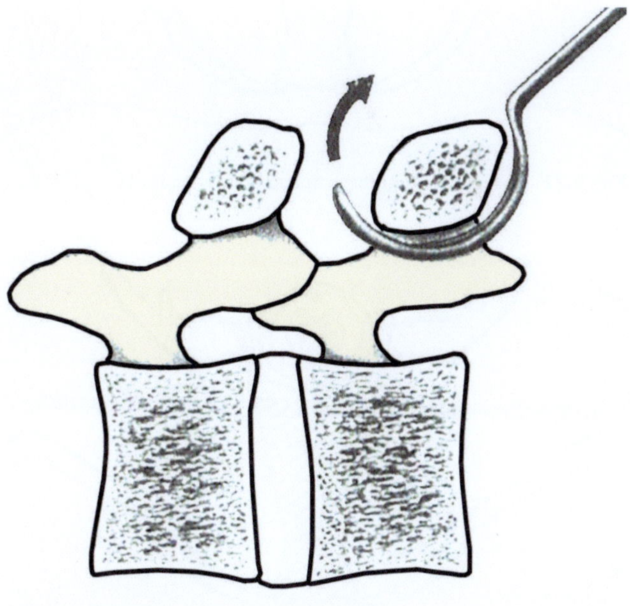

Fig. 9.20 Under the lamina, a steel wire is inserted to fix the separation rod for lateral tension

root and nerve tissue is mechanically stimulated, the patient can timely inform the surgeon of location and degree of numbness and pain, so that surgeons can correct the errors in operation in time. This is more reliable than any wake-up test or intraoperative neurological monitoring.

In these cases, the postoperative incision pain is mild, and the gastrointestinal complications after general anesthesia are avoided. They may ambulate around the bed on postoperative Day 2 and usually recover quickly after operation. There is almost no immediate complication.

There are many advantages of major surgery under local infiltration anesthesia. Especially in spinal surgery, it is of

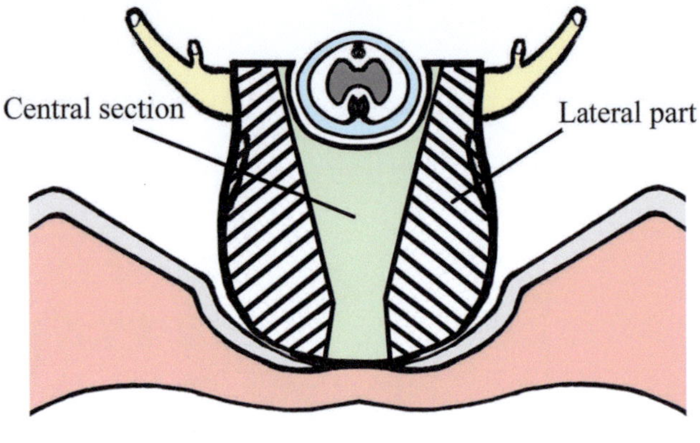

Fig. 9.21 Excision of the lateral portion of the vertebral body (slashed area) by osteotome

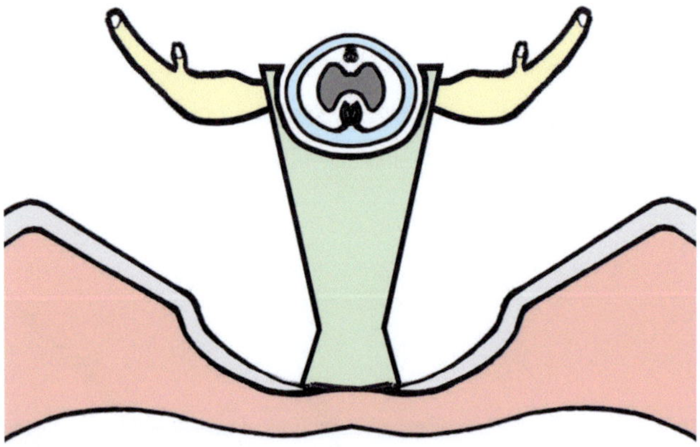

Fig. 9.22 The outer part of the vertebral body is removed

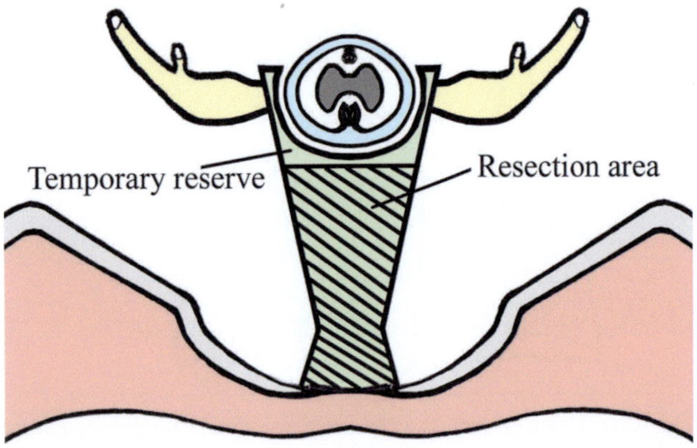

Fig. 9.23 The shadowed area is the central resected part of the vertebral body. The medial edge of the pedicle and the posterior edge of the vertebral body are temporarily preserved

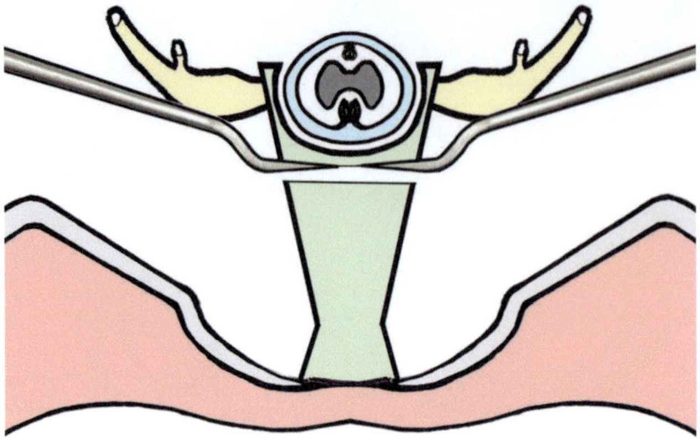

Fig. 9.24 Using a scraper osteotome to resect the posterior portion of the vertebral body

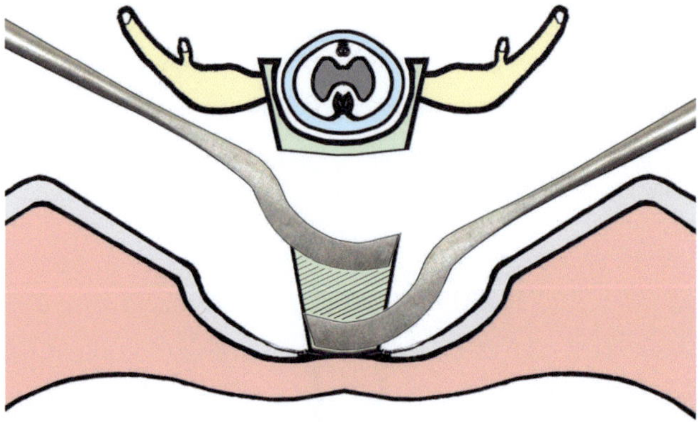

Fig. 9.25 Using the fang blade with the scraper blade to remove the front portion of the vertebral body

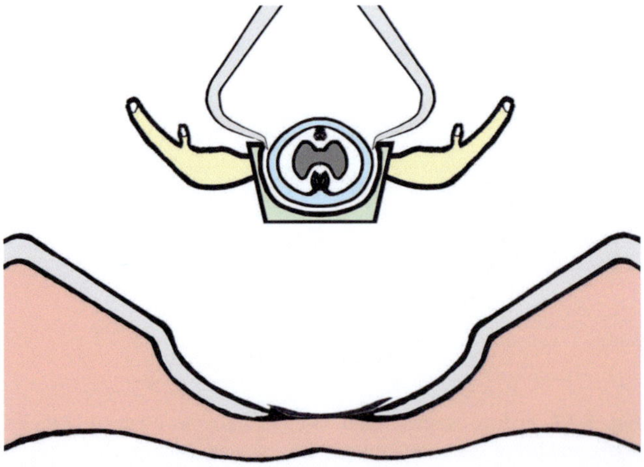

Fig. 9.26 Using the push-down osteotome to remove the medial edge of the pedicle

great significance to use it to retain consciousness and talk with the surgeon to prevent the injury of the spinal cord and nerve tissue during the operation. Local infiltration anesthesia is a perfect anesthetic method that can be achieved by the cooperation of surgeons and anesthesiologists. Intraoperative injection of anesthetics by layers in fractions is done by the surgeons, while intraoperative surveillance and patient management are carried out by anesthesiologists. Therefore, there

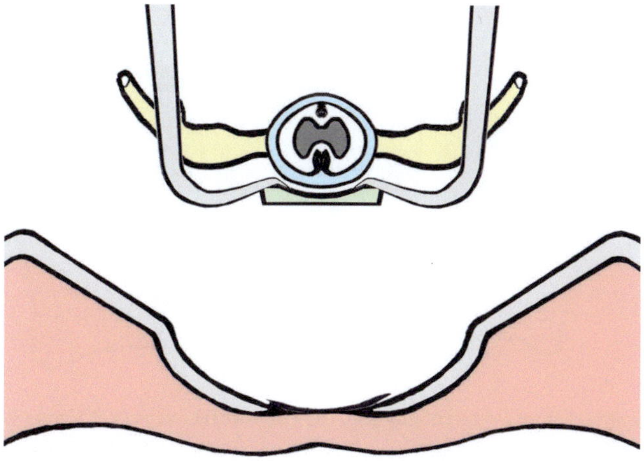

Fig. 9.27 Use the push-down osteotome to remove the posterior edge of the vertebral body

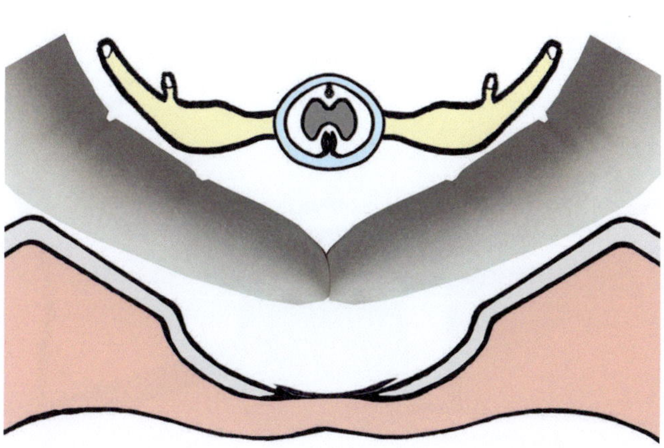

Fig. 9.28 Palpate and ensure no residual bone fragments in the osteotomy gap

must be a tacit understanding between surgeons and anesthesiologists in order to successfully carry out the work of local infiltration anesthesia in major surgery. The concentration and dosage of anesthetic solution must be jointly determined by surgeons and anesthesiologists. The dose of fractional injection by layers must be controlled by the surgeon. Be careful not to overdose or inject the drug into the artery resulting in anesthetic poisoning. Anesthesiologists should carefully and responsibly observe the status of patients to detect abnormalities or drug poisoning in time; otherwise, the delay may cause irreversible brain damage to the patient. Before the operation under local infiltration anesthesia, the detoxification drugs of local anesthetic poisoning should be prepared in advance, such as thiopentone and luminal. The usage of antidote should be well mastered. Once the patient develops convulsion, actions should be taken immediately. Anesthesiologists must have rich theoretical knowledge and practical experience in the rescue of local anesthetic poisoning, so as to avoid anesthetic accidents.

1. Pharmacology of three-caines
   (a) Procaine. It is an ester local anesthetic. Procaine, also known as Novocaine, is one of the earliest synthetic p-aminobenzoate drugs and commonly used local anesthetics because of its low toxicity. This medicine is a short-acting lipid local anesthetic with low lipophilicity and weak penetration of mucous membrane. It is generally not used for topical anesthesia but is often injected locally for infiltration anesthesia, conduction anesthesia, subarachnoid anesthesia, and epidural anesthesia. After injection, the effect will occur in 1–3 min and is maintained for 30–45 min. The maintenance time could be prolonged by 20% with adrenaline co-administration. Procaine is be hydrolyzed by esterase in plasma and converted into p-aminobenzoic acid (PABA) and diethylaminoethanol. The former can resist the antibacterial effect of sulfonamides, so it should not be used simultaneously with sulfonamides. Procaine can also be used for local block treatment in the injured site. Overdose can lead to central nervous system and cardiovascular reactions. Sometimes it can cause anaphylaxis, so a skin allergy test should be done before administration, but anaphylaxis may still occur even when the skin test is negative. Patients who are allergic to this drug can be replaced with chloroprocaine and lidocaine.
   (b) Lidocaine. It is an amide class local anesthetic. lidocaine is also known as serocaine. Because of its definite nerve block effect, rapid onset of action, and moderate action maintenance time, it is still the most widely used local anesthetic. It has obvious biphasic effects of excitation and inhibition on the central nervous system, and there can be no early excitation. When the blood concentration is low, it has the effect of lethargy and increasing the pain threshold; with the increase of the dose, the toxicity increases. The sub-toxic blood concentration has an anticonvulsant effect while convulsions occur when the blood concentration exceeds 5 mg/ml. At low dose, this product can promote the outflow of potassium ion from cardiomyocytes, reduce the automaticity of myocardium, and has the effect of anti-ventricular arrhythmia. At the treatment dose, it had no significant effect on the electrical activity of cardiomyocytes, atrioventricular conduction, and myocardial contraction. Further increase in blood concentration can slow down cardiac conduction, leading to atrioventricular block, inhibition of myocardial contractility, and reduction of cardiac output.
   (c) Bupivacaine. It is an amide class local anesthetic. Bupivacaine, also known as Marcaine, is a butyl derivative of piperidine cyclic hydroxylamide. It is

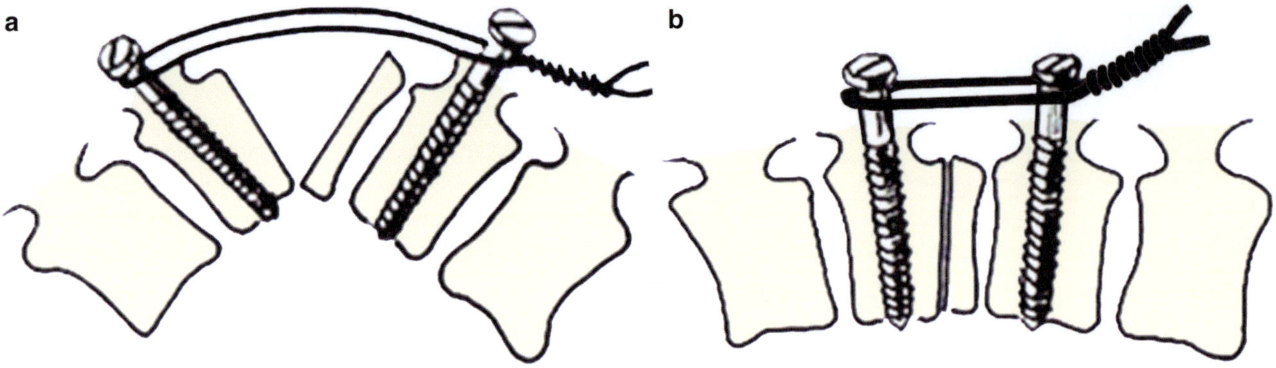

Fig. 9.29 Use pedicle screws with wire for proximal compression. (**a**) Prepare to close the osteotomy gap. (**b**) The wire on the pedicle screws is tightened for closing the osteotomy gap

Fig. 9.30 Closed osteotomy after anterior distraction. After vertebral column resection is performed, the intervertebral space is grafted. The posterior arches are closed to correct kyphosis

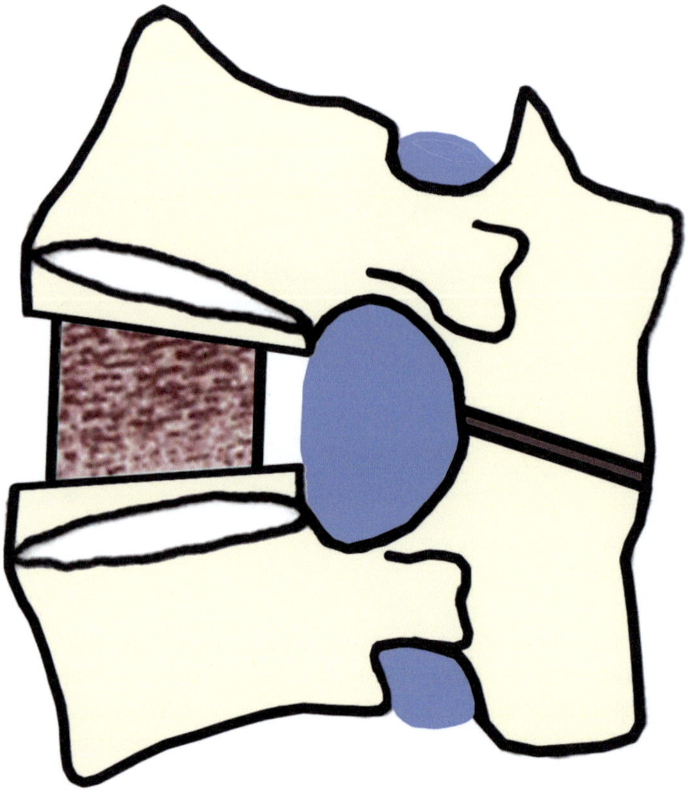

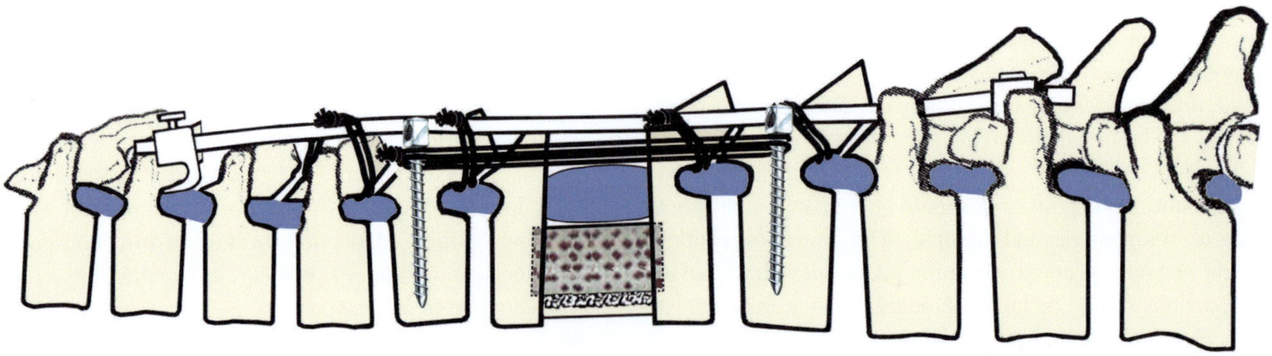

Fig. 9.31 Using the three mechanical effects of proximal compression, distal distraction, and lateral tension to correct kyphosis and straighten the spine

generally used for local infiltration block, peripheral nerve block, spinal epidural space block, and subarachnoid space block, but not for topical anesthesia. The effect of local anesthesia is stronger than that of lidocaine by about four times. The time for 0.25–0.5% solution to take effect is generally 4–10 min, and 0.75% solution takes effect slightly faster. The effect of epidural block anesthesia with 0.5% solution plus epinephrine can be maintained for 5 h. Because of its low concentration in the blood, less accumulation in the body, and long duration of action, this medicine is a safe and long-acting local anesthetic.

2. Preparation and administration of anesthetic solution
   Compound local infiltration anesthetics were used, including 2.5 g procaine hydrochloride, 400 mg lidocaine hydrochloride, 200 mg bupivacaine hydrochloride, 100 mg dolantin, 0.5 ml epinephrine hydrochloride (1:1000), being diluted with normal saline to 1000 ml. It is required to prepare the 1000 ml solution in bulk upfront, and not allowed to prepare it multiple times so as to avoid problems in the proportion of the dosage to affect the effect of the anesthetic or poisoning. Usage and dosage: intradermal, subcutaneous, muscular, and nerve root injections are carried out layer by layer. For adults, the volume of 500–1000 ml should be delivered. The amount of medicine for children under the age of 8 should be halved.

   Preoperative and intraoperative medication: Phenobarbital 30–60 mg is given orally in the evening before the operation and 2 mg/kg of body weight for children. If the patient has unbearable pain during the operation, dolantin intramuscular injection by 50 mg can be given twice in 3–5 h, and the amount of dolantin should be halved in children under 8 years old at 50 mg each time. Together with the 100 mg of dolantin in the local anesthetic solution, up to a total of 200 mg dolantin will be given. Based on the experience in this group, there no adverse reactions during and after the operation. Strong analgesic effect without affecting consciousness is the greatest advantage of dolantin. Patients are able to answer the surgeons' questions at any time. We do not suggest giving drugs that affect the patient's consciousness, such as ketamine.
3. Local infiltration anesthesia technique and surgical operation
   The anesthesiologist monitors the patient, and the surgeon and assistants perform local infiltration anesthesia. The steps are as follows. The patient is put into a prone position. After disinfection and draping, intradermal and subcutaneous infiltration anesthesia is performed along the spinous processes. Then expose the operation field until the posterior layer of the lumbar dorsal fascia, and the paraspinal muscle layer is anesthetized before the fascia is incised. According to the length of the incision, 250–500 ml anesthetic is needed. Next, cut open along the midline, or spinous process and expose the lamina, elevate and remove the soft tissue behind the lamina. Expose the muscle layer with an automatic retractor and then perform the third layer of deep infiltration injection, that is, between the transverse process and adjacent to the transverse process. At the same time, the spinal nerve roots originating from the intervertebral foramen are anesthetized and blocked. Three layers total need local anesthetic solution 500–750 ml (adult dose), and the rest of the solution is reserved for supplementary anesthesia if necessary. Generally speaking, it is better to have more anesthetic solution than is needed to avoid reformulation. Because the local anesthetic solution is injected into the tissue in layers and by fraction, it generally does not cause poisoning due to excessive dosage.
4. Systemic toxicity of local anesthetics
   In the clinic, various toxic reactions caused by local anesthetics are mainly related to the central nervous system (CNS) and cardiovascular system, limited nerve and skeletal muscle stimulation, and some special side effects, such as methemoglobinemia, allergic reactions, and local anesthetic addiction. The toxicity to the cardiovascular and central nervous system and the stimulation to skeletal muscle are determined by the toxicological properties of local anesthetics. Most other adverse reactions are caused by improper medication, such as accidental intravascular or intrathecal injection, or overdose.

   The toxic reactions of local anesthetics to the human body mostly involve the central nervous system while having less inhibition on the cardiovascular system, but once involved the consequences are serious and difficult to deal with.

   The potential toxicity of various local anesthetics to the central nervous system is mainly related to their inherent anesthetic intensity. In cats, for example, injections of procaine about 35 mg/kg can cause convulsions, compared with 5 mg/kg of bupivacaine, and moderate doses of lidocaine, mepivacaine, and procaine. The inherent anesthetic intensity and toxicity of various local anesthetics are different. When bupivacaine is used as local anesthesia, the anesthetic intensity is about eight times higher than that of procaine, and the dose of bupivacaine needed to trigger convulsion in cats is about seven times higher than that of procaine. To cause convulsions in dogs, the dose of lidocaine is about 20 mg/kg, etidocaine is 8 mg/kg, and bupivacaine is 5 mg/kg. As a result, the toxicity ratio of bupivacaine, etidocaine, and lidocaine to the central nervous system is about 4:2:1. The relationship between the anesthetic efficacy of various local anesthetics and the toxic dose of the central nervous system is demonstrated in the study of intravenous injection of volunteers.

There is also a certain correlation between the plasma concentration of convulsions and the anesthetic intensity of various local anesthetics. Bupivacaine could cause convulsions in monkeys when the blood concentration of bupivacaine is about 4.5 μg/ml, and convulsions occurred when the blood concentration of lidocaine is 25 μg/ml. In humans, convulsions can occur when the blood concentrations of bupivacaine and etidocaine are 2–4 μg/ml, while those of less toxic lidocaine need more than 12 μg/ml.

In addition to the correlation between anesthetic intensity and central nervous system toxicity, the injection rate to a specific blood concentration can also affect the toxicity of local anesthesia. For example, Scott pointed out that when volunteers were injected with etidocaine at the rate of 10 mg/min, the average tolerable dose was 236 mg and the intravenous blood concentration was 3.0 μg/ml before onset of central nervous system symptoms. However, when the injection rate increased to 20 mg/min, the average dose tolerated by the volunteers decreased to 161 mg, while the intravenous blood concentration was about 2 μg/ml.

In short, local anesthetics have a significant effect on the central nervous system. Central nervous system excitement leads to convulsions, which is the most common symptom of systemic toxicity of local anesthetics. Excessive injection dose also leads to central nervous system inhibition and respiratory arrest. The potential toxicity of local anesthetics to the central nervous system is related to its inherent anesthetic intensity.

5. Treatment of local anesthetic poisoning
   If respiratory and circulatory functions remain normal, there is no need to take other treatment measures for mild symptoms and signs of poisoning except holding the injection. For early signs of poisoning, keep talking to the patient and monitoring the cardiovascular system, give oxygen, and encourage the patient to breathe normally.
   (a) Convulsion. If local anesthetic triggers convulsion, patients should be sedated immediately to relieve convulsion and relieve respiratory and cardiovascular inhibition to prevent cerebral hypoxia and acidosis.
      I Intravenous injection of barbiturate or sodium thiopental (50–100 mg) quickly inhibits convulsion. But it also has an inhibitory effect on respiratory and cardiovascular function. Therefore, it is necessary to carefully observe the changes in breathing, keep the airway patent and give oxygen. If respiratory depression and apnea occur, endotracheal intubation and artificial ventilation are required.
      II Convulsion can be controlled by intravenous injection of diazepam or midazolam. The time to effect is longer than that of thiopental, but the effect lasts slightly longer. Thiopental sodium or diazepam or midazolam all have the effect of inhibiting convulsion but also cause respiratory and cardiovascular inhibition, so we should be vigilant.
      III Succinylcholine is a neuromuscular blocker and intravenous injection of 50 mg (adult) can inhibit convulsion. However, respiratory muscle paralysis and respiratory arrest may occur after injection, so tracheal intubation and oxygenated ventilation should be given immediately. This drug is only to be used by senior anesthesiologists who master intubation techniques. Succinylcholine inhibits muscle convulsion, but the convulsion process of the brain consumes more cerebral oxygen. However, if respiratory and cardiovascular function restores after oxygen administration, it will not cause harmful sequelae of the central nervous system.
   (b) Cardiovascular inhibition
      If hypotension occurs, hypoxia should be corrected. Legs should be raised. The rate of intravenous infusion should be accelerated. If necessary, vasopressors should be injected intravenously. Since hypotension is usually caused by myocardial inhibition and vasodilation, it is ideal to use drugs that stimulate α and β adrenergic receptors. For example, intravenous injection of ephedrine 10–30 mg or with an increment of 5 mg at a time until a positive reaction is obtained, and atropine 0.4 mg can reverse bradycardia.

      Deep cardiovascular inhibition requires immediate cardiopulmonary resuscitation. Using electric cardioversion to treat ventricular tachycardia or ventricular fibrillation, which requires higher electric energy than normal. It has also been reported that high doses of epinephrine and atropine have the ability to reverse cardiovascular inhibition induced by the injection of bupivacaine in dogs. If circulatory failure occurs, CPR may be required for an hour or more and oxygen-assisted ventilation and injection of sodium bicarbonate were given to correct acidosis.

      Respiratory and vascular inhibition caused by spinal anesthesia can also be treated in the above way. Endotracheal intubation assisted or controlled ventilation should be carried out quickly to prevent hypoxia and acidosis. At the same time, rapid intravenous infusion, vasopressor, and anticholinergic drugs also should be given to treat hypotension and bradycardia. In addition, the extraction of 10–20 ml of cerebrospinal fluid and inject normal saline are helpful to prevent possible nerve injury, especially when chloroprocaine is used for intrathecal injection.

6. Redefining local infiltration anesthesia
    (a) Routine general anesthesia for spinal osteotomy. Since Smith-Petersen used translaminar osteotomy to correct ankylosing kyphosis in 1945 and Harrington used instruments to correct scoliosis in 1962, it has become a convention that correction surgery of spinal deformity only be performed under general anesthesia, and spinal cord function must be monitored indirectly by wake-up test or evoked potential. We did not dare to jump out of the framework of "general anesthesia" in our early stage of spinal correction surgery (1980–1985) and always assumed that only general anesthesia could reduce the contractile force of muscles to straighten the curved spine. Later, through practice, we realized that the contracture of soft tissue has to be solved by preoperative traction (vertical suspension, Halo-Pelvic traction). If the preoperative traction is effective, it means soft tissue of contracture has been released, so operation under local anesthesia also gets satisfactory results. If the effect of preoperative traction is not good, the ideal correction effect may not be obtained even under general anesthesia.
    (b) Redefining anesthesia options. Which anesthetic method should be adopted in the correction of spinal deformity with vertebral column resection and instrumented correction? Endotracheal intubation general anesthesia or epidural anesthesia or local infiltration anesthesia? The author thinks that: (A) general anesthesia intubation can be used for simple instrumented corrections such as the Harrington procedure, bifurcation rod procedure, and other operations that do not directly contact the spinal cord. However, because the monitoring of the spinal cord during total spinal osteotomy and instrumental correction depends on wake-up test or evoked potential monitoring which increases the complexity of the operation, it is more convenient and reliable to rely on patients to answer questions directly under local infiltration anesthesia. (B) Epidural anesthesia for vertebral column resection plus instrumented correction has two disadvantages. First, the range of dissection and exposure was large and the segment of epidural anesthesia is limited, so it is difficult to ensure completely pain-free in the whole incision. Second, the dura mater at the osteotomy site has lost its sensitivity, and the impact or traction of any instrument may easily cause invisible spinal cord injury. (C) Local infiltration anesthesia combined with special surgical instruments and superb surgical skills is the best way to complete total spinal osteotomy.
    (c) Wake-up test and evoked potential monitoring under general anesthesia. The wake-up test is a method that awakens the patient by decreasing the depth of anesthesia and requires the patient to move the lower limbs independently as instructed to evaluate neurological function. It is already too late to find spinal cord injury by this method, and it is actually post hoc because the irreversible degree of spinal cord injury increases with time. Evoked potentials are divided into spinal cord evoked potential (SCEP) and somatosensory evoked potential (SEP). Zhang Guangbo of Beijing China-Japan Friendship Hospital reported that the method of placing the electrode outside the dura mater more accurately reflects the situation of spinal cord ischemia, traction, compression, or decompression, and the maximum pressure that the spinal cord can bear also be measured when the spinal cord is touched during operation. Therefore, evoked potential monitoring is an effective method in spinal surgery, but evoked potentials used in general hospitals often produce false-positive or false-negative results, which makes it difficult to judge. In addition, no matter what kinds of evoked potential, it is presented by image and waveform indirectly. We believe that listen to the patient's direct answer and correct feedback due to the doctor's instructions are the convenient and credible measure in total spinal osteotomy under local infiltration anesthesia.
    (d) Preparation and function of local anesthetic solution. The cocktail anesthetic solution prepared in this group contains three drugs: procaine hydrochloride, lidocaine hydrochloride, and bupivacaine hydrochloride. The formulation increases the toxic threshold of each drug, increases permeability, and prolongs action time. A small amount of epinephrine hydrochloride in the solution shrinks the blood vessels in local tissue, slows down the absorption and metabolism rate of local anesthetic drugs, prolongs the local action time, and reduces the occurrence of poisoning. Putting dolantin 100 mg into medicine solution may antagonize excessive bleeding on the surface of cancellous bone led by the adrenaline induced blood pressure increasing, and at the same time play the role of systemic analgesia. No adverse side effects occurred when adults were given a total dose of dolantin 200 mg in fractions during a 3–5 h operation. However, it should be noted that dolantin is no longer used as an analgesic after operation to avoid addiction.

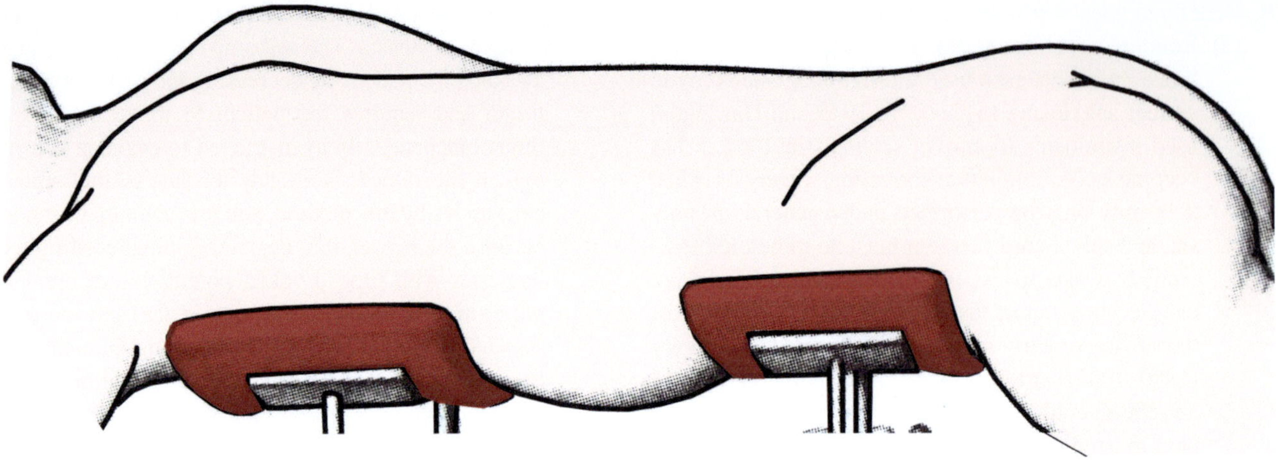

Fig. 9.32 Prone position

9.4.2 Fractional Local Infiltration Anesthesia by Layers

Unlike minor surgery without the assistance of an anesthesiologist, spinal surgery under local infiltration anesthesia requires careful monitoring by anesthesiologists in addition to injection by surgeons. An anesthetic accident occurs during the operation, which delays the rescue time and will have serious consequences. Therefore, anesthesiologists and surgeons need to cooperate skillfully and accumulate experience before they can carry out spinal surgery under local infiltration anesthesia. When performing spinal osteotomy with or without Halo-Pelvic traction under local infiltration anesthesia, the anesthesiologist and the surgeon must decide a surgical scheme together preoperative to confirm how to deal with the procedural accident in time. Given lack of plan B, lack of antidote, being uninformed of the usage and dosage, the delay in rescue time will have serious consequences. So, the monitoring by the anesthesiologist is very important. This section mainly describes the method of local infiltration anesthetic injection by layer.

1. Local infiltration anesthesia through posterior incision along spinous processes:
   The patient takes a prone position (Fig. 9.32). The local anesthetic solution is injected into the skin with a fine needle along the spinous processes until skin bulging is formed. Then inject the anesthetic into the skin, the subcutaneous fat, and the back of the spinous process (Fig. 9.33a–c). Next, cut the skin and subcutaneous tissue along the spinous process until the end of the spinous process is exposed. Temporarily retain the integrity of the posterior layer of lumbar dorsal fascia.
2. The second layer of local infiltration anesthesia:
   Injecting anesthetic solution into muscle layer behind spinous processes, lamina, and articular processes (Fig. 9.34). Cutting longitudinally along the spinous process, and paraspinal muscles are elevated subperiosteally, exposing lamina and articular processes (Fig. 9.35).
3. The third layer of local infiltration anesthesia:
   The local anesthetic solution is injected into the lateral aspects of articular processes, the dorsal side of transverse processes and the space in-between them, and the lateral aspect of intervertebral foramens. After it works, the transverse process is resected and continued to elevate to the lateral side of pedicles and vertebral bodies. Electrocoagulation is performed to stop bleeding from vascular and nerve bundles of the posterior branch of spinal nerves, cut off the posterior branch of the spinal nerves (Fig. 9.36), dissect and expose the intervertebral foramens, and retain the spinal nerve roots exiting neuro foramens.
4. The fourth layer of local infiltration anesthesia:
   Injection around the spinal nerve root (Fig. 9.37). After stratified and fractional local infiltration anesthesia, a completely painless effect can be achieved, and the patient can communicate with surgeons in awake status. But this needs tacit cooperation between the surgeon and the anesthesiologist. Major surgery under local anesthesia is not as simple and easy as endotracheal intubation anesthesia; it is an artistic performance of anesthesiologists and surgeons.
5. Intraoperative complications and notes:
   (a) The process of stratified and fractional local infiltration anesthesia is carried out in parts. Injecting one layer and cutting one layer prolongs the absorption process of anesthetics in the body and reduces the incidence of anesthetic poisoning. It prevents the side effects like convulsions that may occur when blood concentration increases in a short time after once full-dose anesthetic injection.

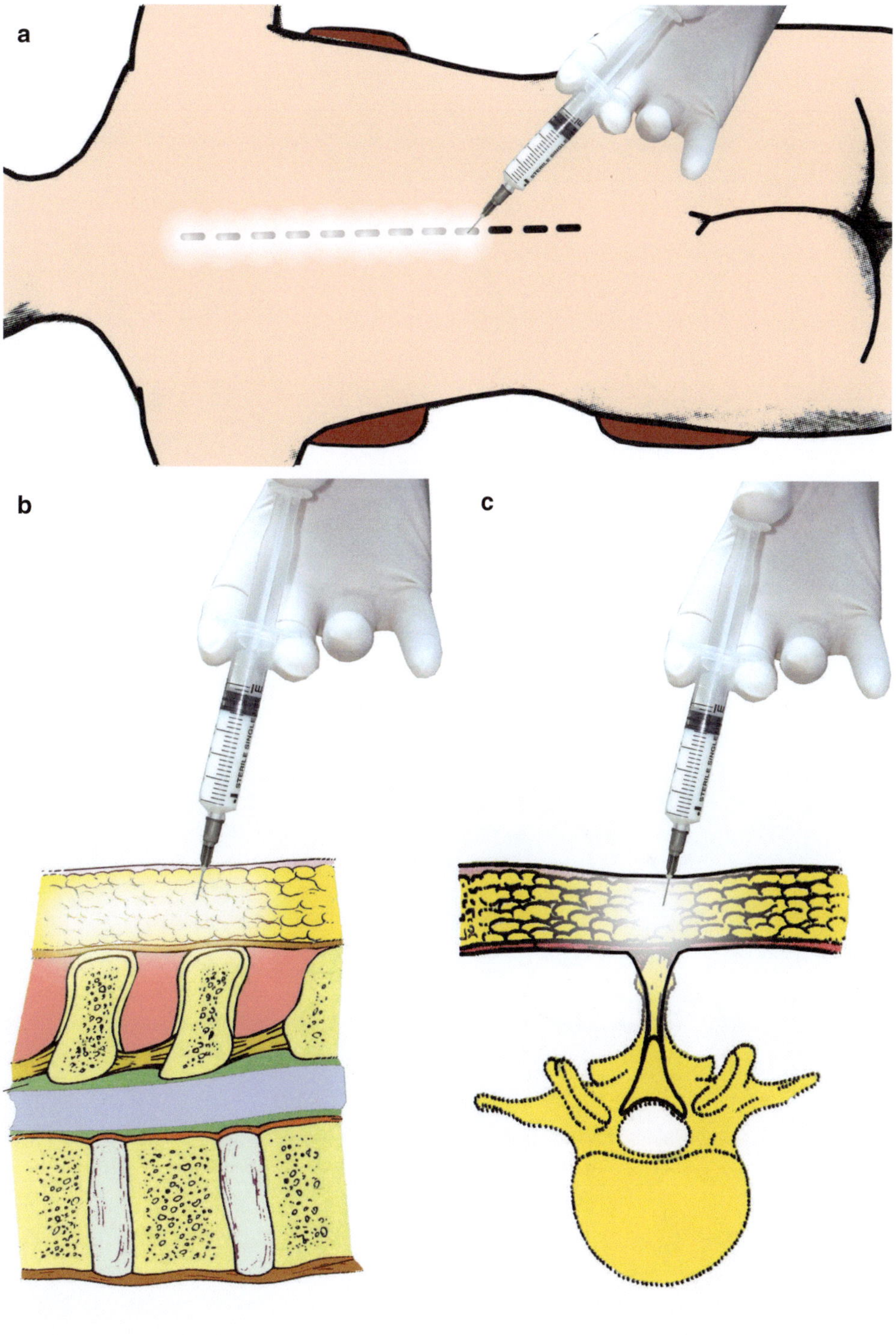

Fig. 9.33 The first layer of local infiltration anesthesia. (**a**) Dorsal view: Intradermal and subcutaneous injection along the spinous processes. (**b**) Lateral view: Intradermal and subcutaneous infiltrative injection. (**c**) Axial view: Intradermal and subcutaneous infiltrative injection

(b) The greatest advantage of major surgery under local infiltration anesthesia is that patient can talk to the surgeon in a conscious state and answer the surgeon's questions, which is more reliable than any wake-up test and evoked potential. Tian Huizhong used local infiltration anesthesia in 185 cases of total spinal osteotomy and 855 cases of spinal deformity correction with Halo-Pelvic traction, deeply realized its superiority in spinal surgery. But the team should remain vigilant against the toxicity of anesthetic drugs.

(c) Tian Huizhong the author applied local infiltration anesthesia in 1040 cases of spinal surgery and achieved excellent results. There were four cases of anesthetic poisoning during the operation, all of which were children under 10 years old. Three cases were rescued by experienced anesthesiologists. Intravenous injection of sodium thiopental and intramuscular injection of sodium phenobarbital were used to control seizure and convulsion, so that breathing returned to normal and hypoxia was relieved. No

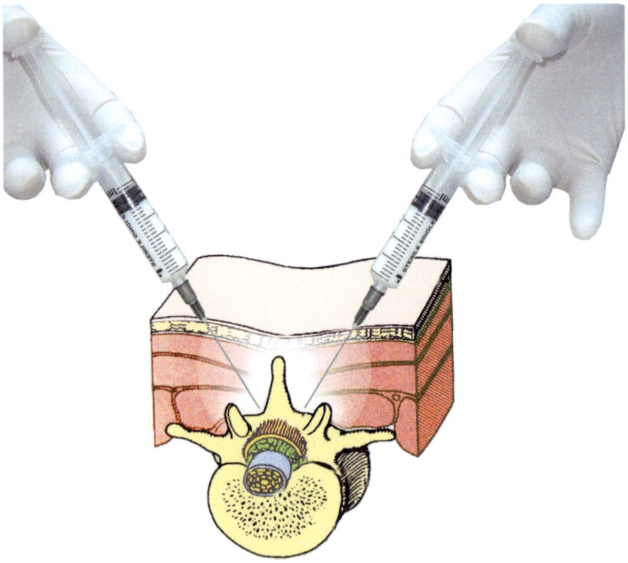

Fig. 9.34 The second layer of local infiltration anesthesia: Injecting muscle layer behind the spinous process, lamina and articular process

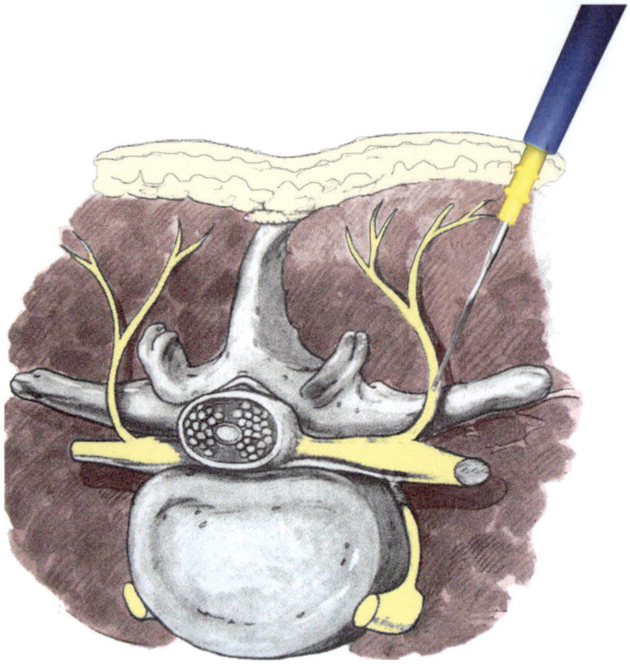

Fig. 9.36 After the third local infiltration anesthesia, cut off the posterior branch of the spinal nerve

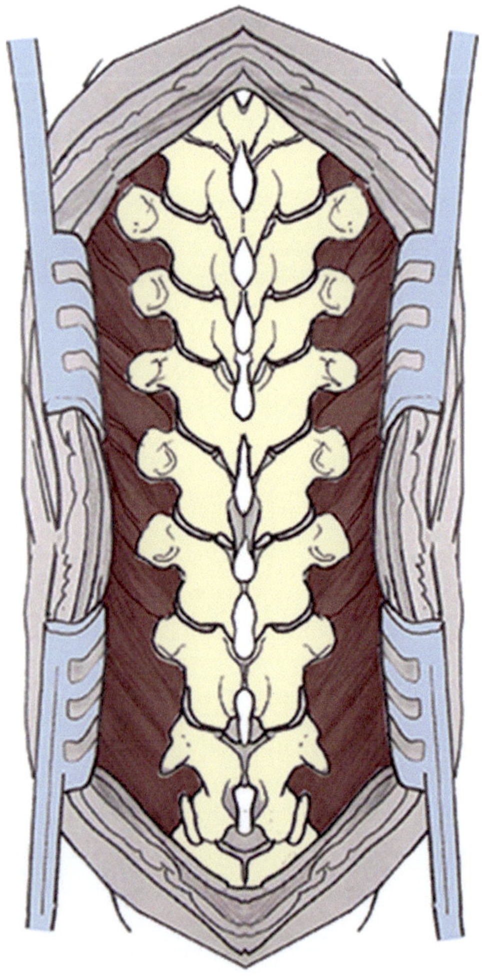

Fig. 9.35 Exposing lamina and articular processes

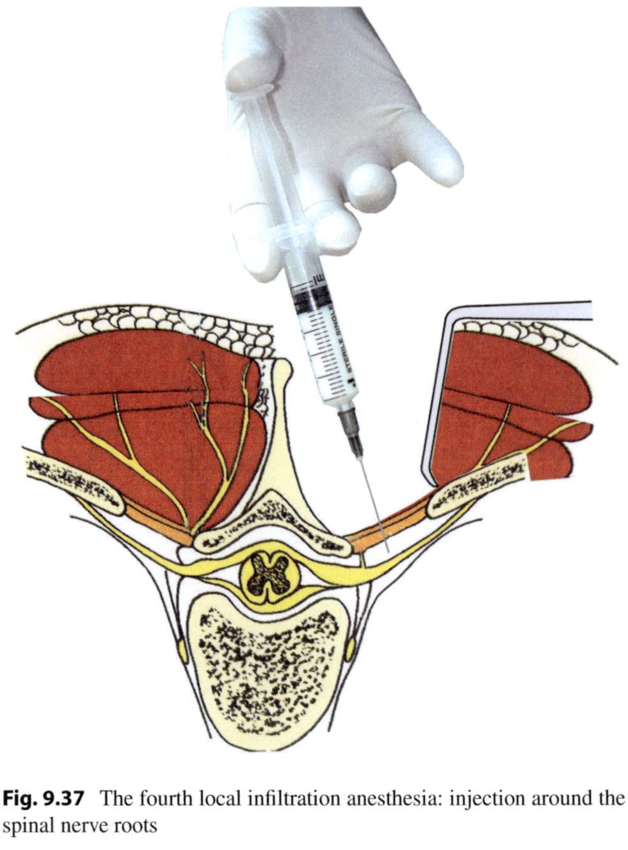

Fig. 9.37 The fourth local infiltration anesthesia: injection around the spinal nerve roots

sequelae were found after the operation. Another 3.5-year-old child had poisoning during the operation with severe seizure and convulsion. Due to lack of experience, the anesthesiologist wasted precious time and failed to give timely rescue and reasonable medication. Phenobarbital sodium was given intramuscular injection, but only a sedative dose was given which did not achieve the anticonvulsant effect. Prolonged hypoxia caused hypoxic-ischemic encephalopathy. This is a pity that the rescue is not timely and is worth drawing lessons from it.

(d) For children less than 10 years old, special attention should be paid to the dose and speed of injection. The concentration of local anesthetic solution must be reduced to half to one-third for adults. Local infiltration anesthesia must be carried out by layer. Timely rescue and anti-convulsion drugs should be given once poisoning symptoms like convulsion occur. No delay, no wait.

(e) Before major surgery under local infiltration anesthesia, it is necessary to organize anesthesiologists and surgeons to have case study together so that they will stay on the same page and prepare the drugs and equipment for intraoperative rescue.

Suggested Reading

1. Tian H. Total spinal osteotomy for the treatment of kyphosis and kyphoscoliosis. In: Japanese Scoliosis Society program of the 25th annual meeting. 1991; 25:23.
2. Tian H. Application of "Tian's spinal bone knife" in orthopaedic surgery. Chin J Orthop. 2003;11(15):1073–5.
3. Tian H. Surgical treatment of kyphosis. Chin J Orthop. 1992;12(3):162–5.
4. Tian H, Lv X, Ma Y. Treatment of severe spinal curvature with total spine osteotomy and internal fixation with head-sleeve ring. Chin J Orthop. 2007;15(3):167–72.
5. Jiang M, Tian H. Clinical application of Tian's pedicle locator. Orthop J China. 2003;11(7):448–50.
6. Tian H, Li F. Spinal deformity and osteotomy. Xi'an: World Book; 2001. p. 377–741.
7. Tian H. Spinal surgeons should be good at using rongeurs and osteotome. Chin J Mod Oper Surg. 2002;6(1):67–8.
8. Tian H, Liu S, Ma Y. Practical spine surgery illustration. Beijing: People's Military Medical Press; 2008. p. 189–385.
9. Chen A, Xu W. Spinal surgery atlas. Beijing: People's Medical Publishing House; 2001. p. 77–233.
10. Tian H, Liu S, Ma Y. Practical spine surgery. Guangzhou: Guangdong Science and Technology Press; 2008. p. 224–75.
11. Tian H, Yuan T, Tian S. Posterior invasion and vertebral osteotomy. Spinal Deformation. 1992;7(1):4–11.
12. Hou S. Spinal surgery. Beijing: People's Military Medical Publishing House; 2005. p. 444–610.
13. Xu S, Ge B, Xu Y. Practice of orthopaedics. 2nd ed. Beijing: People's Military Medical Publishing House; 2003. p. 598–636.
14. Tian H, Bai J, Liu S. Operative orthopaedics gist & atlas. Beijing: People's Medical Publishing House; 2009. p. 93–144.
15. Tian H. History of treatment of spinal deformity in China. Chin J Orthop. 2009;17(9):706–7.
16. Tian H, Wan Y, Li M. Halo-pelvic distraction techniques for the spinal deformity. Guangzhou: Guangdong Science and Technology Press; 2010. p. 3–252.
17. Dang G. Surgical techniques for the spine. Beijing: People's Medical Publishing House; 2004. p. 102–245.
18. Tian H, Alken. Amu D, Du P, et al. Posterior hemiverteectomy for congenital horny kyphosis. Chin J Orthop. 2010;18(15):1250–3.
19. Tian H. Tuberculous kyphosis osteotomy orthopedic surgery. Chin J Orthop. 2011;19(23):1937–40.
20. Tian H, Li M, Ma Y. Spinal deformity osteotomy orthopedics, vol. 5. Beijing: People's Medical Publishing House; 2011. p. 3–339.
21. Standring S. Gray's anatomy. Beijing: Peking University Medical Press; 2006. p. 2–739.
22. Brown DL. Atlas of local anesthesia. Beijing: Science Press; 2008. p. 18–253.
23. Huang W. Local anesthesiology. Beijing: People's Medical Publishing House; 2008. p. 13–174.
24. Meng Q, Liu S, Liu Z. Nerve block. Beijing: People's Medical Publishing House; 2003. p. 1–796.
25. Pan X, Fu Z, Song W. Color atlas of clinical anesthesia and analgesia. Shandong: Shandong Science and Technology Press; 2003. p. 21–273.

Hemivertebra Osteotomy

10

Huizhong Tian, Junjie Cheng, Tao Li, Zhibo Song, Zhiyue Shi, Zhi Zhao, Xu Zhu, Jie Dai, Junyi Ma, Jiangtao Sui, Weibin Sheng, Shaoyu Liu, and Quan Li

10.1 Overview

Children with congenital hemivertebra deformity should be firstly evaluated for its potential progression with X-ray diagnosis (Fig. 10.1a–e). If one or two semi-vertebral bodies are present on the same side (left or right side) on the AP X-ray, it is expected that there will be more serious spinal deformities in the future. If hemivertebra exists on each side of the spine on the AP X-ray, and the distance of the two semi-vertebral bodies is relatively close, the spinal deformity is expected to be self-limited in the future. Conservative observation and external immobilization with bracing may be used instead of surgery immediately. However, single or double hemivertebra ipsilaterally (Fig. 10.2) is an indication of surgery as soon as possible to avoid severe progression in the future.

For the cases of congenital hemivertebra deformity before skeleton maturity with apparent spinal deformity, halo-pelvic traction should be performed if no body connection forms between the vertebral bodies. This is to release the intervertebral tissue of the curved segment. After a period of halo-pelvic traction, hemivertebra osteotomy is be performed to correct the deformity with closing wedge gap after osteotomy in 1 stage. The portable pediatric halo-pelvic traction device, which is designed by the author, can be used for children over 3 years old before and after surgery (Fig. 10.3a–f). With this device to stabilize the spine, long segmental instrumentation is be replaced by a short segment one till fusion of the osteotomy.

Long segmental instrumentation with pedicle screws should not be used in children during early development because internal fixation interferes with the growth and development of the spine. However, Cranial-pelvic traction has the effect of Promoting osteogenesis and correction of spinal deformity in children during early development. Early activity with halo-pelvic traction device promotes longitudinal spine growth. Therefore, halo-pelvic traction combined with short-segment instrumentation is a preferred treatment for hemivertebra deformity in the early stage of development of children.

10.1.1 Formation of Hemivertebra Deformity

The formation of a hemivertebra may be related to embryonic development. During the embryonic period, each vertebra consists of three primary ossification centers including one vertebral ossification center, two pedicles, and a vertebral arch ossification center (bilaterally). In the central part of the vertebral ossification center, there is a trace of the notochord left in the early stage of the embryo. During normal embryo development, the signs of the notochord in the central part of the vertebral body gradually disappear, and the traces of the notochord corresponding to the intervertebral disc extend to the left and right sides, forming an intervertebral space. Therefore, in normal development, the ossification centers located on the left and right sides of the notochord traces are integrated with each other, and the centrally located notochord remains completely disappeared. Thus, the spinal morphology with a series of vertebral bodies and intervertebral discs is established. The pathological causes of the lateral hemivertebra may be related to dysplasia

H. Tian (✉) · X. Zhu · J. Dai · J. Ma · J. Sui
Spinal Surgery, The Sixth Affiliated Hospital of Xinjiang Medical University, Urumqi, China

J. Cheng
Department of Orthopedics, Nanlang Branch, Zhongshan People's Hospital, Zhongshan, Guangdong, China

T. Li · Z. Song · Z. Shi · Z. Zhao · Q. Li
Department of Orthopedics, The 2nd Affiliated Hospital of Kunming Medical University, Kunming, China

W. Sheng
Spinal Surgery, The First Affiliated Hospital of Xinjiang Medical University, Urumqi, China

S. Liu
Spinal Surgery, The Seventh Affiliated Hospital, Sun Yat-sen University, Shenzhen, China

H. Tian et al. (eds.), *Spinal Osteotomy Orthopaedics*, https://doi.org/10.1007/978-981-16-1387-6_10

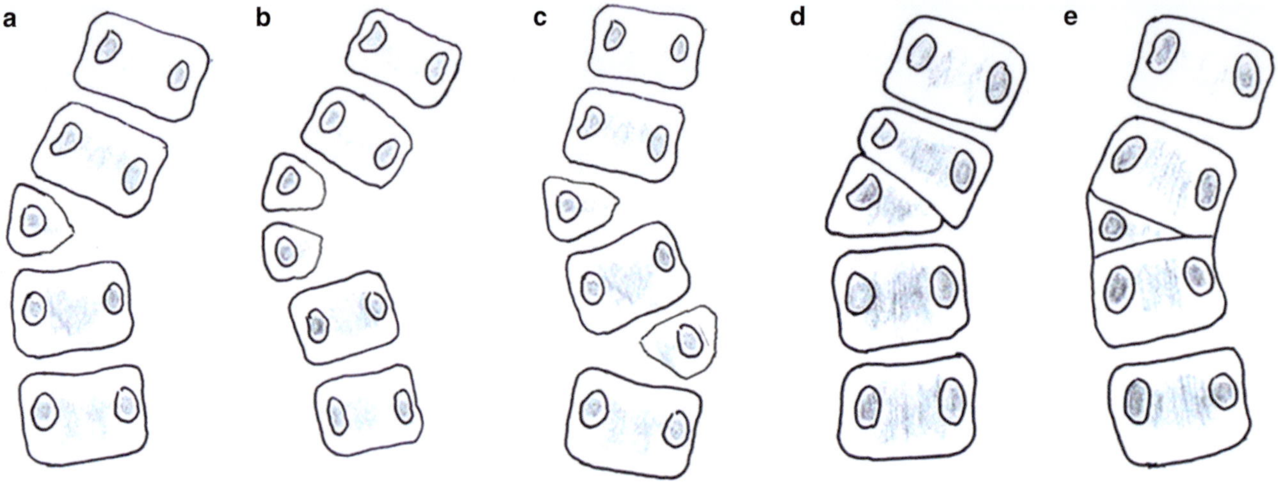

Fig. 10.1 Congenital lateral hemivertebra: (**a**) A unilateral single hemivertebra. (**b**) Unilateral double hemivertebra. (**c**) Bilateral compensated hemivertebra. (**d**) Hemivertebra without segmentation from the upper vertebra. (**e**) Hemivertebra without segmentation from the upper and lower vertebrae

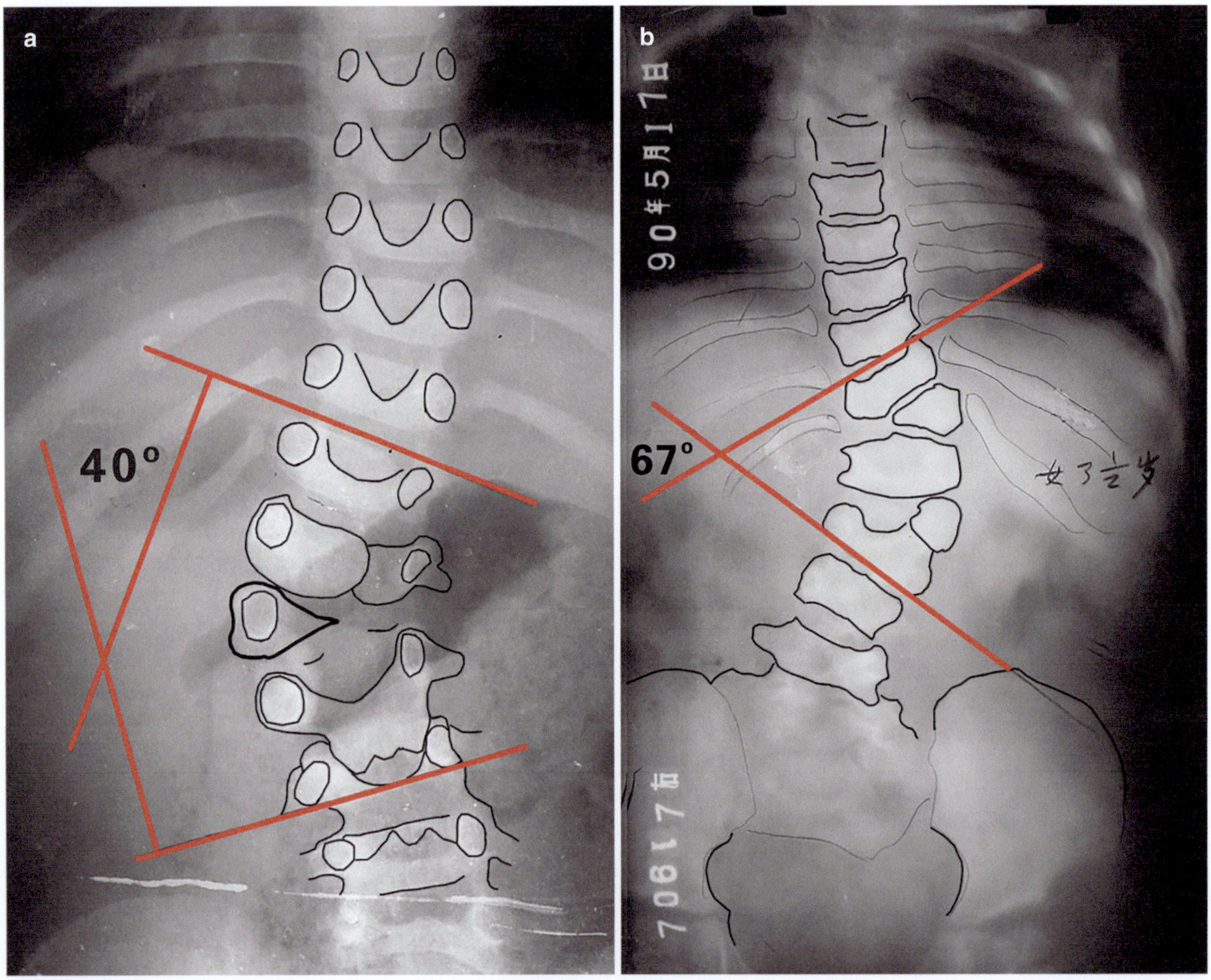

Fig. 10.2 For patients with unilateral single or double hemivertebrae, early surgery is required, as the patient will progress to severe scoliosis in the future. Ideally, preventive hemivertebral resection should be performed before the age of 5 years to have the best prognosis. (**a**) A unilateral single hemivertebra. (**b**) unilateral double hemivertebra on one side

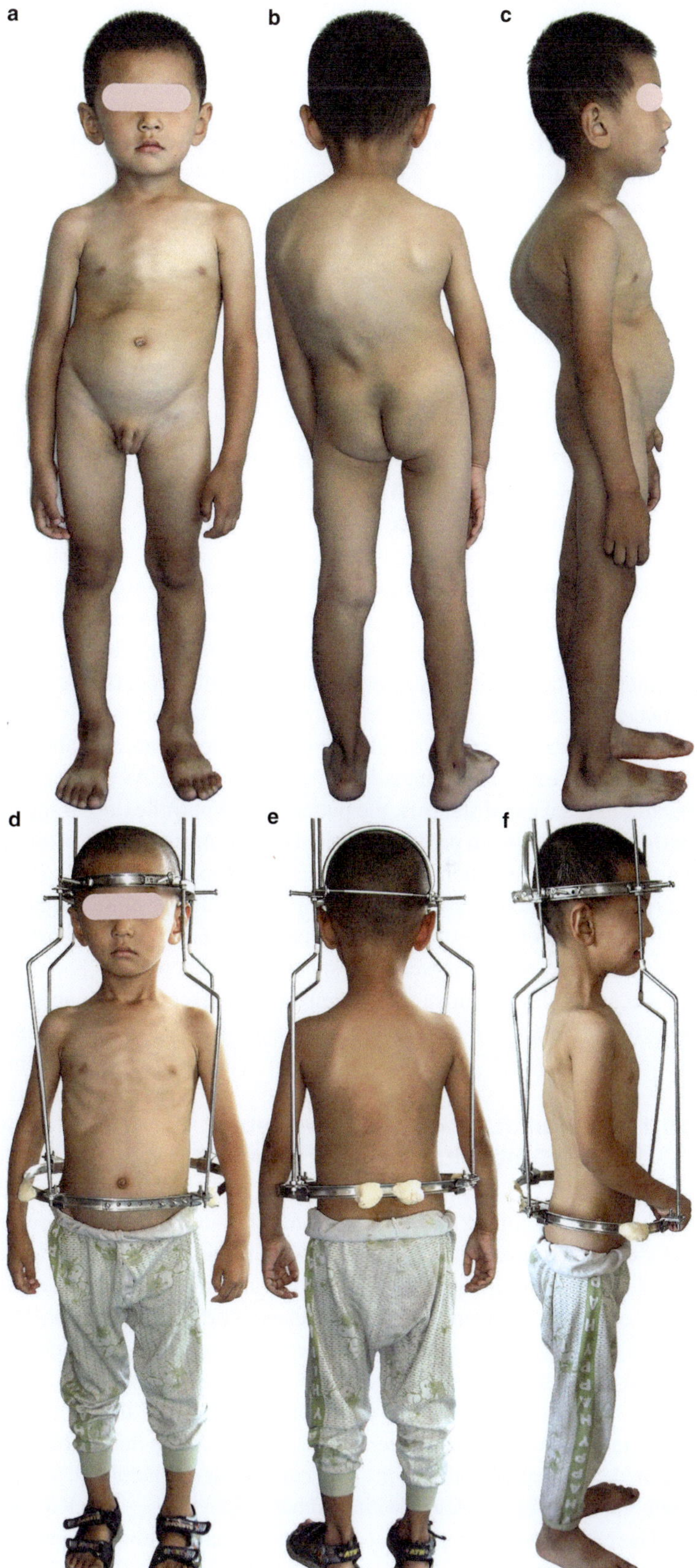

Fig. 10.3 4-year old, congenital hemivertebra, significant kyphoscoliosis. X-ray shows posterior-lateral hemivertebra deformity of the lower thoracic segment. With halo-pelvis traction, the spinal deformity is corrected. Comparison of photo before and after halo-pelvis traction. (**a**) Anterior view. (**b**) Posterior view. (**c**) Lateral view. (**d**) Anterior view. (**e**) Posterior view. (**f**) Lateral view

or underdevelopment of the unilateral (left or right) hemivertebra ossification center, while the other ossification center develops normally, forming a hemivertebra deformity. If the ossification center of both sides (left or right side) of the same vertebral body is underdeveloped, a butterfly vertebra is formed. But generally, it does not cause spinal deformity. The occurrence of double hemivertebra ipsilaterally will aggravate scoliosis. A balanced number of hemivertebra on each side of the spine in a short segment represents a better prognosis. Early resection of the hemivertebra is considered when one or more hemivertebra is present only on one side (left or right).

10.1.2 The Growth and Development of Hemivertebra Aggravates Angular Spinal Scoliosis

Scoliosis formed by congenital lateral hemivertebra progresses most rapidly usually at the age of 10–15 years, with 60–90° Cobb angle on AP X-ray and 30–60° kyphosis on lateral X-ray. Spontaneous osseous fusion often occurs between the angled vertebra laminas, and the disc herniation, which causes spinal canal stenosis, is often seen at the posterior edge of the angled intervertebral space. As a result of spinal canal stenosis, the patient has hyperreflexia with the knee, the sign predicting spinal cord compression. Surgical treatment upon occurrence of myelopathy will increase the difficulty and risk of the operation. For example, complex techniques like VCR for hemivertebral resection is needed to decompress the spinal cord. Therefore, the necessity of preventive early hemivertebra resection is very important.

10.1.3 Congenital Lateral Hemivertebra and Congenital Posterior Hemivertebra

The two most common hemivertebra deformities are seen in the clinical practice: lateral hemivertebra and posterior hemivertebra. The congenital lateral hemivertebral is more common than the congenital posterior hemivertebral. The formation of the congenital posterior hemivertebral may be related to the anterior extension of the bilateral pedicle ossification centers fused with the posterior component of the vertebral body ossification center whose development is thus arrested. Surgical treatment of the congenital posterior hemivertebral body will be described in another chapter.

There are two basic types of abnormal spinal developments: mal-segmentation and mal-formation which rarely stand alone. Almost all patients have a mixture of the two, although one may be outstanding. Mal-segmentation causes scoliosis (unilateral growth and development arrest), and posterior mal-segmentation can cause lordosis (anterior growth and development arrest). Some patients have circumference mal-segmentation. It does not cause deformities but reduces the number of spinal motion segments and shortens spine length.

Mal-formation is the result of an inadequate supply of materials for the normal development of the vertebrae. The deficiency of the posterior component causes spinal bifida. Dysplasia on one side of the vertebrae will form hemivertebrae. Hemivertebrae is not an additional bone of the spine. It is half of the normal vertebrae body and is caused only by deficiency or dysplasia of the contralateral half. If the entire vertebrae body is absent or dysplastic and the posterior component develops normally, it will cause kyphosis. Common mal-formation is usually located on the lateral and anterior sides of the spine. When the posterior-lateral part of the vertebral body is the only bit existing, true kyphoscoliosis can be caused. This is called "1/4 posterior hemivertebrae" (see Fig. 10.1).

There are many forms of hemivertebrae that may coexist. It is important to know that the natural history of each form is different. The hemivertebra does not necessarily create abnormal curvature of the spine, as deformity of the adjacent vertebrae may offset that. This condition is called trapped hemivertebra, or the benign type opposite to the progressive type.

A hemivertebrae may not be separated from one or two adjacent vertebrae. If there is an intervertebral disc separated from the adjacent vertebrae, it is called the hemisegmented hemivertebrae. When being separated from the adjacent upper and lower vertebrae, it is called non-segmented hemivertebrae. When being completely segmented from adjacent vertebrae, it is called free hemivertebrae, or complete hemivertebrae.

Sometimes more than one hemivertebrae may occur at the same time. If both hemivertebrae are on the same side of the spine, the prognosis is poor. The two hemivertebrae can be integrated or completely separated. If each side has a hemivertebrae, the spine may be more balanced, or two progressive curves may occur. Hemivertebra and mal-segmentation can occur simultaneously, such as unilateral arrested vertebrae, which is the most severe type of scoliosis.

10.1.4 Inspection Method

Routine AP and lateral X-ray of the spine should be taken to observe the segments and parts of the hemivertebral deformity, any scoliosis, the side of hemivertebra, number of hemivertebras on the same side, or compensation by balanced distribution of hemivertebra across the two sides. It is highly associated with the decision-making process of surgery. Once hemivertebra is found, CT, MRI, or myelography should be ordered to exclude spinal cord compression or diastematomyelia.

10.2 Hemivertebra Osteotomy Under Halo-pelvic Traction

1. Anesthesia: local infiltration anesthesia or intubated general anesthesia
2. Positioning: In the prone position under pelvic traction, four rods are loosened by 5 cm (cranial end), and one rod can be removed if necessary.
3. Procedure:

   The skin incision is made along the spinous process for 10–15 cm, and the lamina and transverse process are exposed on both sides. In the case of lateral hemivertebra or posterolateral hemivertebra, the transverse process of the hemivertebra is truncated from the convex side. The lamina of the hemivertebra is removed by osteotomy, followed by elevation along the pedicles and the waist of the vertebral body to the anterolateral side of the vertebral body. Use a retractor to retract the surrounding soft tissue and segmental blood vessels to expose the side of the whole hemivertebra (Fig. 10.4).

   Use a straight osteotome to remove the pedicle and the lateral part of the hemivertebra (Fig. 10.5). A pedicle screw or extra-pedicle screw is placed intrapedicle above and below the hemivertebra (Figs. 10.6 and 10.7). They are used for compression on the near side, after the hemivertebral resection.

   Use a crescent osteotome and a shovel osteotome to remove the central part of the hemivertebra (Fig. 10.8). Before the central part of the hemivertebra is removed, the temporary protective wire is applied to pull screws close to each other and fixed (Fig. 10.9) in order to avoid the detachment of the broken end of osteotomy due to the retractive force of the pelvic ring after the hemivertebral osteotomy is completed. After the hemivertebra is completely resected, close the osteotomy space and reduce it, and change over to a titanium cable for fixation

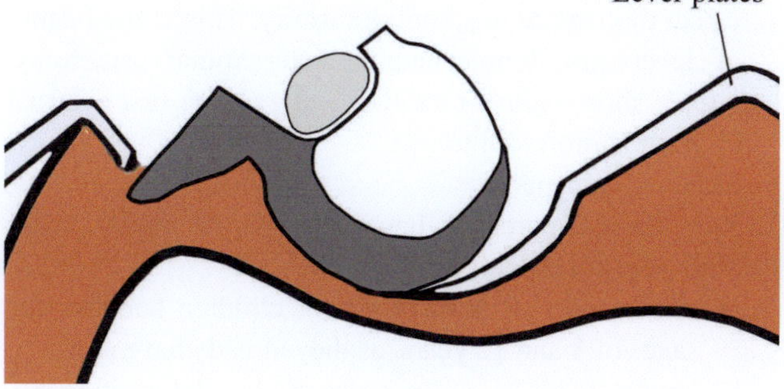

Fig. 10.4 Insert the retractor to completely expose the lateral surface of the hemivertebra

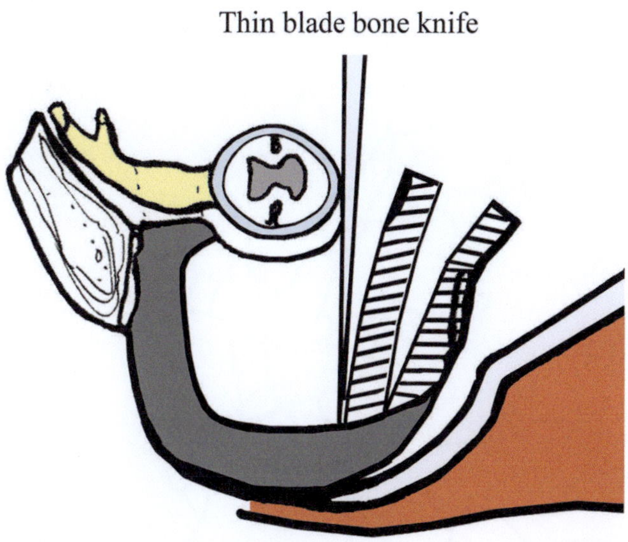

Fig. 10.5 Delaminated excision the lateral part of pedicle and centrum with thin-blade straight osteotome

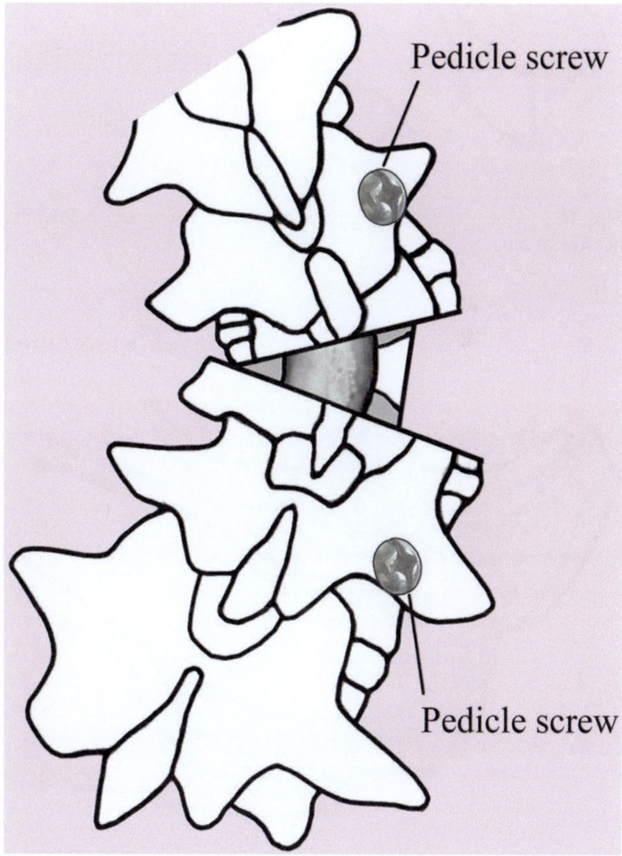

Fig. 10.6 One screw is placed in the pedicle above and below the hemivertebra before resecting the central part of the hemivertebra

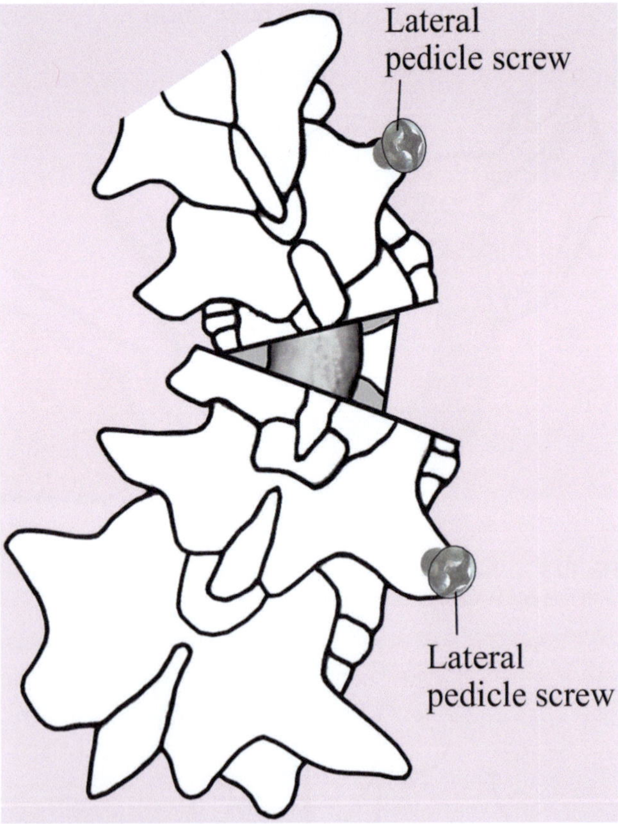

Fig. 10.7 One extra-pedicle screw is placed above and below the hemivertebra

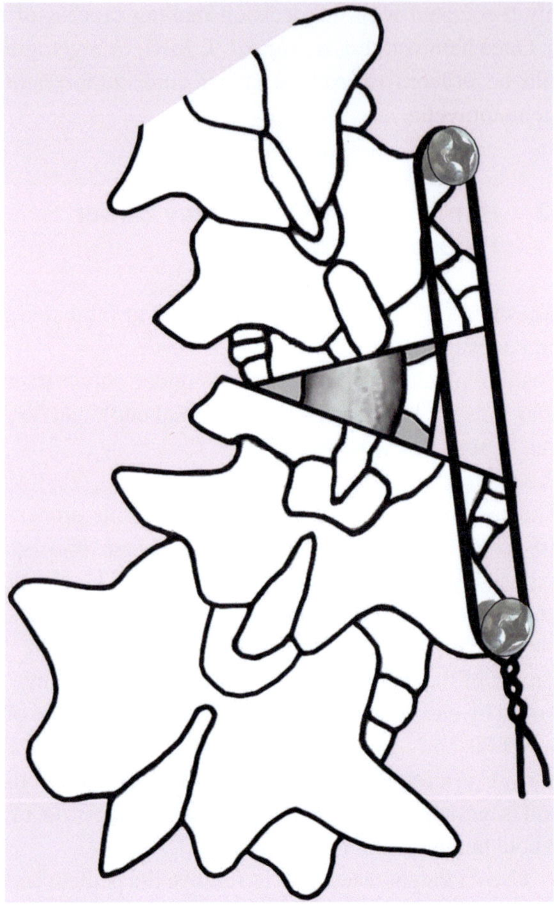

Fig. 10.9 Before the central part of the hemivertebra is removed, the temporary protective wire pulls screws together and fixes them

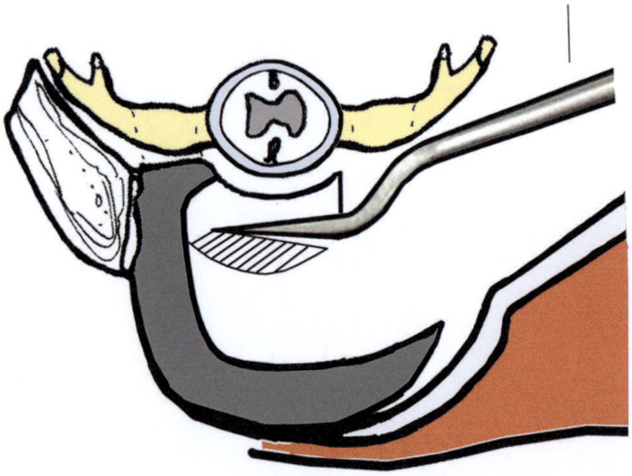

Fig. 10.8 Use a crescent osteotome and a shovel osteotome to remove the central part of the hemivertebra

(Fig. 10.10a, b). Strict electrocoagulation is used to stop bleeding, a drainage tube is placed, the incision is closed by layers to complete the operation.

4. Postoperative management: As the patient is managed by halo-pelvic traction before, during, and after the operation, only compression on the near side fixation is performed during the operation without distraction on the opposite side. Three weeks after the operation, the halo-pelvic traction is replaced by a plaster vest for immobilization, which is sufficient to maintain the alignment of the spine until bony fusion occurs. Hence, long instrumentation with rods and screws is spared to save cost and avoid complications caused by internal fixation. Simple internal fixation is used to replace complex and expensive internal fixation, with the same effect of correcting spinal deformity. This is the beauty of leveraging biomechanics. After spinal osteotomy, simple short-segment fixation and gypsum vest external fixation is preferred to use.
5. Expert comments:

   The main features of hemivertebral osteotomy under halo-pelvic traction:

   (a) Indications: It is intended for children between the ages of 8 and 12 years, as they already have apparent scoliosis based on the hemivertebra deformities. So, hemivertebral resection should be performed under halo-pelvic traction.

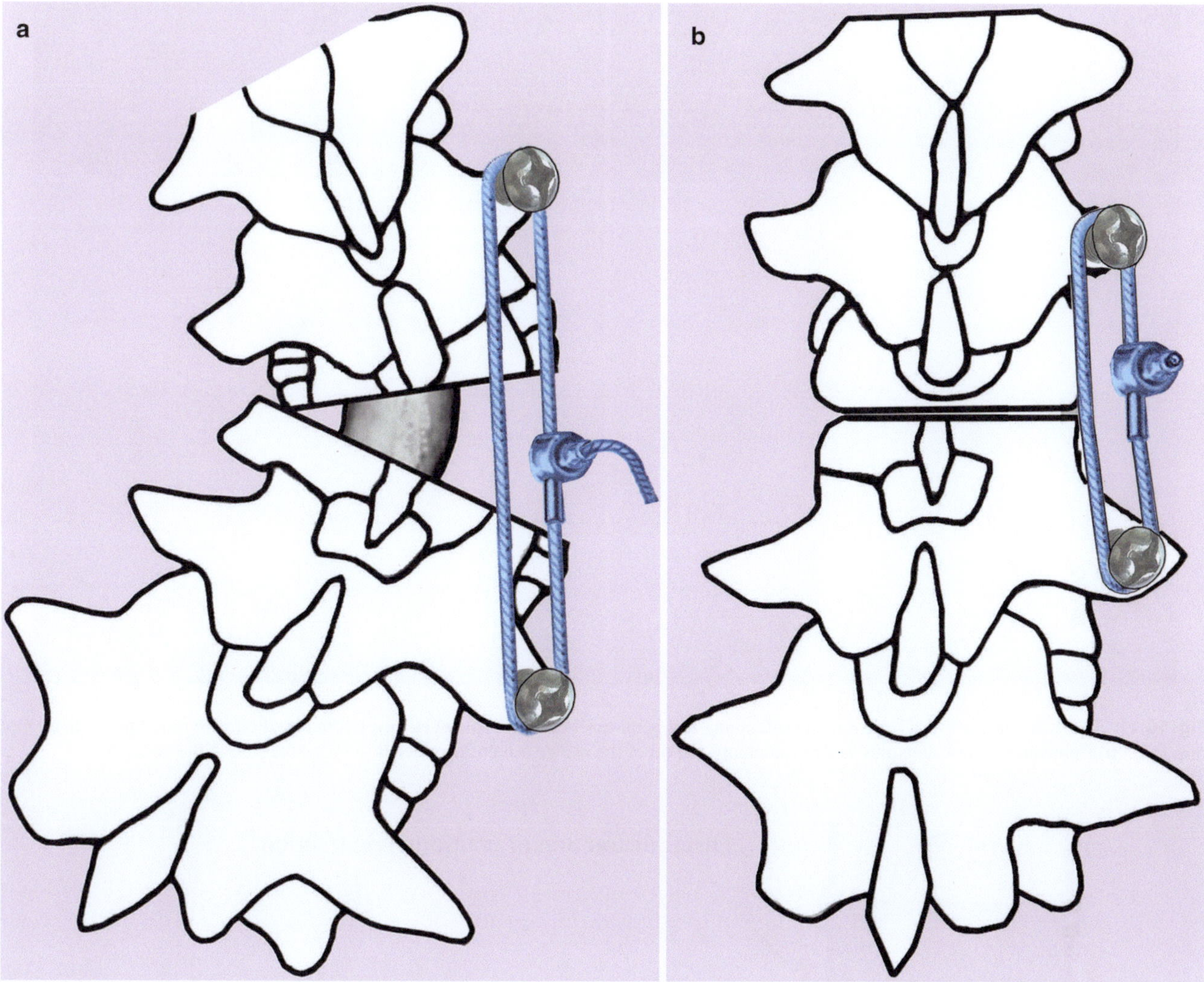

Fig. 10.10 Close and reduce it after osteotomy and replace it with titanium cable for fixation. (**a**) Tighten the titanium cable to close the osteotomy space. (**b**) By tightening the titanium cable and closing the osteotomy space, the scoliosis is corrected

(b) Halo-pelvic traction lengthens the trunk, loosens soft tissue in contracture, corrects the scoliosis, improves the shape of the human body, and brings convenience to surgical removal of hemivertebrae and reduction of the osteotomy gap. And before, during, and after surgery are performed under pelvic traction, it is of great benefit to patients to get out of bed early and maintain the correct position of the spine.

(c) The difference between hemivertebrae osteotomy and hemivertebrae resection. The former involves wedge-shaped osteotomy in addition to the removal of the hemivertebrae. The tip of the osteotomy must reach the contralateral side of the vertebrae (Fig. 10.11a, b).

(d) Screw and wire internal fixation spanning the osteotomy level instead of long instrumentation achieves the same effect of correcting deformities and straightening the spine (Figs. 10.12 and 10.13).

(e) Short segment fixation retains the activity and function of each vertebra.

(f) Halo-pelvic ring is replaced by plaster vest to maintain the extension of the spine until healing. It is a noninvasive protection.

10.3 Hemivertebrae Osteotomy and Instrumentation with Extrapedicle Screw and Rod System

10.3.1 Indications

1. Congenital scoliosis with hemivertebra: As the congenital lateral hemivertebrae makes the development of the two sides of the spine asymmetrical, and the resulting scoliosis is aggravated year by year, it is an indication of oste-

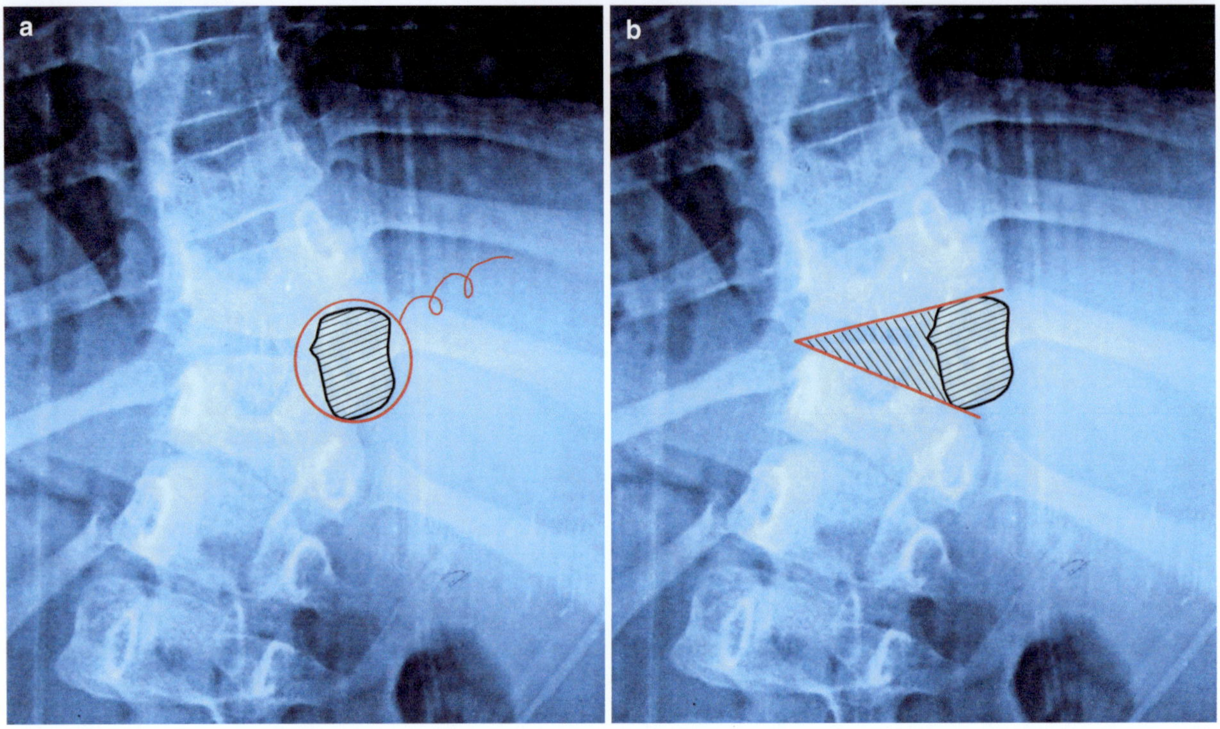

Fig. 10.11 The difference between hemivertebra osteotomy and hemivertebra resection. (**a**) Hemivertebra resection with only one hemivertebra removed. (**b**) Hemivertebra resection plus wedge osteotomy, the tip of the wedge osteotomy reaches the opposite side of the vertebra

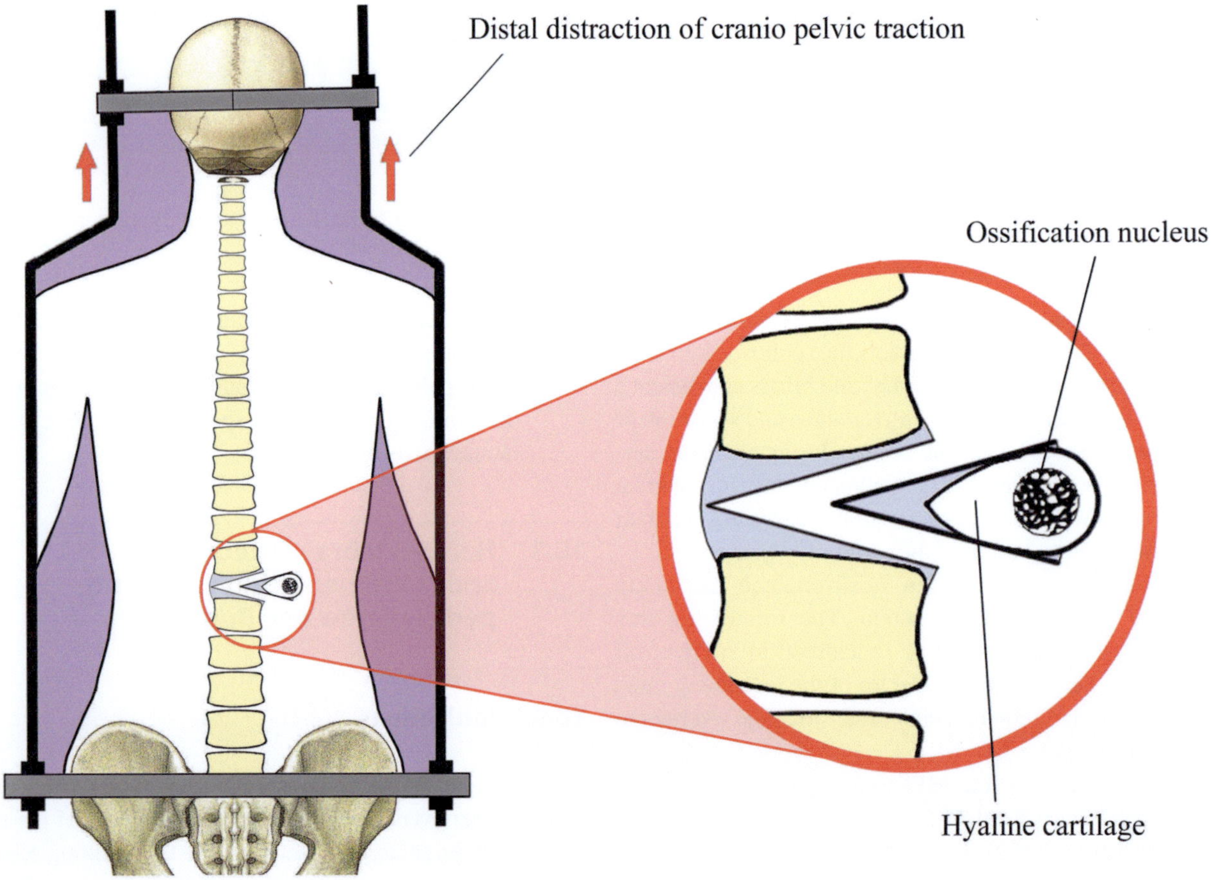

Fig. 10.12 Hemivertebra osteotomy under halo-pelvic traction. The tip of the wedge osteotomy reaches the contralateral edge of the vertebra. The resection area includes the ossified nucleus of the vertebra and the hyaline cartilage

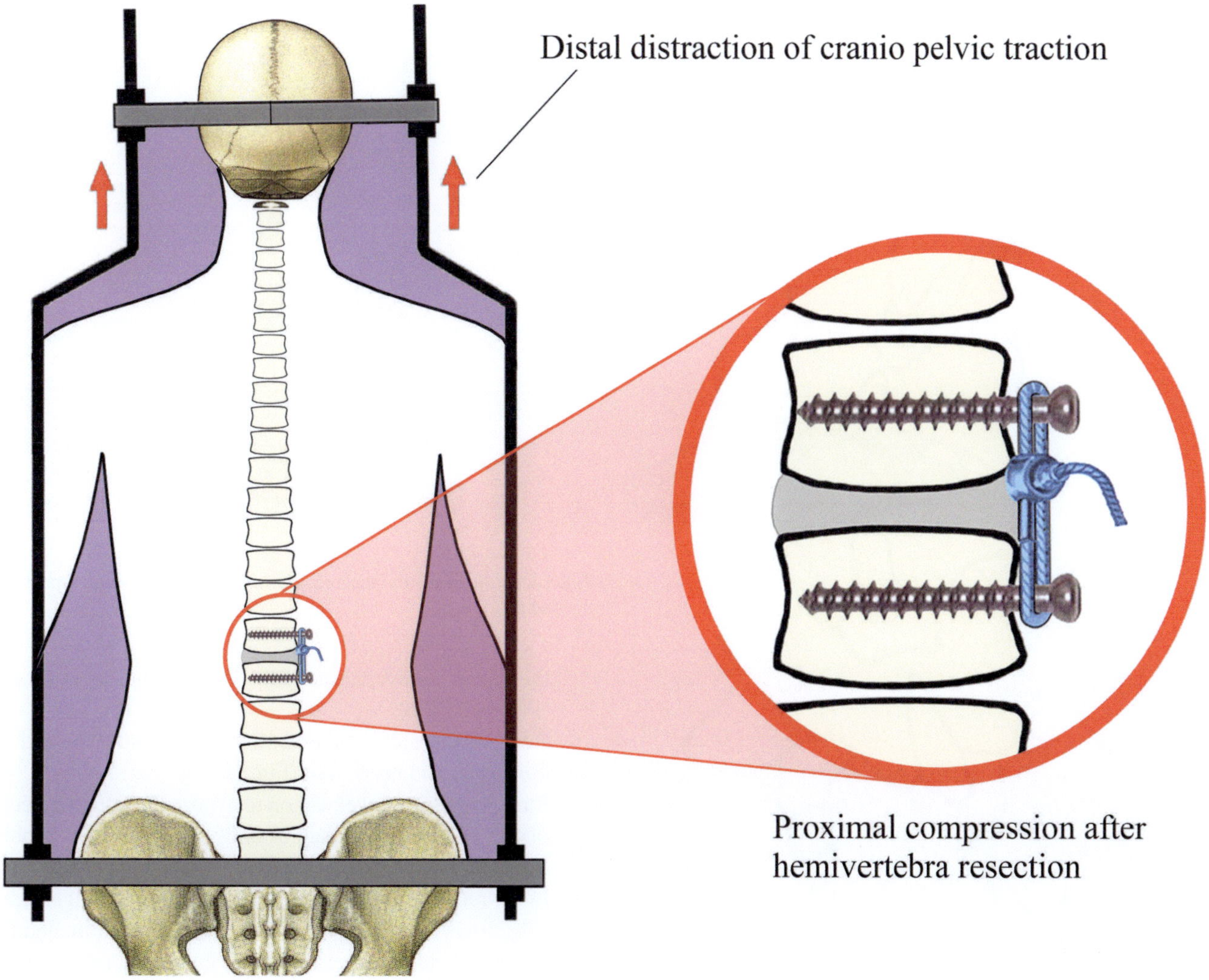

Fig. 10.13 After hemivertebral osteotomy under halo-pelvic traction, short-segment fixation with extra-pedicle screw and titanium cable are used for internal fixation

otomy to remove the hemivertebrae and fix with extra-pedicle screw and rod system.

2. Patients over 8 years of age with lateral hemivertebrae: Apparent scoliosis deformity following the development of lateral hemivertebrae. Simple preventive osteotomy to remove hemivertebrae is no longer suitable. It is necessary to have total vertebral column resection to remove the hemivertebrae followed by fixation with an extra-pedicle screw and rod system, in order to completely correct scoliosis.
3. Congenital lateral hemivertebra deformity brought to adult stage, given sound correction and restoration of alignment to allow for the alignment of extra-pedicle screws.
4. Same indication for hemivertebral osteotomy and screw–wire fixation for children aged 3–7 years old.

10.3.2 Contraindications

1. Severe congenital scoliosis which is not able to be completely corrected and realigned by halo-pelvic traction and osteotomy
2. Over 25 years of age, multi-segmental facet joint stiffness
3. Congenital scoliosis with severe thoracic deformities
4. Concomitant congenital heart disease or other visceral dysfunctions

10.3.3 Surgical Procedure

1. Anesthesia: general anesthesia with tracheal intubation
2. Positions: prone or lateral

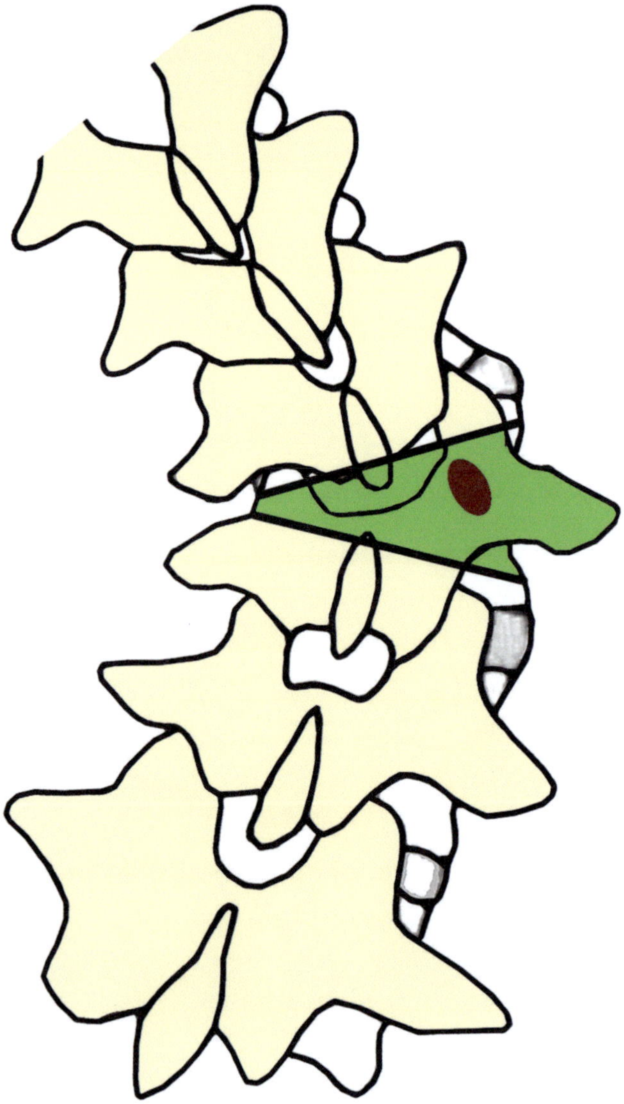

Fig. 10.14 Posterior exposure of spinous processes, lamina, articular processes, and transverse processes. Determine the scope of lamina resection

3. Incision: about 10–15 cm along the spinous process
4. Exposure: First expose the concave side of the scoliosis spine, perform a thorough subperiosteal exfoliation release between the intervertebral, interarticular and transverse processes, and then expose the lamina, articular processes and transverse processes on the side of the hemivertebrae (Fig. 10.14). Then locate the hemivertebrae position with C-arm.
5. Truncate the transverse process of the hemivertebrae (Fig. 10.15) along the lateral of the pedicle and the convex side of lateral vertebrae, then dissect to expose the entire hemivertebrae and its upper and lower discs (Fig. 10.16a, b).

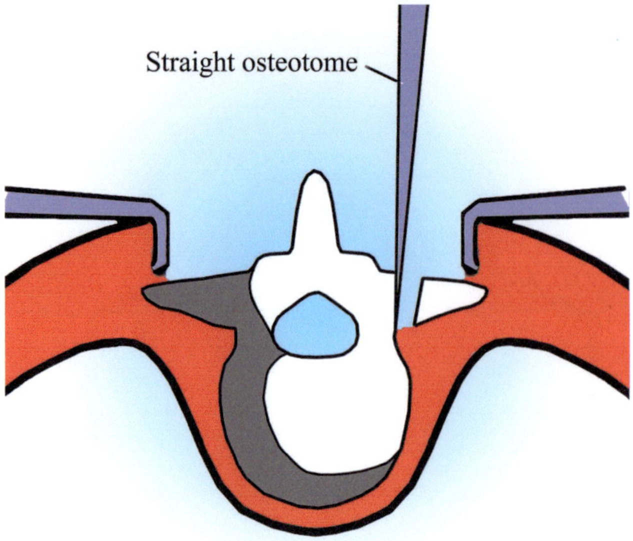

Fig. 10.15 Truncate the transverse process along the lateral aspect of the pedicle

6. Remove the arch of the hemivertebrae and expose the dural duct and nerve root (Fig. 10.17).
7. Strict subperiosteal elevation to expose the lateral aspect of the pedicle and vertebral body (Fig. 10.18) without ligation of segmental vessels.
8. Insert retractor below the anterior longitudinal ligament (Fig. 10.19) to retract soft tissue, expose the entire hemivertebrae and its upper and lower intervertebral space.
9. Cutting bone to remove the lateral part of the pedicle and vertebral body (Fig. 10.20), then remove the medial part of the vertebral body. The wedge osteotomy should reach directly to the contralateral side of the vertebral body (Fig. 10.21a, b).
10. Keep the thin layer of bone at the posterior edge of the vertebral body temporarily, so as not to cause bleeding of the epidural vein and impact the operation (Fig. 10.22).
11. Use a push-down osteotome to remove a thin layer of bone at the posterior edge of the vertebrae as quickly as possible (Fig. 10.23). Use finger to palpate the presence of residual bone fragments in the osteotomy space (Fig. 10.24). If no residual bone fragments are present, the osteotomy gap should be closed immediately.
12. Install the upper and lower pedicle lateral screws before the vertebrae is fully truncated (Fig. 10.25), for rapid reduction and internal fixation of the gap after the completion of the osteotomy.

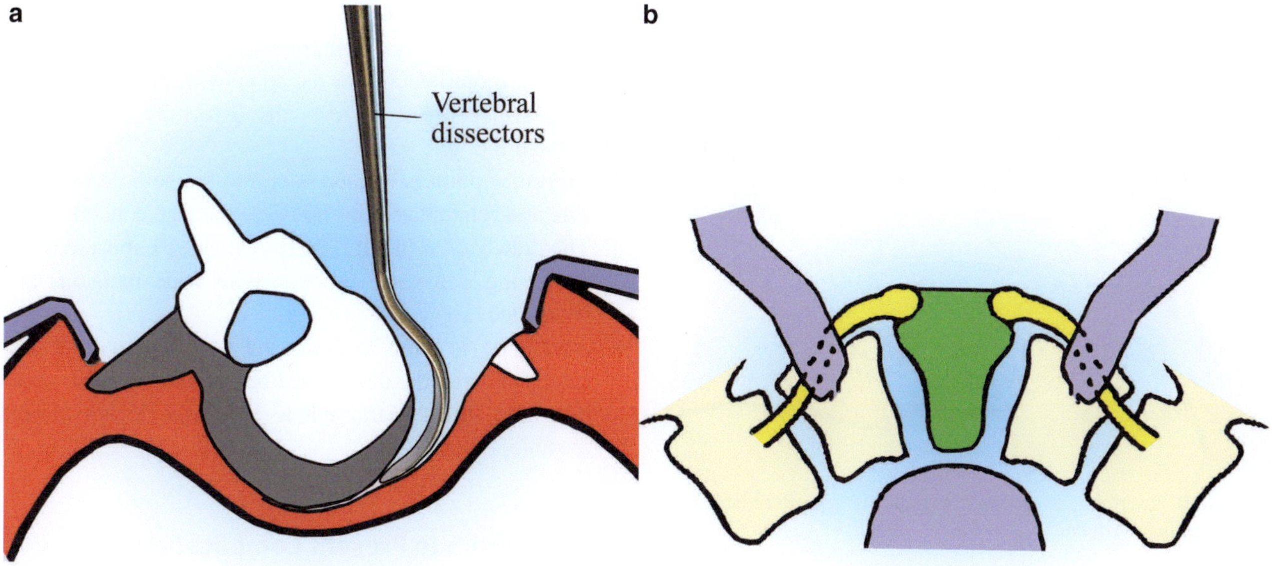

Fig. 10.16 (**a**) Along the lateral aspect of the pedicle and vertebral body, elevate to the anterior until being underneath ALL. (**b**) Elevate to the anterior along the pedicle and lateral aspect of the vertebral body to expose the entire hemivertebra and disc up and down

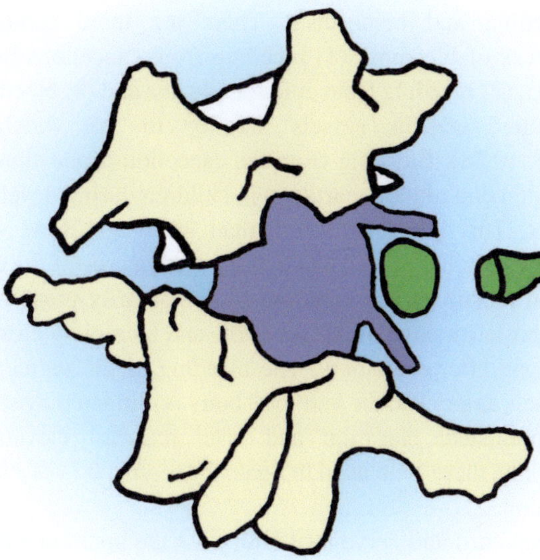

Fig. 10.17 Wedge osteotomy of the lamina cap, expose dura, nerve roots, and pedicle of the hemivertebra

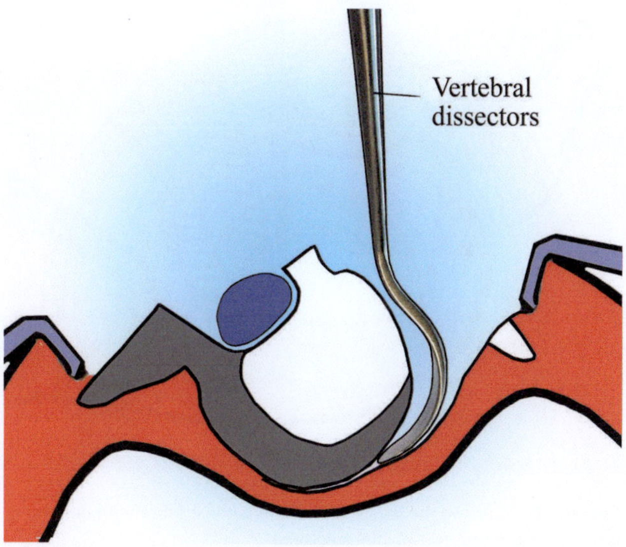

Fig. 10.18 Strict subperiosteal dissection can expose the lateral surface of the semi-vertebral body without damaging segmental blood vessels

13. Closed the osteotomy gap and internal fixation: Capture the adjacent screw head with a bone holding forceps to close the osteotomy gap, and correct scoliosis by tensioning the wire and closing the osteotomy temporarily (Fig. 10.26).
14. After closing the gap of cutting bone, the shortened epidural tube expands and compresses the epidural venous plexus. Bleeding will stop spontaneously.
15. Reduce the concave rod first and then the convex rod. Cut and remove the temporary wire. Alternatively, compress the convex side and distract the concave side to correct scoliosis while tightening and locking the set screws (Fig. 10.27).
16. Inspect the wound, thoroughly electric coagulate for hemostasis. Place the rubber drainage tube and close by layers.

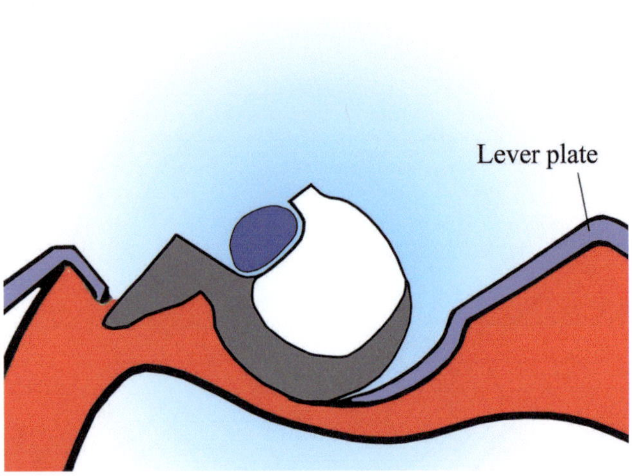

Fig. 10.19 Insert the Lever plate to completely expose the lateral surface of the hemivertebra

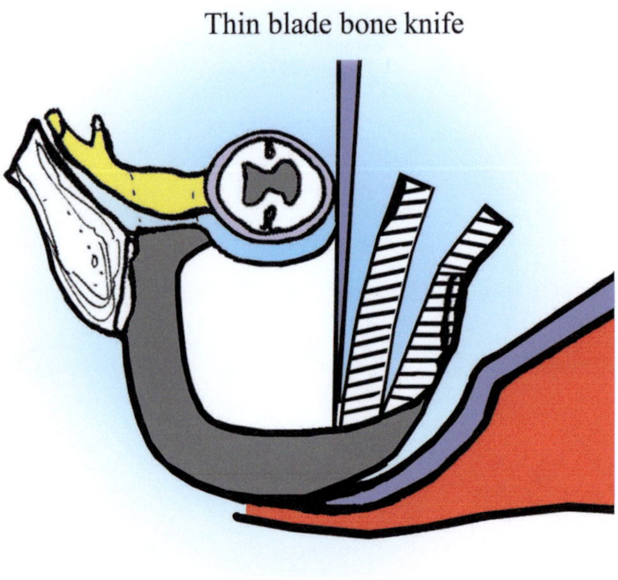

Fig. 10.20 Remove the lateral part of the hemivertebra with delamination technique and thin-blade osteotome

17. Postoperative management: Lie flat after returning to ward, body turning over, suture removal on day 10. A bracing or plaster vest is applied as appropriate to promote bone fusion.

10.3.4 The Advantages and Disadvantages of Fixation with Extra-pedicle Screw and Rod System

1. For idiopathic scoliosis with a degree within 80° and good compliance before skeleton maturity, the extra-pedicle screw and rod system performs well in correcting the main curve, while outperforms the pedicle screw system.
2. Extra-pedicle screws produce more distraction force on the concave side and compressive force on the convex as they sit more laterally to the spine with the longest lever arm. Especially it corrects the deformity of the main curve directly.
3. The entry point is located lateral to the pedicle, which is safe and reliable and has no nerve damage concern.
4. The drawback is that it requires extensive exposure to the tip of the transverse process, with wide incisions and more bleeding.
5. As L4–L5 is more lordotic, the lateral transverse processes fall into the deep space behind the posterior superior iliac spine, extra-pedicle technique is not always feasible.

10.3.5 Tactics to Prevent Complications

1. Hemivertebrae osteotomy is usually performed in children before skeleton maturity. The vertebral arch and vertebral body have more cartilage components which makes them suitable for resection with a thin-blade osteotome or sharp knife. Burr does not work well in this situation.
2. Bleeding and hemostasis: There are three common sources of bleeding: (1) bleeding from cancellous bone sinus; (2) bleeding from epidural plexus; and (3) bleeding of the segment vessels anterior to the vertebrae (Fig. 10.28). Bleeding from the cancellous bone sinuses is often due to more cartilage in children during development. This bleeding is less than in adults. Bone wax application helps with hemostasis. Hemostasis of the epidural plexus can be achieved by temporarily preserving the posterior edge of the vertebrae and by rapidly closing the gap after osteotomy. The bleeding of the segmental vessels anterior to the vertebral body is mitigated by strict subperiosteal elevation and level retractor elevation. Usually, there is no need to ligate the segmental vessels in general.
3. Spinal cord and nerve root injury: As the operator's anatomical concept is not clear, or the operative skill is not good, injuring the spinal cord nerve by mistake or cutting the spinal nerve root will cause the damage of irreversible nerve function. The effective action to avoid the injury is to study the local anatomy carefully and improve proficiency of local anatomy. When performing the osteotomy around the epidural tube and the nerve roots, care must be taken to avoid carelessness and avoid error in operation.
4. When removing the bone tissue around the epidural tube with a rongeur, make sure that the dura is not caught by the jaw, to prevent epidural tear and "sticking thread phenomenon." CSF leakage causes trouble for postoperative recovery.

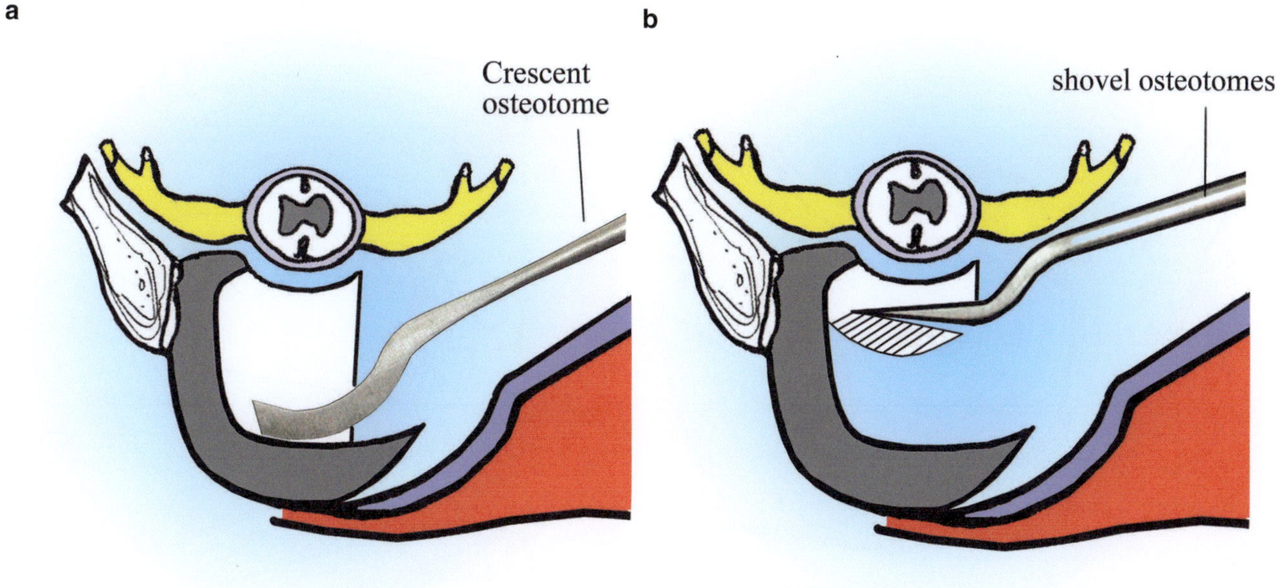

Fig. 10.21 Crescent osteotome and shovel osteotome are used to remove the medical part of the hemivertebra

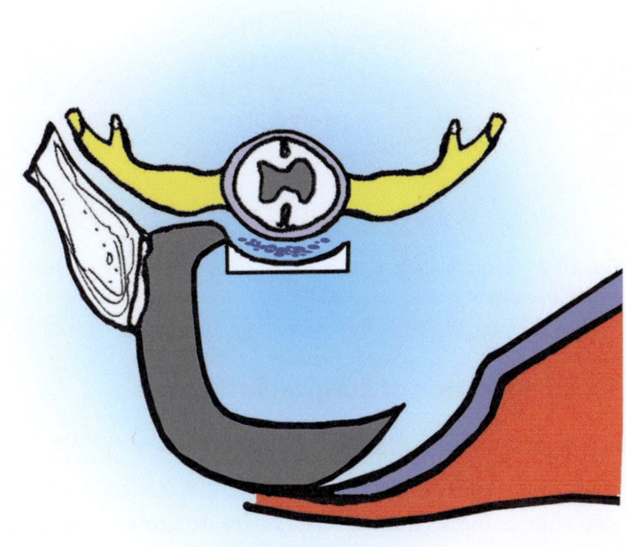

Fig. 10.22 Temporary preservation of thin bone fragments at the posterior edge of the vertebral body, so as not to cause the bleeding of anterior dural venous plexus, which makes the operation difficult

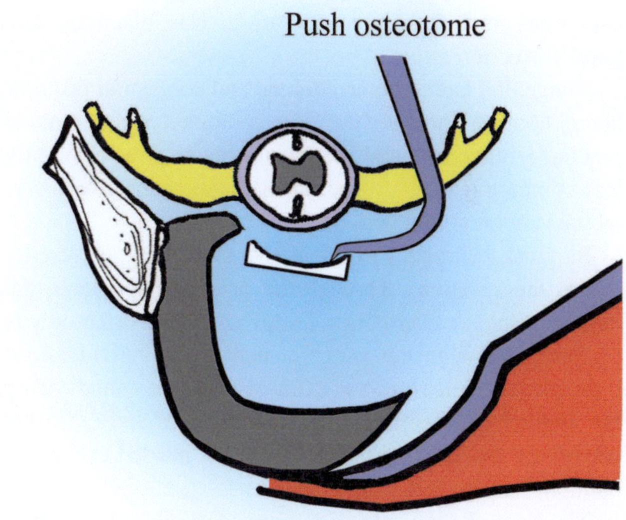

Fig. 10.23 Remove the posterior edge bone sheet with push-down osteotome

10.4 Preventive Osteotomy for Lateral Hemivertebra

Congenital hemivertebrae deformity is based on the site of the hemivertebrae to cause the direction of spinal curvature that formation. Scoliosis will be formed based on the underlying lateral hemivertebra. Kyphosis will be formed based on the underlying posterior hemivertebra. Kyphoscoliosis will be formed based on the underlying posterior lateral hemivertebra. But anterior hemivertebrae deformity is rare in clinical practice. The surgical treatment effect of congenital hemivertebrae deformity is better in the early stage rather than late, so the author advocates preventive hemivertebrae osteotomy between the age of 3 and 7

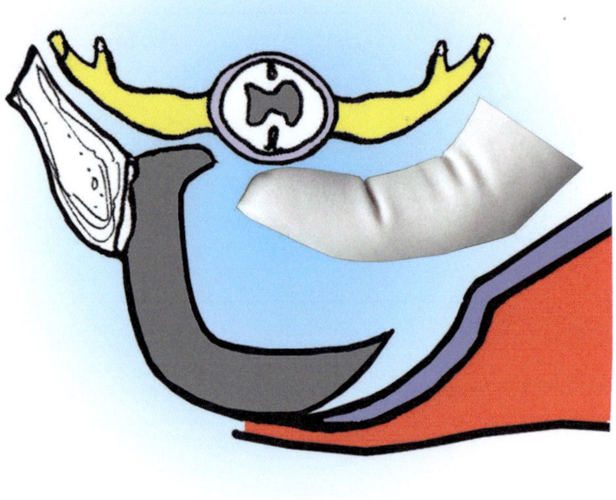

Fig. 10.24 Palpitate the anterior aspect of the dura to check any residue bone chips. The osteotomy space is closed once the space is clear

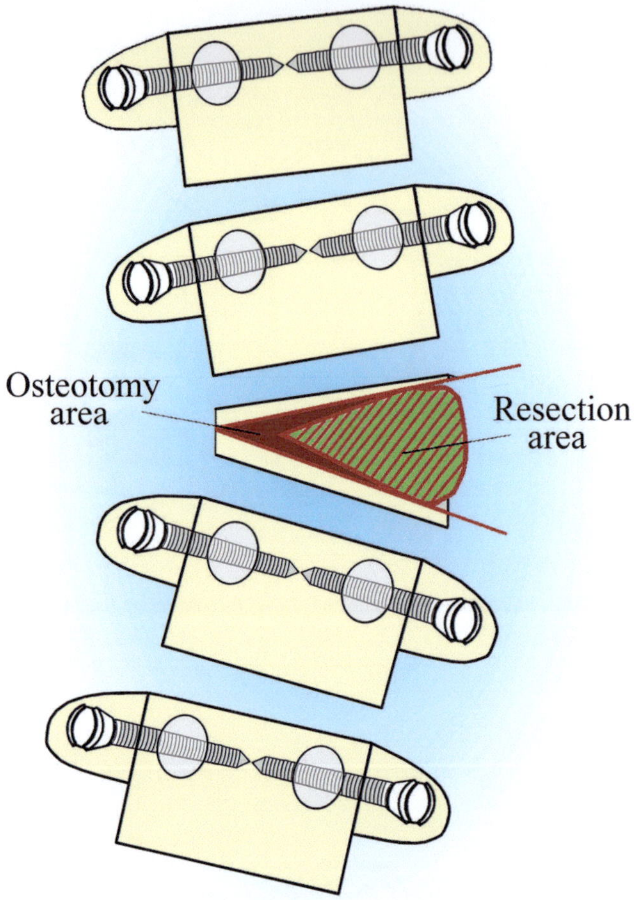

Fig. 10.25 Extra-pedicle screws placed up and down before osteotomy is completed

years. The advantages of preventive (early) hemivertebrae osteotomy include simple operation, less bleeding, and good correction effect.

Congenital lateral hemivertebrae and congenital posterolateral hemivertebrae are the more common types in clinical practice while congenital posterior hemivertebrae is slightly less common (Fig. 10.29a–c). Congenital anterior hemivertebrae is not reported yet.

Surgical techniques of preventive osteotomy are similar across the spectrum. Through the posterior approach, the lamina of the hemivertebra is removed. Wedge osteotomy is performed through the vertebral body with individualized directions. Pedicle screws or extra-pedicle screws and wiring are applied as internal fixation to compress and close the osteotomy space. Long instrument is not needed except for children over 8 years of age

The base of the wedge osteotomy for lateral hemivertebrae should be toward the lateral side. The internal fixation should use an extra-pedicle screw with wiring (Fig. 10.30). The base of the wedge osteotomy for posterior-lateral hemivertebrae should be toward the posterior-lateral side. The internal fixation should use unilateral pedicle screws (Fig. 10.31). The base of the wedge osteotomy for posterior hemivertebrae should be toward the posterior side. A bilateral approach is needed and the internal fixation should use the bilateral pedicle screw plus wiring to close the osteotomy space (Fig. 10.32).

10.4.1 Selection of Surgical Technique

It is difficult to restrict the aggravation of scoliosis year after year simply with concave side distraction and convex side compression. Conservative treatments such as brace and traction do not solve the problem. Only early hemivertebral osteotomy, compression, and fixation are effective. The younger the patient is, the less bleeding and easier periosteum elevation. The difference lies in surgical instruments and the techniques of osteotomy. Children are cartilage-rich before skeleton maturity on the vertebral arch and vertebra body which are similar to the hardness of hard rubber. It responds poorly to a burr. Thin-blade osteotome and sharp osteotome is the only choice, which is very capable of removing bone at this hardness level such as wedge osteotomy of the hemivertebra. The tip of

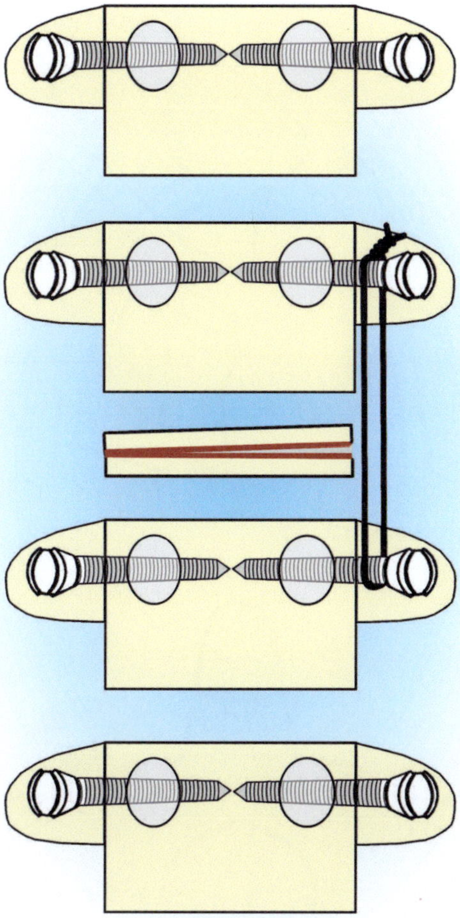

Fig. 10.26 Upon completion of hemivertebra resection, tension is applied to the wire to drag screw heads closer as temporary protection and closure of the gap

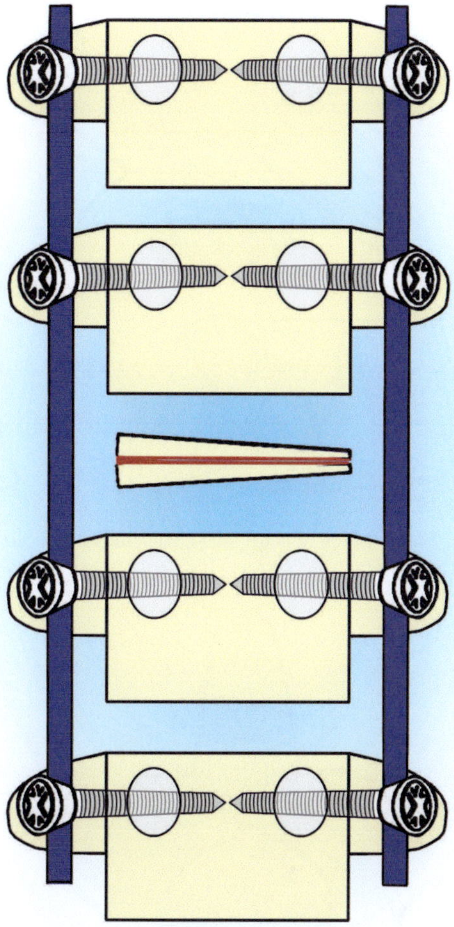

Fig. 10.27 Once the rods are reduced and fixed, cut and remove the temporary wire

the wedge must reach the opposite side of the vertebrae and not just dig out a sphere of hemivertebrae; otherwise, gap closing will be more difficult. For all cases of this group treated with sharp thin-bladed osteotome for hemiverteral osteotomy, no one had spinal cord injury. The operation time is 1–2 h. Removing a rigid rub-like hemivertebra is faster, easier than removing the same hemivertebrae in an adult with less bleeding. The objective of the osteotomy is to make the wedge tip cross the contralateral side of the vertebrae. Simple resection of the hemivertebra without osteotomy set the barrier to correct angular scoliosis of the spine.

10.4.2 Selection of Instrumentation

After hemivertebrae resection for children below the age of 8 years, the wiring on top of the screws to close the space corrects the scoliosis deformity with no need of distraction and

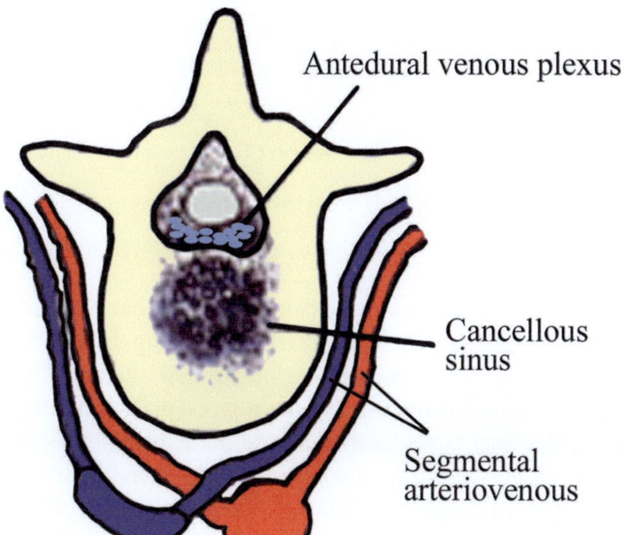

Fig. 10.28 There are three common sources of bleeding: (1) bleeding from cancellous bone sinus; (2) bleeding from epidural plexus; (3) bleeding of the segment vessels anterior to the vertebrae

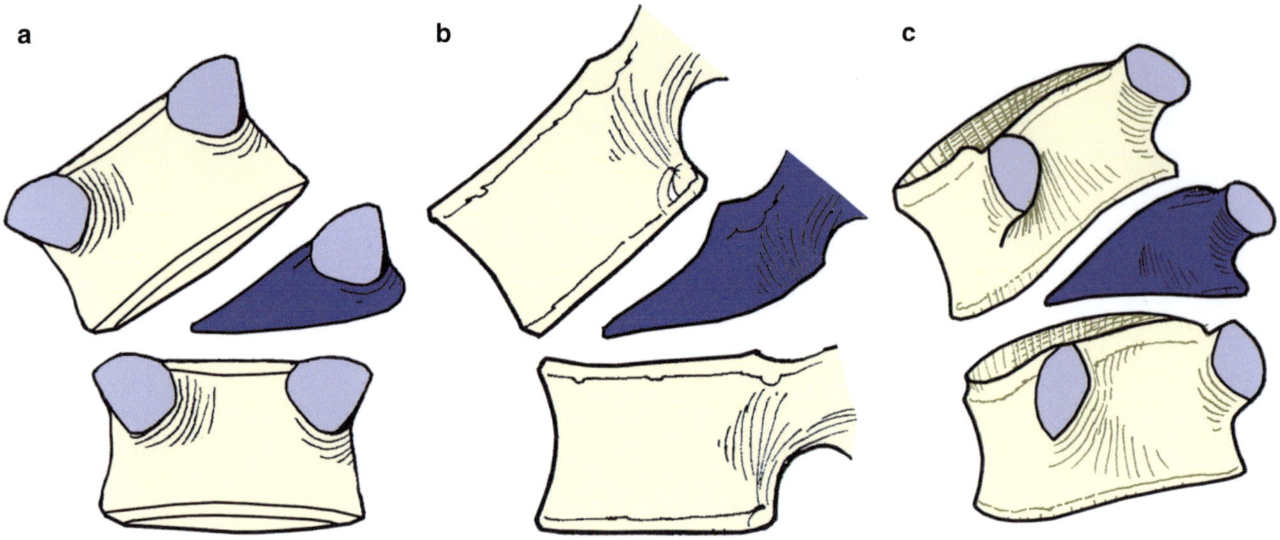

Fig. 10.29 Classification of congenital hemivertebra. (**a**) Lateral; (**b**) posterior; (**c**) posterior-lateral

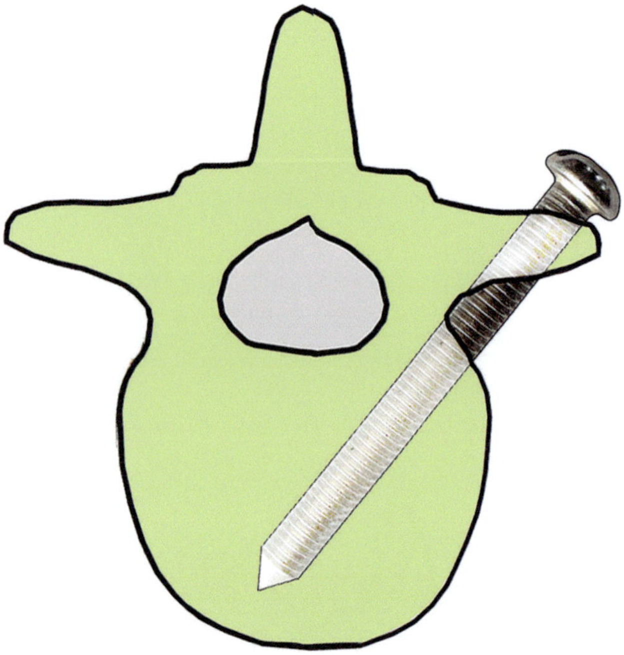

Fig. 10.30 Extra-pedicle screw for lateral hemivertebra

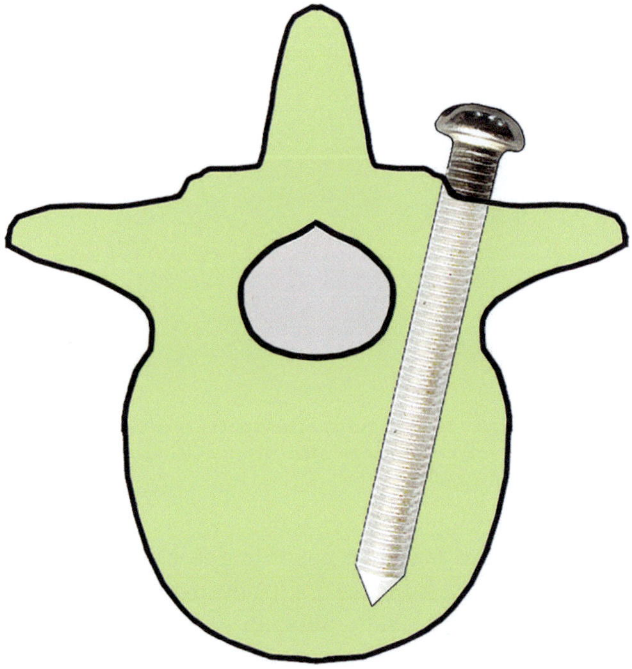

Fig. 10.31 Unilateral pedicle screw for posterior lateral hemivertebra

fixation on the other side as children below the age of 8 years respond well to conventional screws and wiring. If the tip of the wedge-shaped osteotomy reaches the opposite side of the vertebral body, gap closing is not a problem. If just lateral hemivertebrae is resected and close the gap solely by the force of the instrument, it will be difficult. Therefore, hemivertebral osteotomy and hemivertebral resection have different clinical relevance.

10.4.3 Indications

1. Period of 3–8 year-old is the intended time window of preventive osteotomy for lateral hemivertebra resection with pedicle or extra-pedicle screw and wiring or titanium cable fixation technique.
2. The younger the preventive osteotomy performed, the simpler the operation and the better the effect.

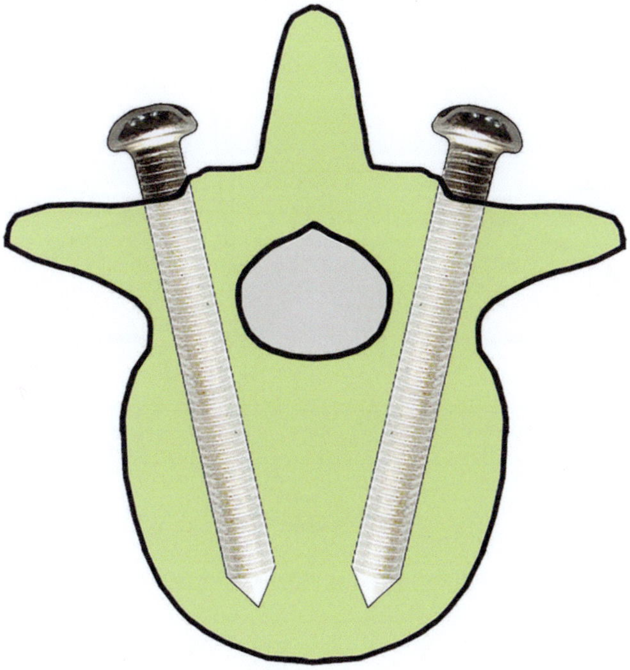

Fig. 10.32 Bilateral pedicle screw for posterior hemivertebra

3. X-ray finding of single or double hemivertebra on the same side constitutes indications for preventive resection, regardless of spinal mal-alignment.
4. Consent should be obtained from the family members of the patient to perform preventive surgery.

10.4.4 Contraindication

1. Beyond the age of 8 years, with a big curve, with prior history of hemivertebra resection, failure of wiring on the screws.
2. Congenital heart disease or other severe congenital organ malformations
3. Diplomyelia, syringomyelia, and meningocele as found by radiology
4. Cases without consent and signature by the family

10.4.5 Surgical Technique

1. Preoperative preparation: Preoperative X-ray is used to determine the position and number of hemivertebrae and analyze the progress of lateral curvature deformity. Prepare surgical instruments for hemivertebral resection and vertebral column resection (Fig. 10.33) and the internal fixation instruments for near side compression. As it is a preventive operation, it should be explained in detail with the family members and obtain the consent and signature of the family members.
2. Anesthesia: Local infiltration anesthesia or tracheal intubation anesthesia may be used according to the age and degree of the child.
3. Position: prone position.
4. Operation procedure:

   Step 1: The patient is in a prone position. After disinfection and draping, a posterior median incision is made along the spinous process. Expose bilateral lamina, articular process, and transverse process. First, release the ligaments and soft tissue attached to the contralateral transverse process, and then completely expose the lamina, articular process, and transverse processes on the side of the hemivertebra (Fig. 10.34).

   Step 2: Cut off the transverse process of the hemivertebrae (Fig. 10.35) and detach forward along the pedicle and vertebral body waist (Fig. 10.36). Directly get to the anterior longitudinal ligament. Expose the entire hemivertebrae. Lever the whole hemivertebrae up with a lever retractor (Fig. 10.37).

   Step 3: Osteotomy to remove the lamina and pedicle of the hemivertebrae and expose the epidural sac, nerve root, and pedicle of hemivertebrae (Figs. 10.38 and 10.39).

   Step 4: Before hemivertebrotomy, place extra-pedicle screws into the levels above and below the hemivertebrae (Fig. 10.40a, b).

   Step 5: Use straight osteotome to cut off pedicle and lateral part of the vertebral body layer by layer (Fig. 10.41), then cut off the inside part of the vertebra body with crescent osteotome and shovel osteotome (Figs. 10.42 and 10.43).

   Step 6: Temporarily retain a thin bone sheet at the posterior edge of the vertebral body to avoid bleeding from the epidural venous plexus. Finally, the posterior wall of the vertebral body is quickly removed by a push-down osteotome to complete the resection operation of the whole hemivertebrae (Figs. 10.44 and 10.45).

   Step 7: The operator touched if bone fragments in the osteotomy space with his finger (Fig. 10.46a, b). After hemivertebrotomy, the lateral pedicle screw and wire are used to close the gap of the osteotomy quickly, then lead to the epidural sac expansion to contact the epidural venous plexus and the bleeding would stop

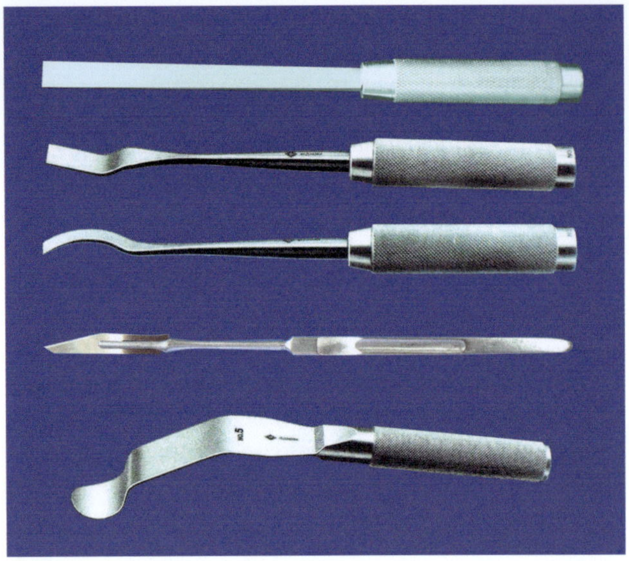

Fig. 10.33 These five tools are what hemivertebra resection needs

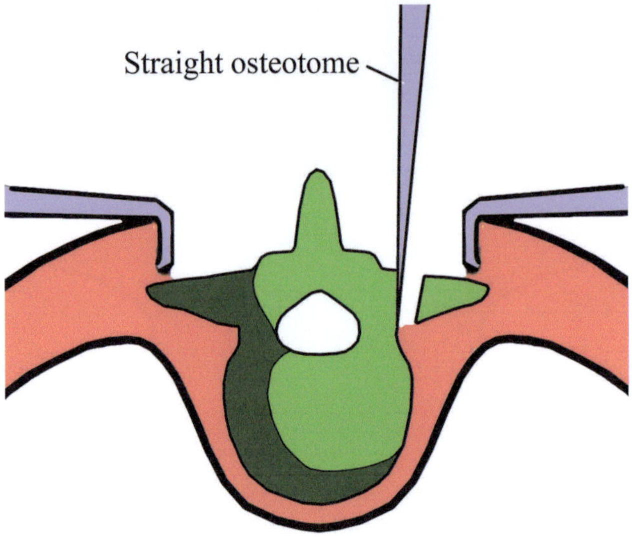

Fig. 10.35 Cut off the transverse process of the hemivertebrae

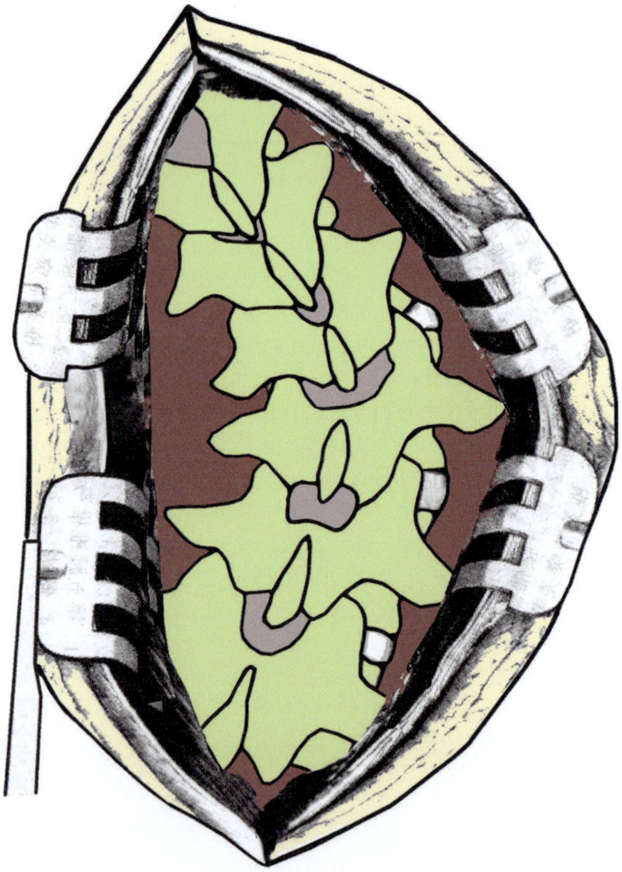

Fig. 10.34 Expose lamina cap and bilateral transverse processes through posterior approach

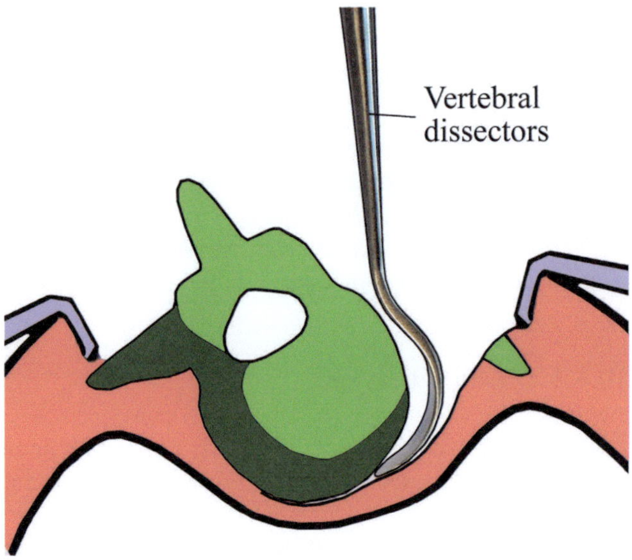

Fig. 10.36 Detach forward along the pedicle and vertebral body waist. Directly get to the anterior longitudinal ligament

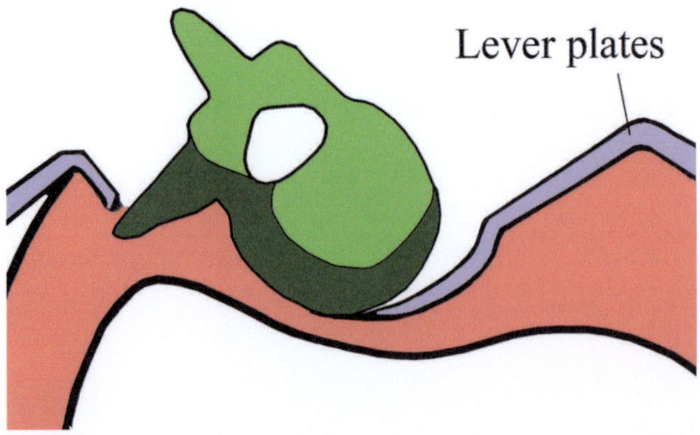

Fig. 10.37 Lever and expose the whole hemivertebrae up with a lever retractor

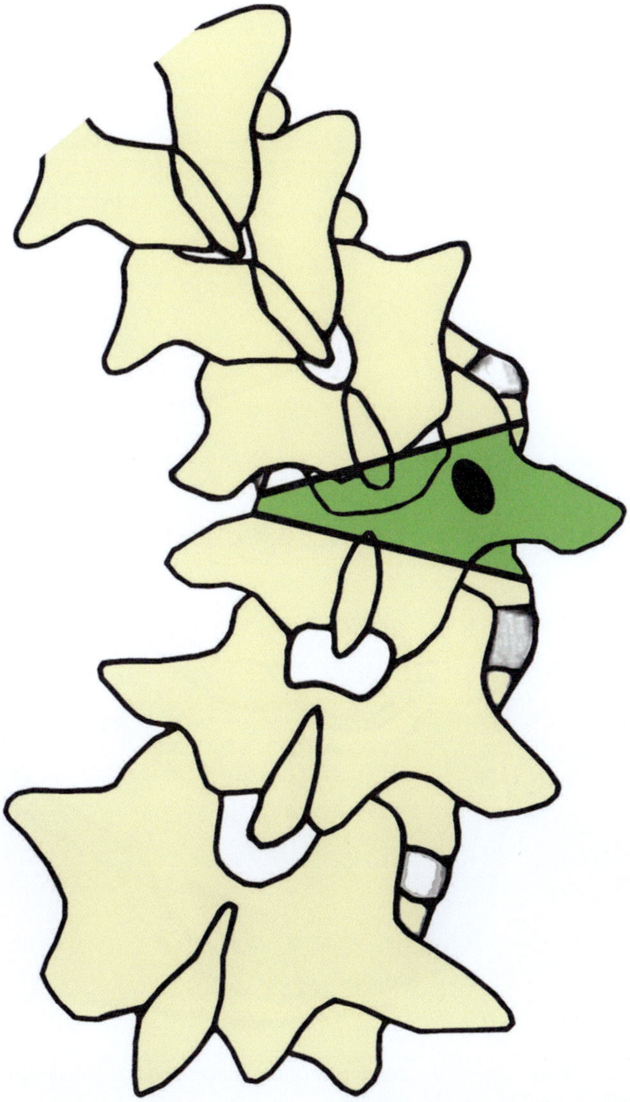

Fig. 10.38 Scope of laminectomy in wedge osteotomy

naturally (Fig. 10.47a, b). Alternatively, an extra-pedicle screw with titanium cable may be used (Fig. 10.48a, b).

5. Postoperative treatment:
   Flatbed rest in the ward. Remove the negative pressure drainage tube in 24–48 h. After removing the suture, patients should wear a brace or plaster vest as external immobilization for 4–6 months.

10.4.6 Advantages of Preventive Surgery and Instrumentation with Screw and Wiring

1. The advantages of early preventive osteotomy to remove the lateral hemivertebrae: simple operation, less bleeding, short operation time, and quick recovery.

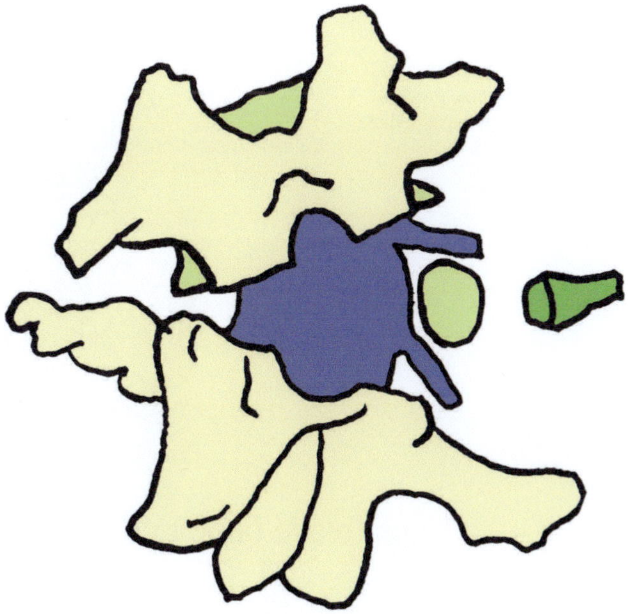

Fig. 10.39 Osteotomy for hemivertebra arch, expose the dural sac, nerve roots, and pedicles of the hemivertebra

2. Simple instrumentation: After hemivertebra resection, a lateral extra-pedicle screw with wire or titanium cable fixation (Fig. 10.49) will be sufficient to close the gap of the osteotomy without long segmental instrumentation.
3. The long-term effect of preventive hemivertebral osteotomy and instrumentation with screw and wiring is better than the epiphyseal arrest technique of compressing convex side only without hemivertebra osteotomy. The simple epiphyseal arrest technique is prone to fracture of wire or screw, and it is also difficult to prevent further progression of scoliosis.

10.4.7 Prevention of Complications

1. We should be careful about if there have a recessive lamina crack during elevation to avoid spinal cord injury.
2. The contralateral paravertebral soft tissue should be released first to create conditions to facilitate reduction after osteotomy.
3. The probability of excessive bleeding and hemorrhagic shock during the operation caused by prophylactic osteotomy is very small. Generally, the procedure does not require a large amount of intraoperative blood transfusion. Blood transfusion may even be spared.
4. The vertebral body in children is mostly composed of cartilage, so high-speed burr or electric saw is not good. Only sharp, thin-edged osteotomes are handy tools.
5. If the operation can be carried out by thin-blade osteotome and sharp osteotome, there is little damage to the

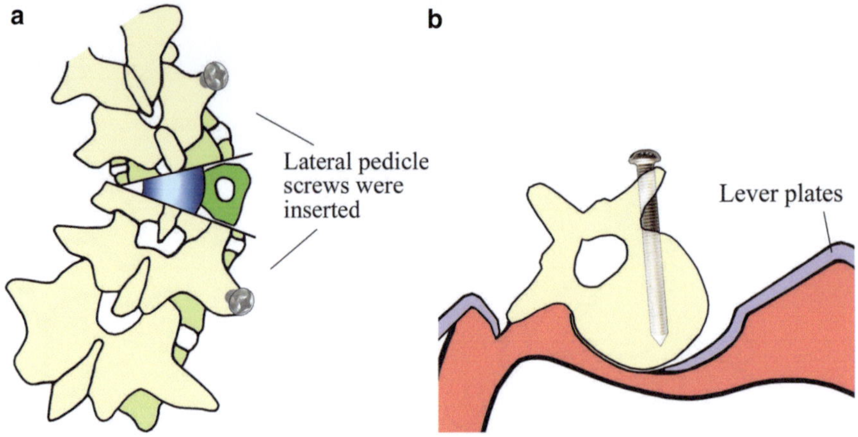

Fig. 10.40 Extra-pedicle screw technique. (**a**) Entry point of extra-pedicle screw: tip of the transverse process. (**b**) Trajectory of extra-pedicle screw

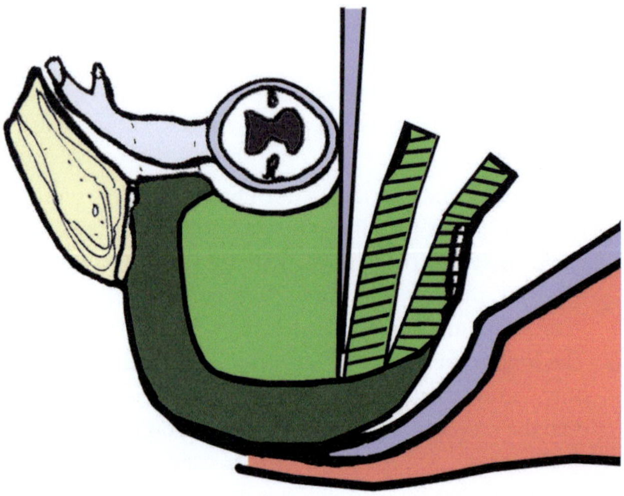

Fig. 10.41 Use straight osteotome to cut off pedicle and lateral part of the vertebral body layer by layer

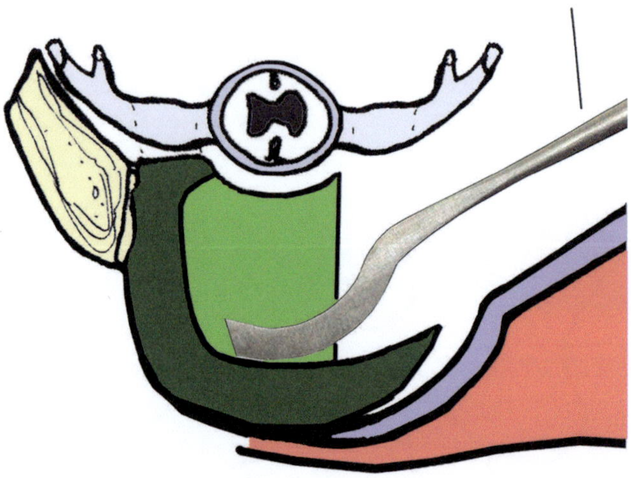

Fig. 10.42 Cut off the inside part of the vertebra body with crescent osteotome and shovel osteotome

spinal cord or nerve root under the circumstances of the operation skill and anatomical basis are available.

6. The possibility of accidentally injure of dural sac to cause "thread phenomenon" and cerebrospinal fluid leakage is also reduced because we do not use lamina rongeur to bite the bone tissue near the dural sac during the operation.
7. In order to avoid spinal cord injury due to instability after osteotomy, pedicle screws or extra-pedicle screws should be inserted first above or below the gap of the osteotomy.
8. Hemivertebra resection is not adequate. We should perform a wedge-shaped osteotomy to make the tip of the wedge reach the contralateral side of the vertebra, so that we can close the osteotomy space to correct the deformity smoothly when we place compression internal fixation.
9. The segmental vessels anterior to the vertebrae do not need to be ligated. Strict subperiosteum elevation with a lever retractor is helpful to achieve hemostasis.
10. Controlling epidural venous plexus bleeding can be achieved by compression of the epidural venous plexus by shortening and widening dural sac by rapidly closing the gap after osteotomy.
11. With an extra-pedicle screw and wiring to close the osteotomy gap, the closure of the osteotomy space can be properly approximated to avoid nonunion after operation.
12. Pedicle screws and wiring is suitable for younger patients who only need convex side compression without concave side distraction. For older children, concave distraction and convex compression are required simultaneously.

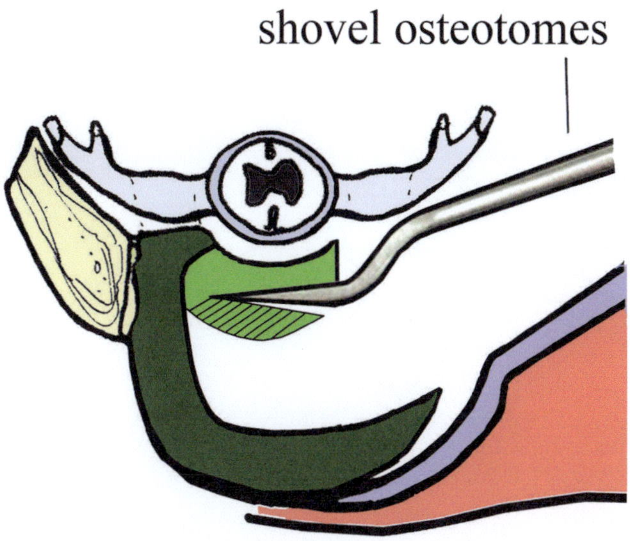

Fig. 10.43 Resect the central part of vertebral body with a shovel osteotome

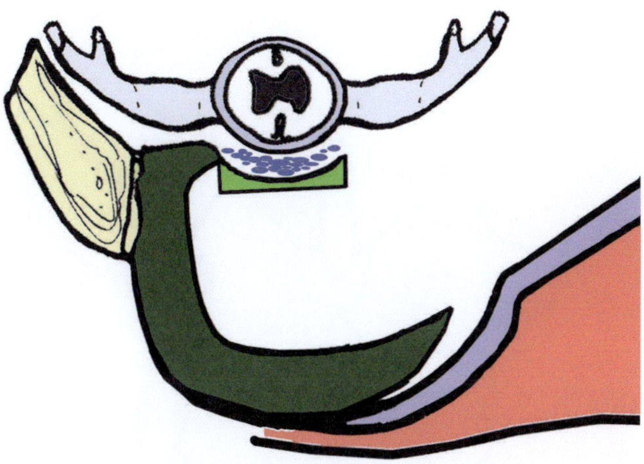

Fig. 10.44 The posterior margin of the vertebral body was preserved temporarily

10.4.8 Conclusion

Early preventive osteotomy for congenital hemivertebrae prevents the progression of spinal curvature. The treatment will be more difficult upon progression. Extra-pedicle screw and wiring simplifies the operation process and improves the biomechanical effect of scoliosis correction.

10.5 Posterior Hemivertebral Osteotomy

The formation of the congenital posterior hemivertebrae may be related to the forward extension of the bilateral pedicle ossification centers which fuse with the posterior part of the vertebral ossification center and related to the developmental

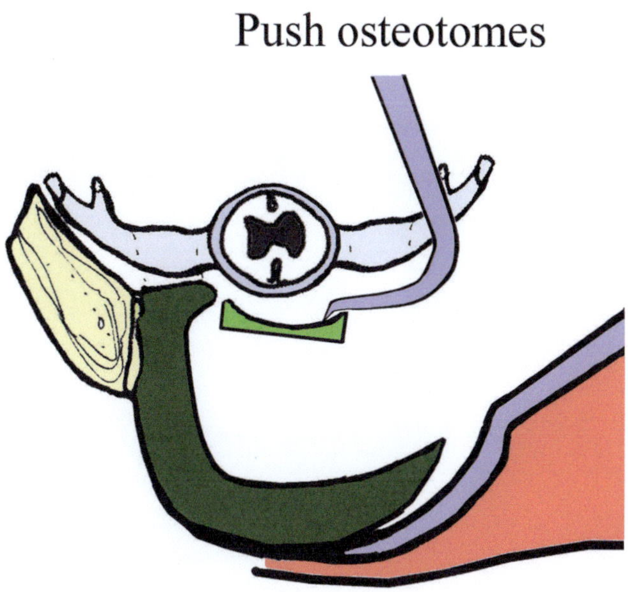

Fig. 10.45 Rapid reduction of the posterior margin of the vertebral body with a push-down knife

disorder of the ossification center of the vertebral anterior part. The spinal deformity caused by the congenital posterior hemivertebral body is angular kyphosis, which should be distinguished from spinal tuberculosis in X-ray diagnosis. There is no paravertebral abscess on coronal X-ray, and there is no narrowing of the intervertebral space on the lateral view, no vertebral bone destruction and the presence of dead bone, and its angular kyphosis are generally less than 90° Cobb angle. On the lateral view, the posterior hemivertebrae usually looks round, and the anterior edge of the upper and lower vertebrae is often present fish-mouth signs (Fig. 10.50). The type of surgery that treats congenital posterior hemivertebral deformity is to retain the upper and lower bilateral endplate, and resect through the waist of the vertebra or whole hemivertebra. With additional internal fixation, the result is usually satisfying. As the kyphosis angle caused by congenital posterior hemivertebrae is smaller than that caused by tuberculous kyphosis, there are fewer adhesions in the epidural space, and the bleeding during operation is relatively limited. Thus, the posterior hemivertebra is the absolute indication for vertebral column resection through the posterior route.

10.5.1 How the Posterior Hemivertebra Is Formed

Clinically, the congenital posterior hemivertebrae is less common than the congenital lateral hemivertebrae. According to the author, the formation of the posterior hemivertebrae may be associated with embryonic development. Each vertebra consists of three primary ossification centers: primary

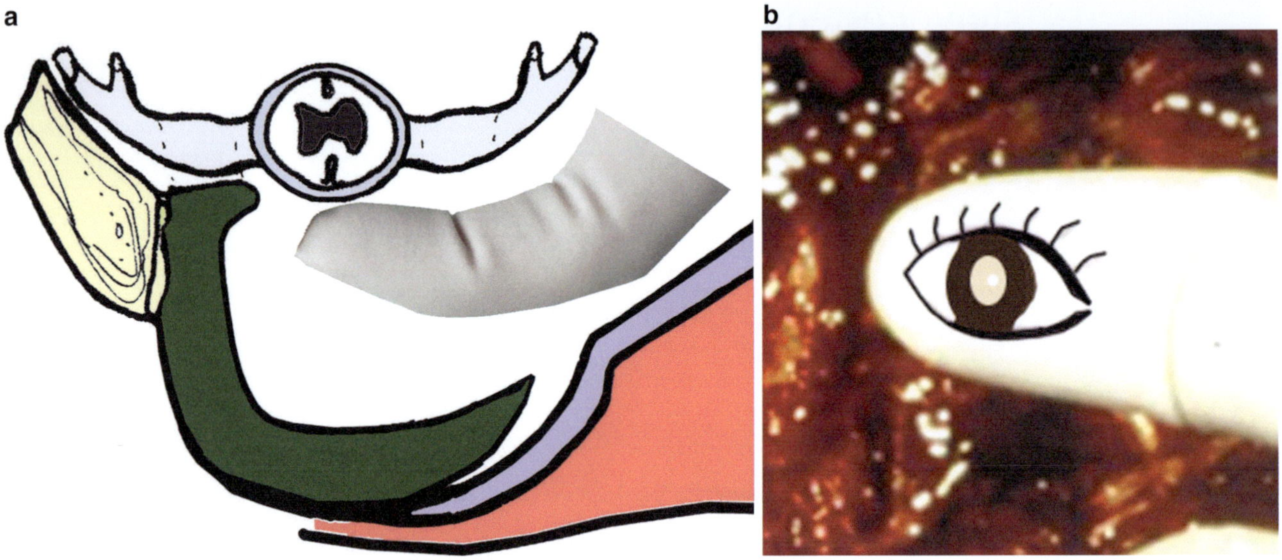

Fig. 10.46 Palpate the presence of bone fragments in the osteotomy space. (**a**) Palpitation for bone fragments in the osteotomy gap. (**b**) Check bone fragments with palpitation instead of visual inspection

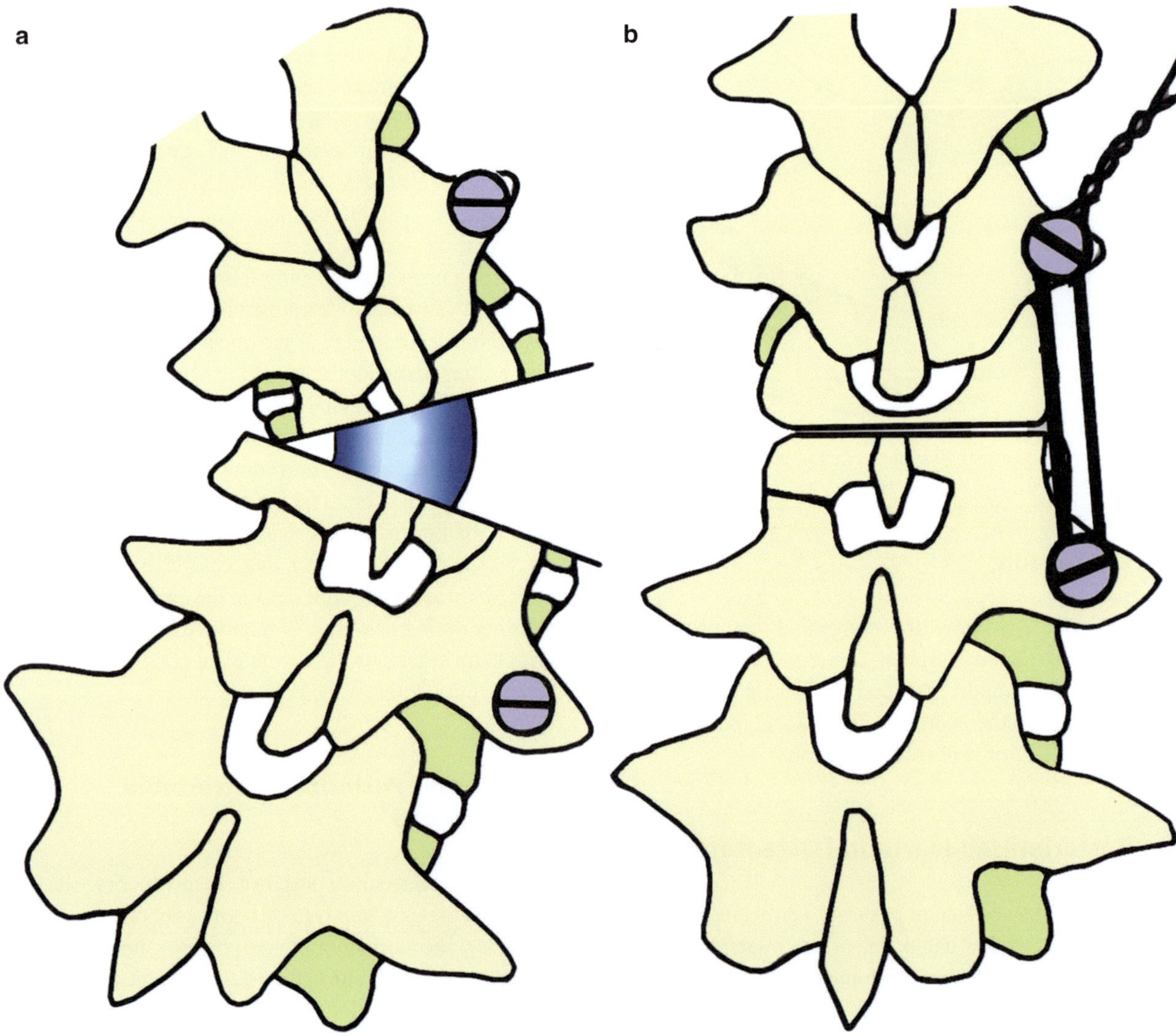

Fig. 10.47 Extra-pedicle screw with wiring. (**a**) After osteotomy, (**b**) after compression with wiring

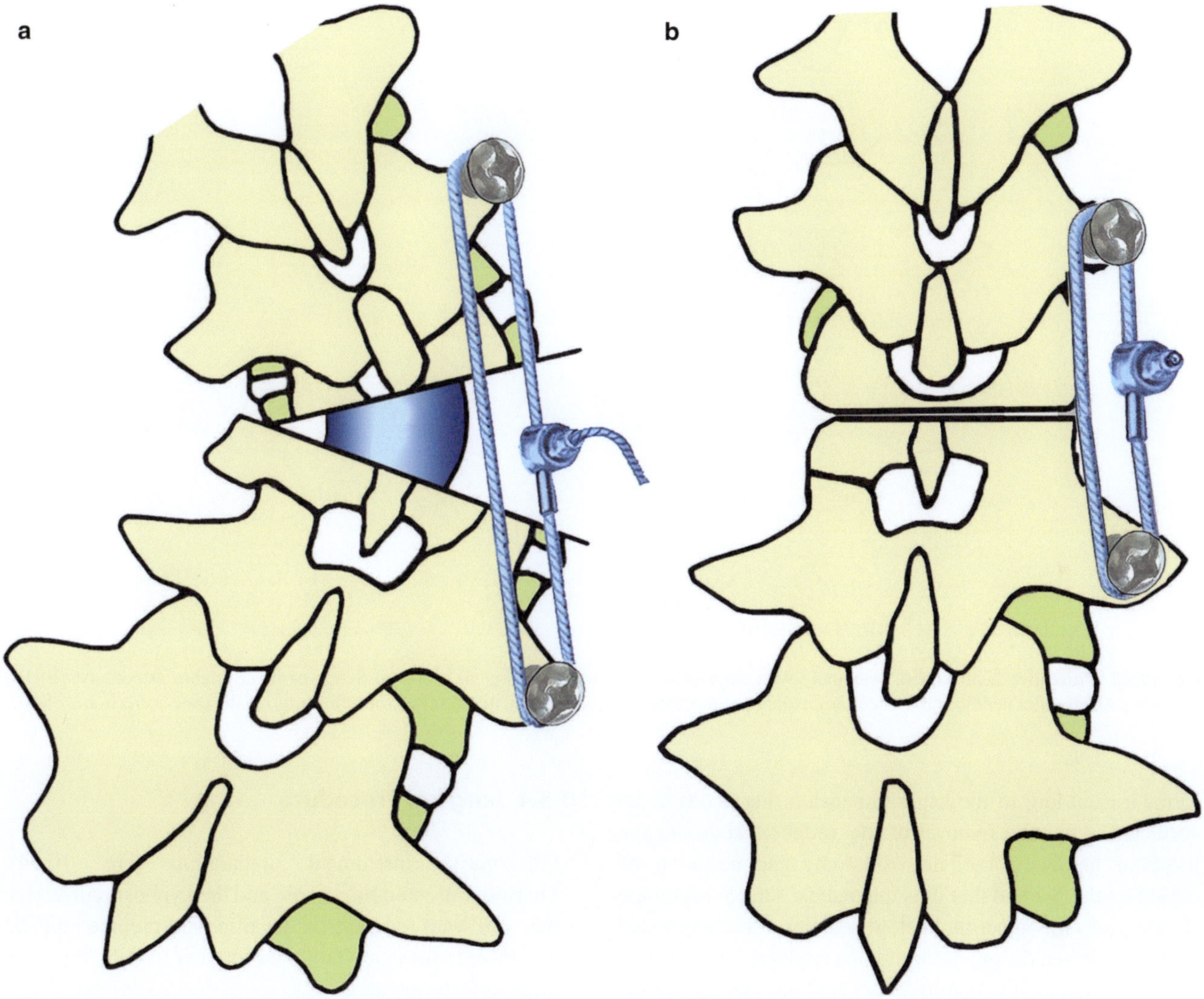

Fig. 10.48 Extra-pedicle screw with titanium cable fixation. (**a**) Titanium cable applied. (**b**) Titanium cable tensioned

vertebral body ossification center; left and right primary vertebral arch and pedicle ossification center. When the posterior part of the vertebral body ossification center develops vigorously with the vertebral arch and the pedicle ossification center, the two form one body. While the anterior part of the vertebral body ossification center develops with dysplasia or absence, the posterior hemivertebra and an extra vertebral arch form. With the development of posterior hemivertebrae and an extra vertebral arch, angled kyphotic deformity will be aggravated year by year. By the age of 15–18, kyphosis of 60–90 Cobb degree is often seen.

10.5.2 Examination Method

Anterioposterior and lateral X-ray film of the spine is performed to determine the segment of the posterior hemivertebral deformity and the extent of angular scoliosis (Fig. 10.51a–c), and whether there are symptoms and signs of spinal cord compression. If necessary, spinal angiography, MRI examination, and CT examination should be performed to illustrate the relationship between kyphosis and spinal canal.

10.5.3 Osteotomy and Instrumentation

It is the most effective technique to remove the extra vertebral arch and posterior hemivertebrae with a thin-blade sharp osteotome. As the vertebral arch and vertebral body of children are mostly composed of cartilage tissue and bone tissue, its texture is similar to hard rubber. It is very suitable for cutting with a thin-blade osteotome. Tian's set of osteotome is used to remove the pedicle and posterior half of the vertebrae, which can easily solve the problems. Total posterior hemivertebral resection or subtotal excision can be per-

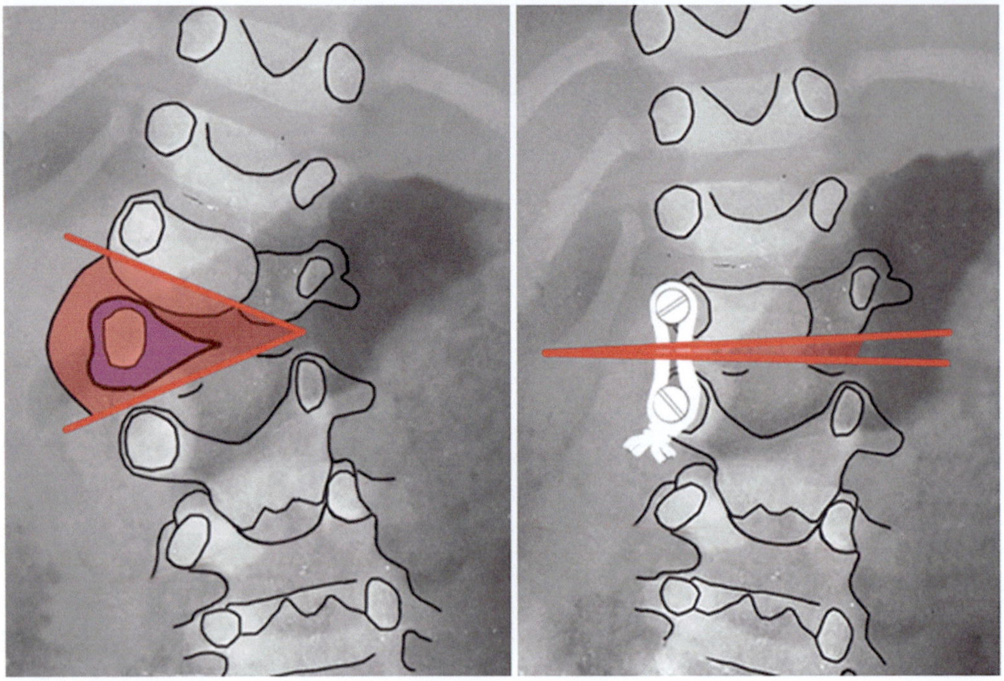

Fig. 10.49 Preventive hemivertebra osteotomy with extra-pedicle screw and wiring fixation. (**a**) Scope of hemivertebra osteotomy; (**b**) For younger patients, after hemivertebra osteotomy, compression wiring fixation is adequate to correct the deformity, ideally over-correction by 5–10°

formed according to the angle dimension that needs to be corrected. After the removal of the vertebral arch and the posterior hemivertebrae, the osteotomy gap needs to be closed by the method that uses the pedicle screws which are inserted into the upper and below pedicles and compressed with rods. When the gap is closed, the epidural tube is shortened and expanded to compress the epidural venous plexus. Bleeding from epidural venous plexus will stop. For younger patients, in order not to avoid restricting growth and development, proximal compression can be used to close the osteotomy gap, and using a growth rod to maintain straightness of the spine can make the growth of the spine unrestricted. This method can also replace the surgical method of internal fixation of the posterior screw–rod system.

To children younger than 8 years old with light kyphosis deformity, we can use pedicle screws and wire to compress and fixate the vertebra without opening the distal end after posterior hemivertebral excision (Fig. 10.52a, b), and use a plaster vest to immobilize the patient postoperatively. To the children over 8 years old with obvious kyphosis deformity, we should distract the distal end and compress near the end to fixate the vertebra after posterior hemivertebral resection (Fig. 10.53a, b), and use a plaster vest to immobilize postoperatively.

10.5.4 Surgical Procedure

1. Preoperative instrument preparation (Fig. 10.54): Measure the osteotomy angle and the kyphosis correction that you want to reach on the film, and prepare surgical instruments for osteotomy and internal fixation type and internal instruments.
2. Anesthesia: Endotracheal intubation general anesthesia
3. Body Position: The patient takes the prone position, lying on the Hall–Relton frame, make the abdomen unsupported to reduce abdominal pressure and venous bleeding. The upper arm and elbow should be carefully padded and the shoulder abduction should not exceed 90°. The upper two points of the 4 point bracket hold the chest, not the armpit. The lower two points should support the anterior superior iliac spines, do not hold in the abdomen
4. Operation procedure:
   Step 1: Patient takes prone position. After disinfecting and draping, the incisions are made in the midline along the spinous processes, exposing the bilateral lamina, articular processes, and transverse processes. Identify the bilateral transverse processes of posterior hemivertebrae. And remove the transverse process. Perform subperiosteum elevation along the lateral edge of pedicles to the

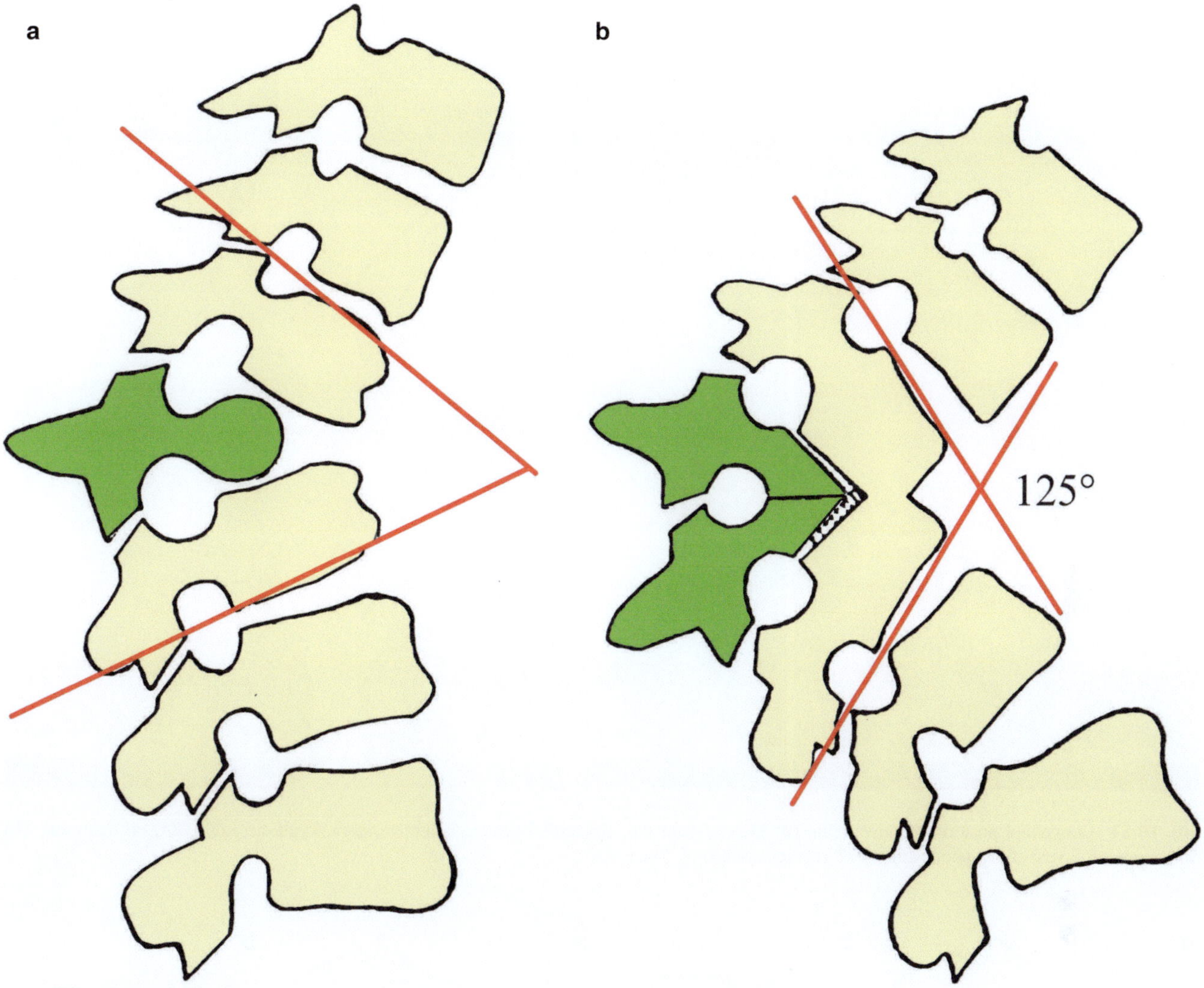

Fig. 10.50 Differential diagnosis for congenital posterior hemivertebra and TB angular kyphosis: (**a**) Congenital posterior hemivertebra deformity, roundish hemivertebra, protruding to the posterior, fish-mouth relation between the upper and lower vertebra. No bony fusion in the disc space. The kyphotic angle is less than 90°. (**b**) The angle of TB angular kyphosis is usually more than 90°, with 3–4 vertebra involved in the apex. Interbody bony fusion commonly exists

hemivertebra and anterior-lateral edge of vertebral bodies up and down. Insert lever retractor bilaterally to expose the vertebral body (Fig. 10.55).

Step 2: Remove the entire lamina of the hemivertebrae with an osteotome or rongeurs. And expose the dorsal side of the bilateral pedicle, epidural tube, and spinal roots (Fig. 10.56a, b).

Step 3: To identify the upper and lower edges of the hemivertebra from its bilateral sides. Using an osteotome to mark a scope of osteotomy, that is, a wedge with its base toward the posterior. Its wedge tip reaches the anterior longitudinal ligament, its base reaches the posterior longitudinal ligament, and its bilateral wedge-shaped osteotomy lines align with each other (Fig. 10.57).

Step 4: Resect layer by layer with an osteotome from the lateral edge of the pedicle and vertebrae, to the medial edge of the pedicle, and after excision of the medial edge of the pedicle, expose the lateral of epidural tube (Fig. 10.58).

Step 5: Before the vertebrae is fully resected, the pedicle screws are placed in the upper and lower pedicle first to avoid spinal cord injury caused by instability after vertebral body truncation (Fig. 10.59).

Step 6: Before resecting the posterior edge of the vertebrae, use a wire or rod for temporary fixation to prevent spinal cord injury caused by instability (Fig. 10.60). Excision of the posterior edge of the hemivertebrae requires a posterior longitudinal ligament elevator, push

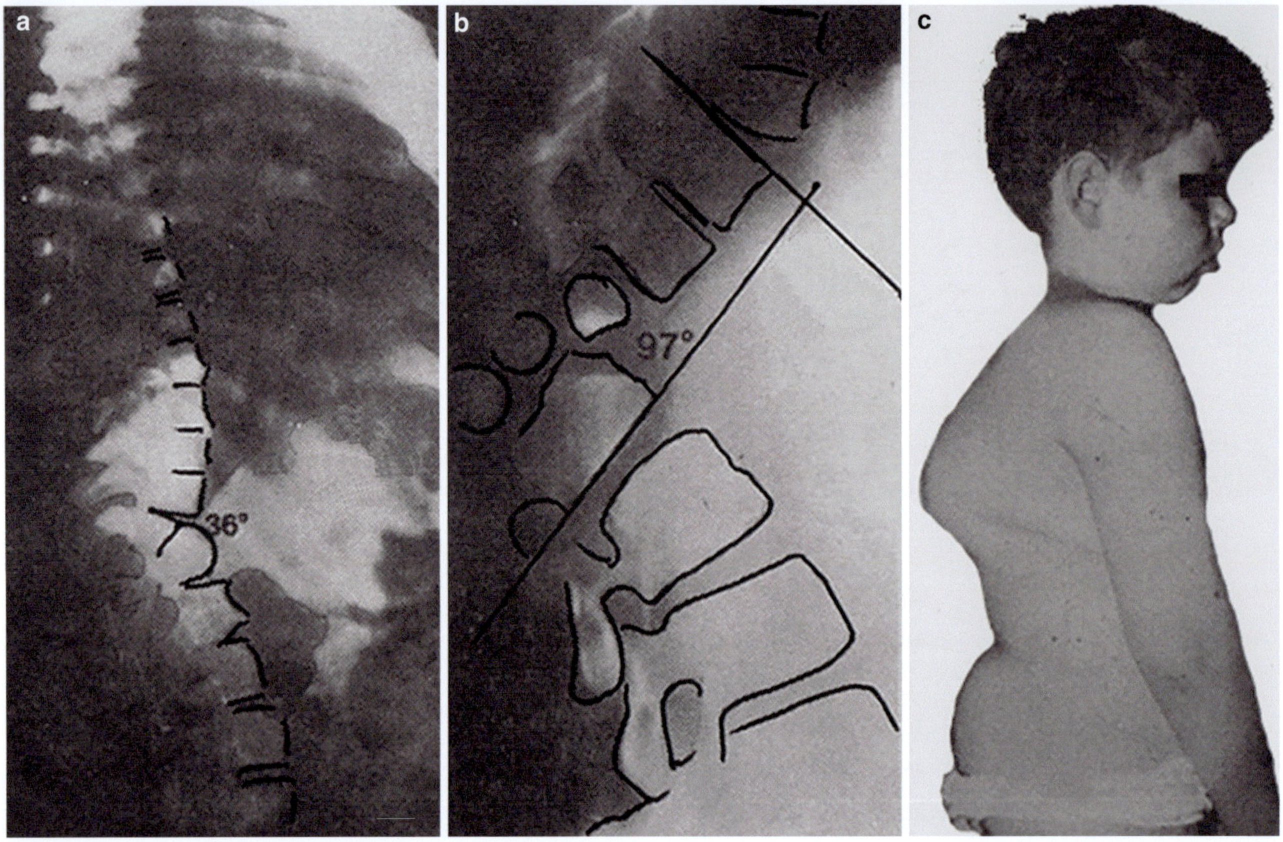

Fig. 10.51 Congenital posterior hemivertebra: (**a**) Male, 1-year-old, congenital posterior hemivertebra, kyphotic angle 36°, no treatment. (**b**) Same patient, 7-year-old kyphotic angle 97°. (**c**) Appearance of 7-year-old

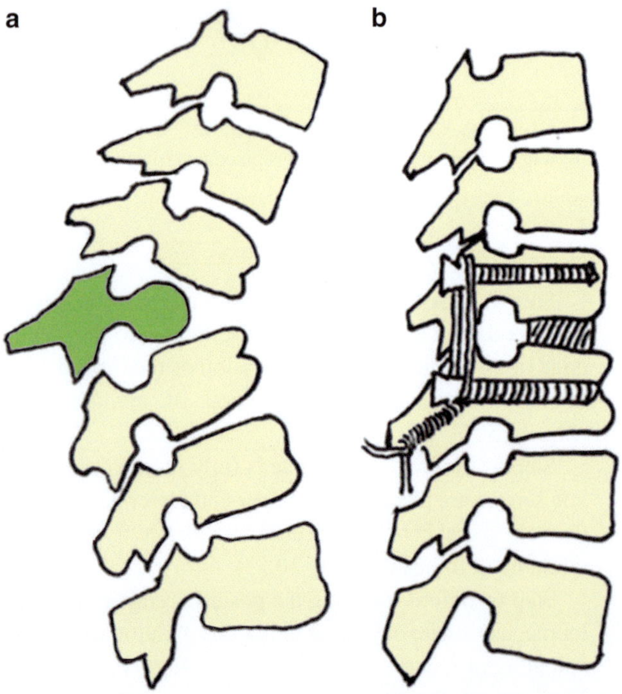

Fig. 10.52 (**a**) Congenital posterior hemivertebra, round shape, fish-mouth sign of anterior vertebral bodies up and down. (**b**) After posterior hemivertebra resection for children below 8, deformity is corrected with compression only

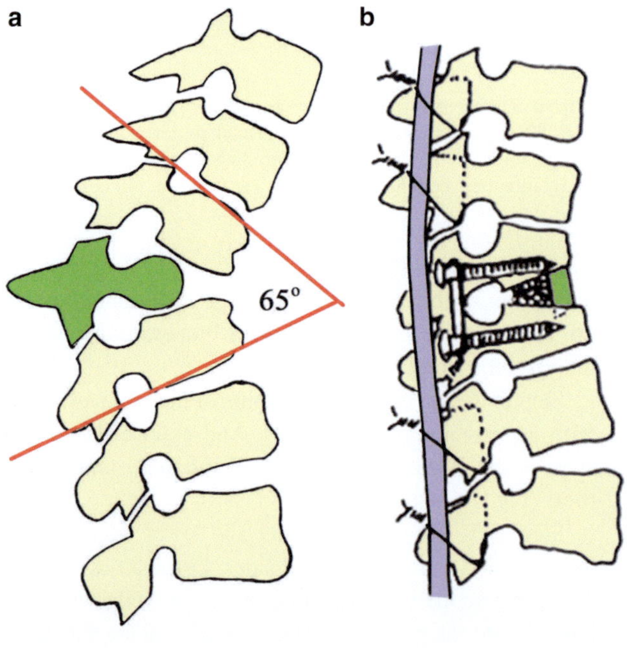

Fig. 10.53 (**a**) Congenital posterior hemivertebra, Cobb angle 60–90°. (**b**) After posterior hemivertebra resection for children above 8, distal distraction and proximal compression is preferred

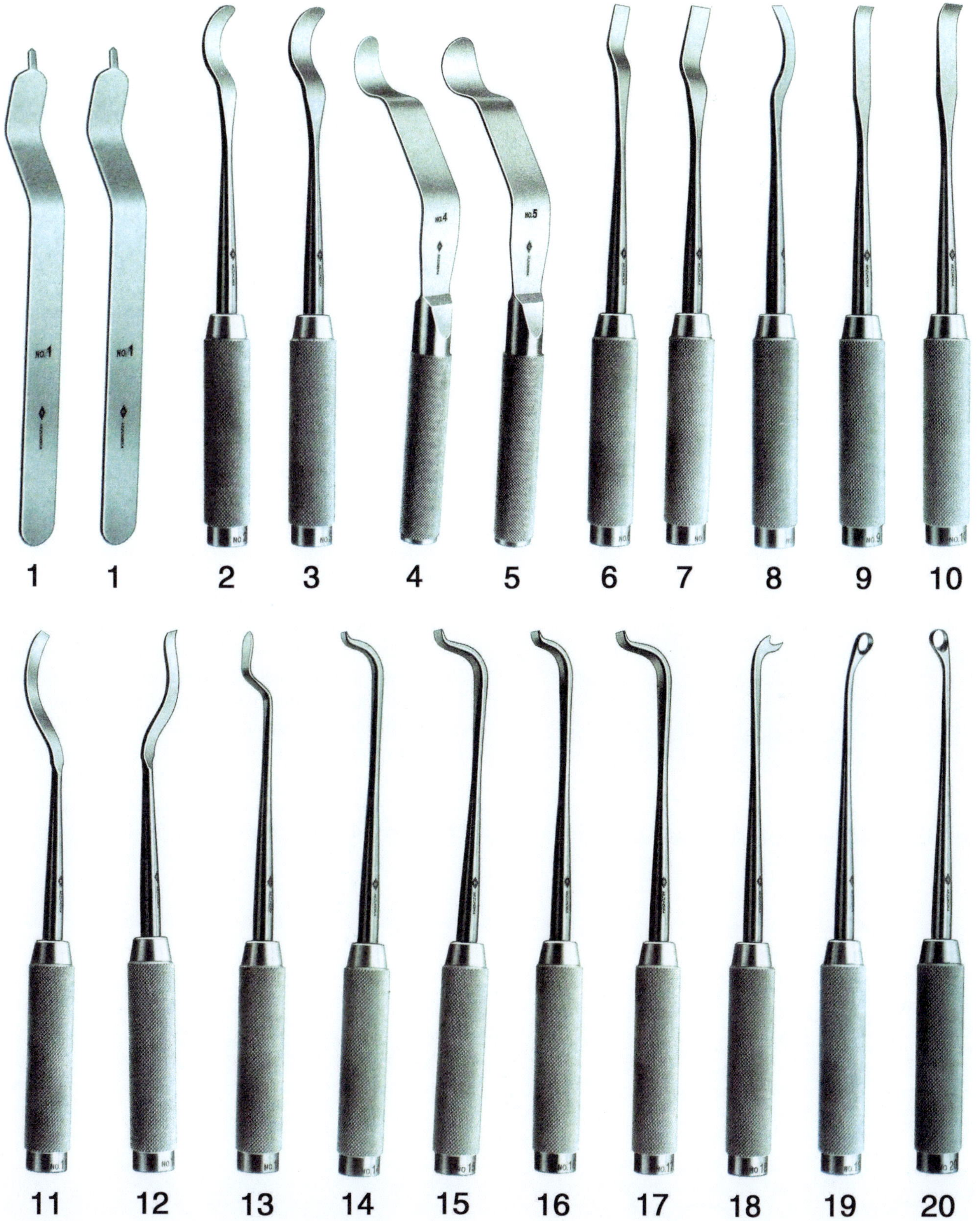

Fig. 10.54 A set of Tian's osteotomes with various angles

the posterior longitudinal ligament and epidural venous plexus, then push the thin layer bone at the posterior edge of the vertebral body with a push-down osteotome. The fragments are removed with medullary forceps (Fig. 10.61a, b). Until after bilateral osteotomy is completed, the fingers can touch each other in the front of the epidural tube and palpate for the presence of any residual bone fragments within the osteotomy space (Fig. 10.62).

Step 7: After complete excision of the pedicle and posterior hemivertebrae, then perform reduction and internal fixation (Fig.10.63a, b). The bleeding can be controlled due to the epidural tube is shorten and expansion so that compress the epidural venous plexus.

5. Postoperative management:
   Younger patients without cranial pelvic ring traction lie on flatbed after returning to the ward and the negative pressure drainage tube is removed after 24–48 h. Plaster-of-Paris jacket external fixation should be used for 6–10 months after taking out the suture (Fig. 10.64a, b), and come to the hospital regularly for re-examination of X-ray films.

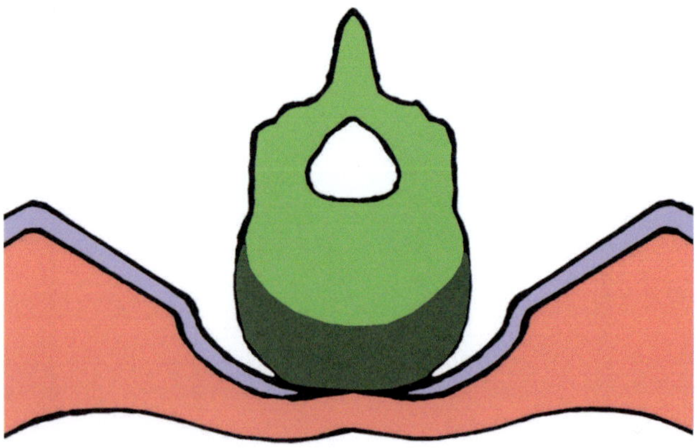

Fig. 10.55 Bilateral exposure of posterior hemivertebra

10.5.5 Key Points for Prevention of Complications

1. Clarify the diagnosis that whether congenital posterior hemivertebrae or tuberculous kyphosis before the operation. Because the congenital posterior hemivertebrae is the absolute indication of this operation, its operation is not difficult. And it is more difficult to perform total spinal osteotomy with tuberculous angular posterior convexity. If not prepared enough, to treat tuberculous kyphosis as a congenital posterior hemivertebrae is likely to encounter difficulties.
2. You should be careful to determine the hemivertebrae lamina during the operation, and must not recognize the wrong one. Only resect one hemivertebrae lamina is sufficient. If necessary, you can determine the position of the hemivertebra with C-arm.
3. The posterior edge of the vertebral body should be retained when excising vertebra, so as not to cause difficulty in operation by the turbulent bleeding of the epidural venous plexus.
4. When the adhesion between the posterior edge of the vertebral body and the dural sac is too close, it can be treated with the method of thin bone fragment floating, but there is no difficulty in congenital patients.
5. Protective measures for temporary internal fixation of pedicle screws and wire or rod should be done first before vertebral column resection is done to prevent the instability of the spine.

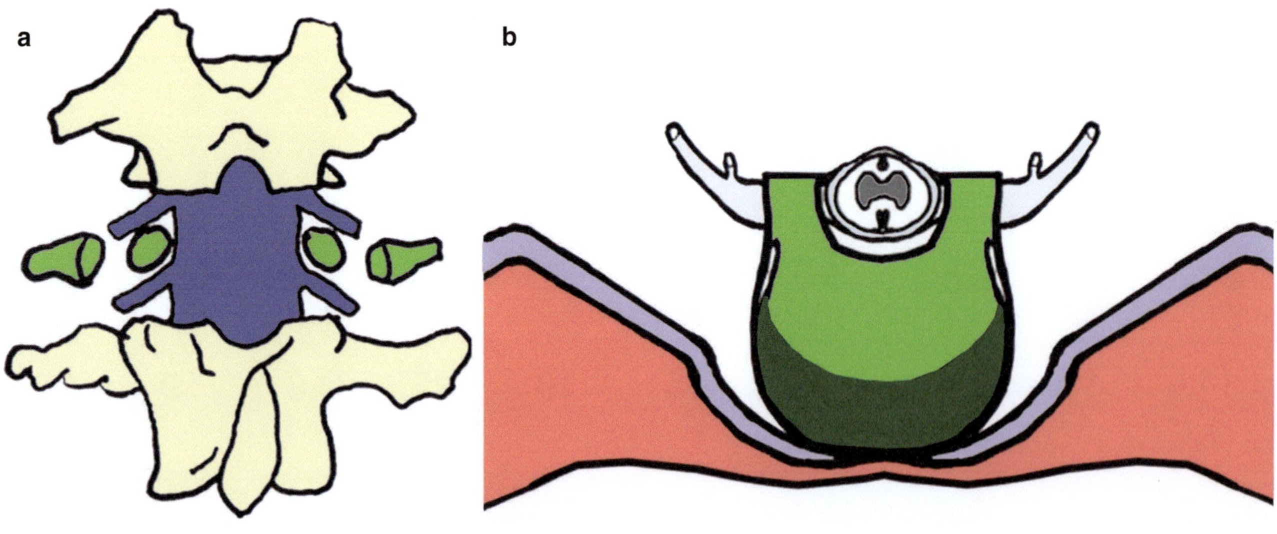

Fig. 10.56 (**a**) Posterior view, arch is removed. (**b**) Axial view, arch is removed

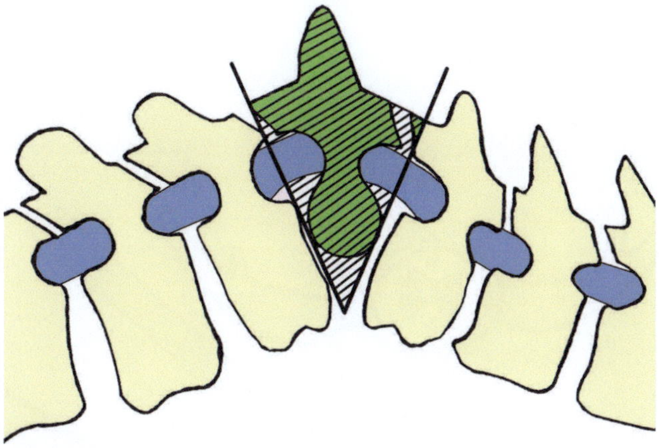

Fig. 10.57 Scope of wedge osteotomy

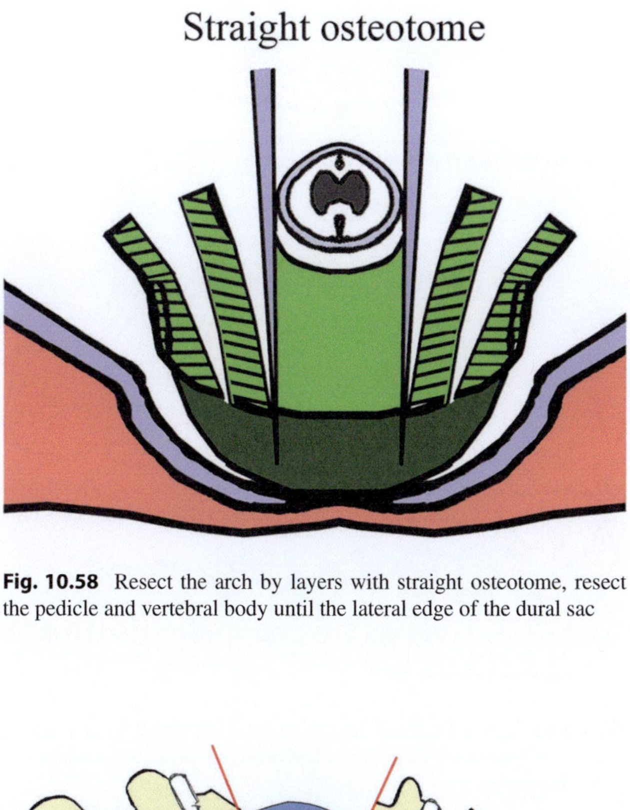

Fig. 10.58 Resect the arch by layers with straight osteotome, resect the pedicle and vertebral body until the lateral edge of the dural sac

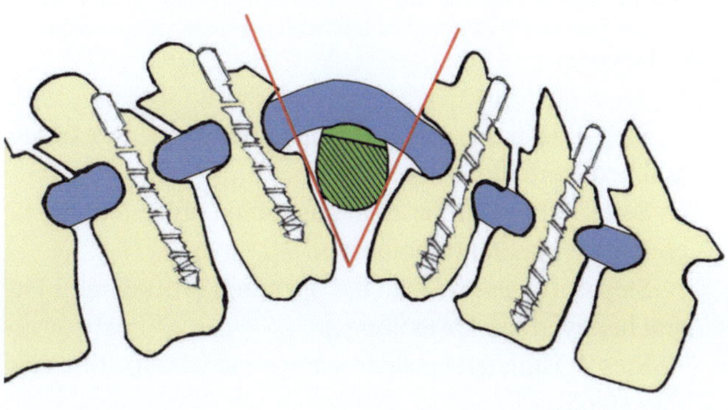

Fig. 10.59 Pedicle screws inserted before truncating the spine

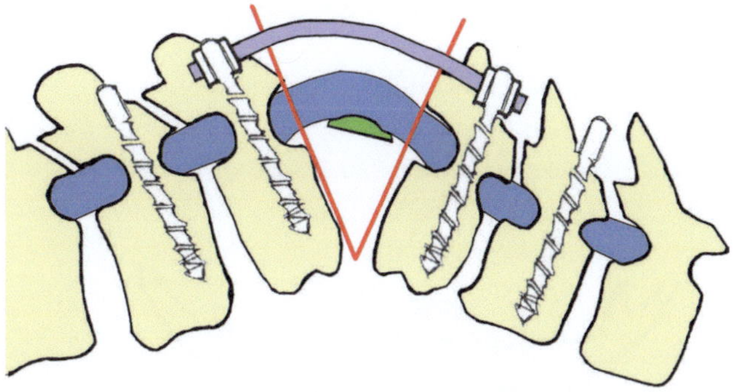

Fig. 10.60 Temporary rod inserted and ready to remove the posterior bone sheet

10.6 Posterolateral Hemivertebral Osteotomy

The operation procedures of congenital posterolateral hemivertebral osteotomy and congenital lateral hemivertebral osteotomy are similar. It is also through the posterior approach, dissecting and exposing from one side to the anterior. Wedge osteotomy is performed on the posterolateral vertebra, and the tip of the wedge osteotomy should reach the contralateral side of the vertebra; otherwise, it will bring difficulties to close the osteotomy gap and correct deformity if hemivertebra is the only structure to be resected. As the base of the wedge gap faces on the posterolateral side of the spine, so it is suitable to use unilateral pedicle screws for internal fixation (Fig. 10.65a–e). This is different with paralateral hemivertebra about the method that using extra-pedicle screws for internal fixation. The rest of the procedure is close to lateral hemivertebra osteotomy.

10.6.1 Surgical Procedure

1. Preoperative preparation: Preoperative imaging to locate the anatomical position of the hemivertebra, whether the wedge base of the hemivertebra is toward the posterolateral side, and analysis of the direction of the osteotomy. Determine fixation techniques such as pedicle screw or extra-pedicle screw. As the operation is a preventive operation, the family should be interviewed in detail to obtain the consent and signature of the family.
2. Anesthesia: According to the cooperativeness of the kid, choose the appropriate anesthesia such as endotracheal intubation general anesthesia or local infiltration anesthesia.
3. Position: Prone position is general used.
4. Operation procedure:

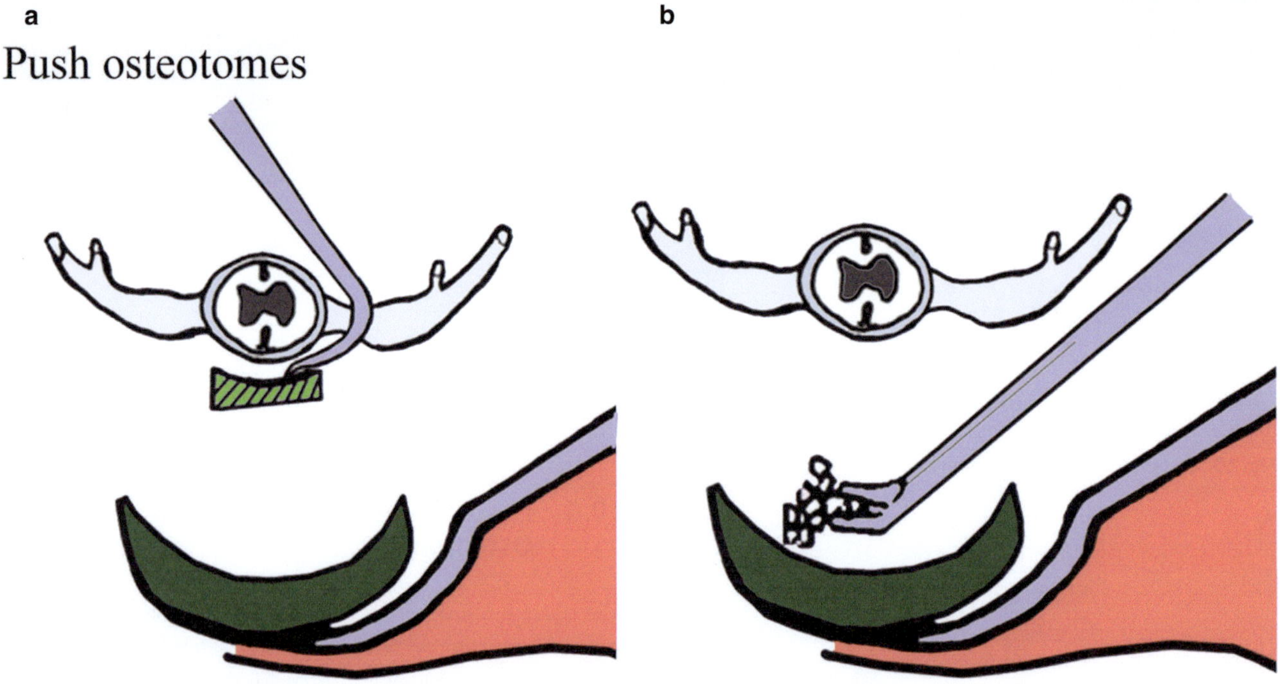

Fig. 10.61 (**a**) Push down the posterior bone sheet with push-down osteotome. (**b**) Remove bone debris with forceps

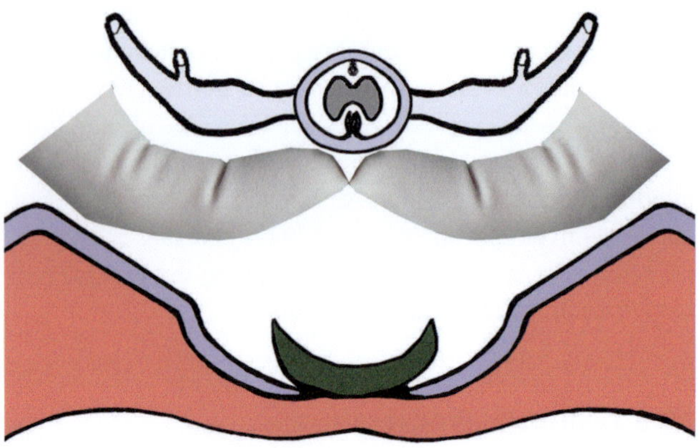

Fig. 10.62 Explore the osteotomy gap with fingers for any residue bone debris

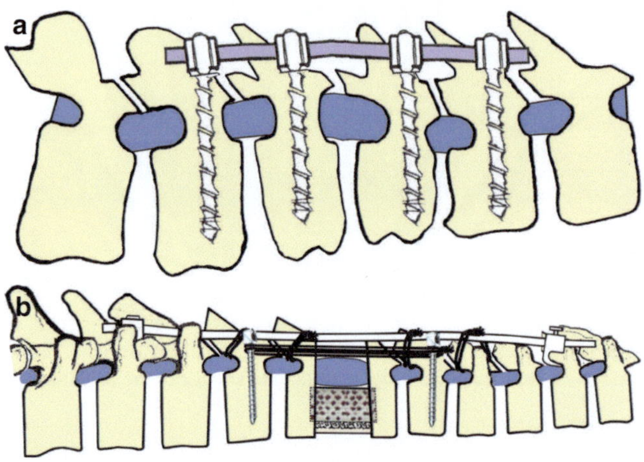

Fig. 10.63 Internal fixation. (**a**) The method of internal fixation with a screw–rod system. (**b**) Internal fixation with proximal compression and distal distraction

Step 1: After disinfecting and draping, make a longitudinal incision along spinous processes to expose the bilateral lamina and transverse process. Release contralateral soft tissue first, and then expose the lamina, articular processes, and transverse processes of one side of the hemivertebrae. (Please refer to the operation procedure of lateral hemivertebral osteotomy.)

Step 2: (Please refer to the operation procedure of lateral hemivertebral osteotomy.)

Step 3: (Please refer to the operation procedure of lateral hemivertebral osteotomy.)

Step 4: (Please refer to the operation procedure of lateral hemivertebral osteotomy.)

Step 5: (Please refer to the operation procedure of lateral hemivertebral osteotomy.)

Step 6: (Please refer to the operation procedure of lateral hemivertebral osteotomy.)

Step 7: Unilateral pedicle screws and wire fixation (see Fig. 10.65).

5. Postoperative management: Same as the postoperation procedure of lateral hemivertebral osteotomy.

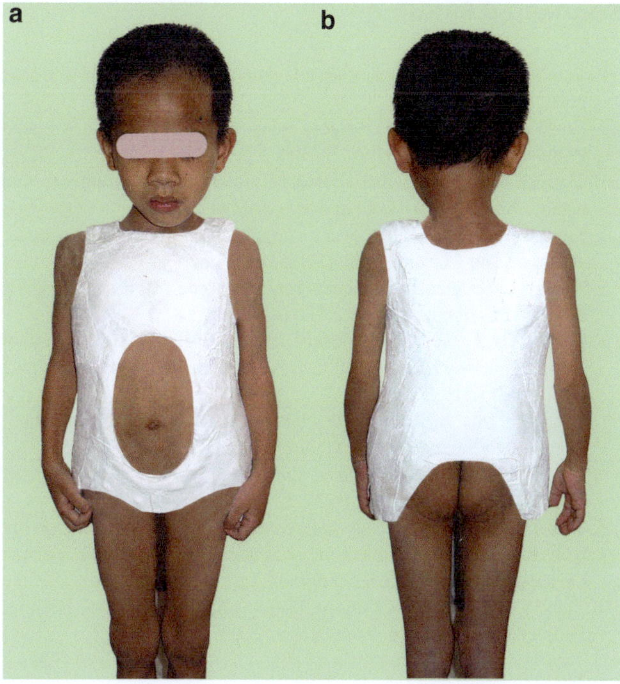

Fig. 10.64 Plaster vest immobilization is very important for postoperative management over any potential bone growth. Internal fixation only without external is wrong. Postoperative immobilization should last for 8–10 months. (**a**) Frontal view. (**b**) Back view

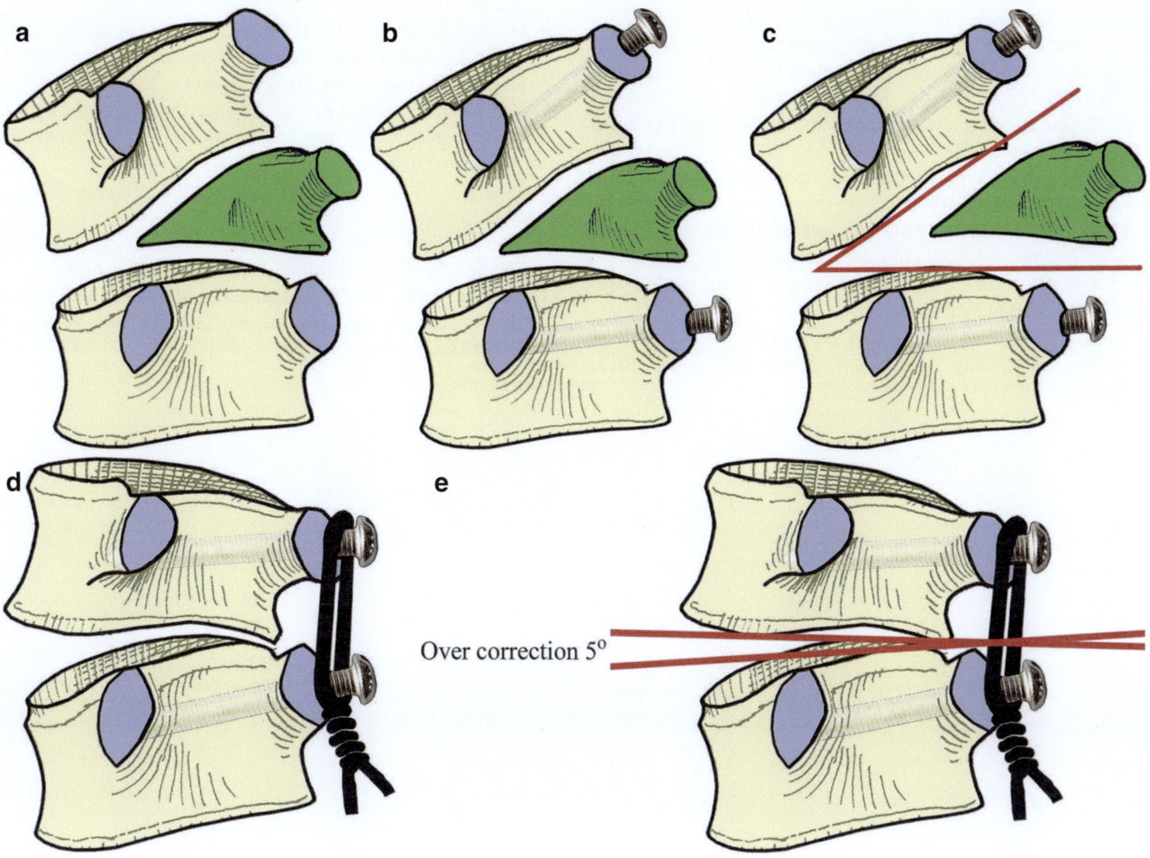

Fig. 10.65 Intersection view of posterior-lateral hemivertebra: illustration of posterior-lateral hemivertebra osteotome. (**a**) Posterior-lateral hemivertebra. (**b**) Unilateral pedicle screw insertion before osteotomy. (**c**) Wedge hemivertebra osteotomy. (**d**) Unilateral pedicle screw and wiring fixation. (**e**) Overcorrection by 5–10°

Suggested Reading

1. Tian H, Li F. Spinal deformity and osteotomy. Xi'an: World Book; 2001. p. 377–519.
2. Chen A, Xu W. Spinal surgery atlas. Beijing: People's Medical Publishing House; 2001. p. 77–300.
3. Tian H. Spinal surgeons should be good at using rongeurs and osteotome. Chin J Mod Oper Surg. 2002;6(1):67–9.
4. Tian H. Application of "Tian's spinal bone knife" in orthopaedic surgery. Chin J Orthop. 2003;11(15):1073–5.
5. Dang G. Surgical techniques for the spine. Beijing: People's Medical Publishing House; 2004. p. 102–245.
6. Tian H, Lv X, Ma Y. Treatment of severe spinal curvature with total spine osteotomy and internal fixation with head-sleeve ring. Chin J Orthop. 2007;15(3):167–72.
7. Tian H, Liu S, Ma Y. Practical spine surgery. Guangzhou: Guangdong Science and Technology Press; 2008. p. 87–285.
8. Tian H, Liu S, Ma Y. Practical spine surgery illustration. Beijing: People's Military Medical Press; 2008. p. 152–546.
9. Tian H, Ma Y, Lv X. Halo pelvic distraction and elastic growing rods fixation for treatment of scoliosis during growing period. Orthop J Chin. 2008;16(21):1660–3.
10. Tian H, Bai J, Liu S. Operative orthopaedics gist & atlas. Beijing: People's Medical Publishing House; 2009. p. 93–144.
11. Tian H. History of treatment of spinal deformity in China. Chin J Orthop. 2009;17(9):706–7.
12. Tian H, Wan Y, Li M. Halo-pelvic distraction techniques for the spinal deformity. Guangzhou: Guangdong Science and Technology Press; 2010. p. 3–252.
13. Vaccaro AR, Albert TJ. Spinal surgery tricks of the trade. 2nd ed. Shenyang: Liaoning Science and Technology Press; 2010. p. 229–32.
14. Tian H, Alken A, Du P, et al. Posterior hemiverteectomy for congenital horny kyphosis. Chin J Orthop. 2010;18(15):1250–3.
15. Tian H, Alken A, Ma Y. Prophylactic osteotomy for the treatment of congenital lateral paravertebral vertebral body. Chin J Orthop. 2011;19(07):541–4.
16. Tian H. Pedicle lateral screw-rod system for the treatment of scoliosis. Orthop J China. 2011;19(13):1135–9.
17. Tian H. Tuberculous kyphosis osteotomy orthopedic surgery. Chin J Orthop. 2011;19(23):1937–40.
18. Tian H, Li M, Ma Y. Spinal deformity osteotomy orthopedics, vol. 5. Beijing: People's Medical Publishing House; 2011. p. 3–339.
19. Xu S, Ge B, Xu Y. Practical orthopedics, vol. 2. 3rd ed. Beijing: People's Military Medical Press; 2011. p. 1776–7.
20. Tian H, Zhang H, Liang Y. Surgical treatment of spinal deformity. Guangzhou: Guangdong Science and Technology Press; 2012. p. 1–483.
21. Tian H, Li M, Wang Z. Key points and diagrams of thoracolumbar surgery. Beijing: People's Medical Publishing House; 2012. p. 1–470.
22. Errico TJ, Lonner BS, Moulton AW. Surgical management of spinal deformities. Beijing: Peking University Medical Press; 2011. p. 1.133–5.
23. Leong JCY, Day GA, Luk KDK, Freedman LS, Ho EKW. Nine-year mean follow-up of one stage anteroposterior excision of hemivertebrae in the lumbosacral spine. Spine. 1993;18(14):2069–74.
24. Wang L, Liu S, Huang C, et al. Surgical techniques for children's spinal deformity correction. Beijing: People's Military Medical Press; 2014. p. 1–415.
25. Tian H, Lv X, Tian B. Halo pelvic distraction in combination with total spine osteotomy and internal fixation for treatment of severe scoliosis. Orthop J China. 2006;1(1):11–6.
26. Tian H, Qu L, Lu X, et al. Application of traction osteogenesis technique in spinal deformity during development. Orthop J China. 2006;14(13):969–71.
27. Tian H. Surgical treatment of congenital scoliosis. Chin J Orthop. 1999;5:223.
28. Tian H. Surgical treatment of kyphosis kyphosis. Chin J Orthop. 1992;12(3):162–5.
29. Tian H, Yuan T, Tian S. Posterior invasion and vertebral osteotomy. Spinal Deformation. 1992;7(1):4.
30. Tian H. Treatment of kyphosis and kyphoscoliosis with combined vertebrae and vertebral arch osteotomy. Chin J Orthop. 1989;9(5):321–4.
31. Hu Y, Dang G, Tang T. The textbook of spinal surgery. 2nd ed. Beijing: People's Medical Publishing House; 2000. p. 1591–848.
32. Li M, Hou T. The basic principles and techniques of scoliosis surgery. Shanghai: Second Military Medical University Press; 2001. p. 27–116.
33. Ouyang L, Qian J, Xu H, et al. Anatomy of the extraspedicular screw fixation through costotransverse unit of thoracic vertebrae. Chin J Clin Anat. 2009;27(4):397–400.
34. Yan J, Huan J, Zheng Z, et al. CT measurement of the upper-middle thoracic pedicle-rid unit and its significance. Chin J Clin Anat. 2007;25(6):636–9.
35. Zhong S, Jin D. Spinal internal fixation. Beijing: Science Press; 2012. p. 438–54.
36. Tian H, Wang Z, Wang C. Pediatric operative orthopaedics. Beijing: People's Medical Publishing House; 2014. p. 1–640.
37. Tian H, Li F, Tan J. Children's spinal operative orthopaedics. Guangzhou: Guangdong Science and Technology Press; 2016. p. 1–443.

11 Osteotomy for Tuberculosis Angular Kyphosis

Huizhong Tian, Sikandaer Siyiti, Quan Li, Zhiyue Shi, Jie Dai, Xu Zhu, Yingsong Wang, Ni Bi, and Li Li

11.1 Overview

11.1.1 Objective and Clinical Relevance

According to the conventional treatment strategy, once the spinal tuberculosis lesion is debridement, followed by grafting and stabilization, the disease is considered cured even though kyphosis remains. From 1980 to 2006, the author carried out Posterior Vertebral Column Resection (PVCR) and correction in 305 cases with angular kyphosis, including 85 patients with tuberculous kyphosis. These patients achieved satisfactory results. The objective of this chapter is to promote the surgical technique, and overwhelm the perception of tuberculous angular kyphosis as an "incurable disease" into a "curable disease."

Conventionally, surgical treatment of spinal tuberculosis only involved lesion debridement and grafted fusion (Fig. 11.1a, b). However, for the sequelae kyphosis deformity after the tuberculosis lesion is controlled, spine surgeons often deemed it as a problem that does not require treatment and cannot be treated. Patients were often informed that "your tuberculosis is stabilized, with grafted fusion, and it is the end. Without spinal cord compression and early paralysis symptoms, it's not necessary and impossible to deal with the kyphosis." However, spinal tuberculosis in childhood mainly violates the vertebral body and intervertebral disc, usually two bodies and one disc. It causes the destruction and collapse of the intervertebral disc and the bone tissue of the vertebral body, leaving behind a cheese-like mass and an abscess. After anti-tuberculosis drug treatment and surgical removal of the lesion and bone graft fusion, most patients' tuberculosis lesions can be stabilized, so that the remaining vertebral bodies and pedicles are brought together to form bone fusion. As a result, the development of the anterior vertebral body is arrested, while the posterior vertebral arch and lamina continue to grow. As a result, the kyphosis deformity increases year by year. After the age of 10, the kyphotic deformity often goes beyond 90°, so that these patients confront the need to correct kyphosis.

Some surgeons attempt to perform anterior distraction and bone grafting, and some perform two-stage anterior and posterior surgery to correct the severe angular kyphosis caused by spinal tuberculosis. However, the extent of correction is not satisfying. Therefore, in the field of spine surgery, by now it is still a challenge.

From 1980 to 2006, in the course of 26 years, the author personally performed 305 cases of PVCR, including 85 cases of tuberculous kyphosis. It is believed that PVCR is effective in correcting tuberculous kyphosis. However, the large curve of tuberculous kyphosis and epidural adhesions are the main challenges of surgery (Fig. 11.2a, b). Due to the epidural venous plexus embolism caused by tuberculous epidural adhesions, there is not much bleeding in the epidural venous plexus. However, the adhesion between the dura mater and the osseous spinal canal is severe. When dissecting around the dura mater, the spinal cord can be damaged even though the surgeon does not directly work on the dura, or causing cerebrospinal fluid leakage. In the author's 85 cases, complications of neurological injury and cerebrospinal fluid leakage did not occur.

11.1.2 Why Tuberculosis Kyphosis Was Seen as "Incurable" in the Past

Tuberculosis kyphosis was seen as an "incurable disease," mainly because tuberculous kyphosis was treated only by debridement and grafted fusion, while PVCR was not yet introduced. Since Professor Hui-zhong Tian of the Xinjiang Spine Surgery Research Institute introduced PVCR to treat

H. Tian (✉) · S. Siyiti · J. Dai · X. Zhu · L. Li
Spinal Surgery, The Sixth Affiliated Hospital of Xinjiang Medical University, Urumqi, China

Q. Li · Z. Shi · Y. Wang · N. Bi
Department of Orthopedics, The 2nd Affiliated Hospital of Kunming Medical University, Kunming, China

H. Tian et al. (eds.), *Spinal Osteotomy Orthopaedics*, https://doi.org/10.1007/978-981-16-1387-6_11

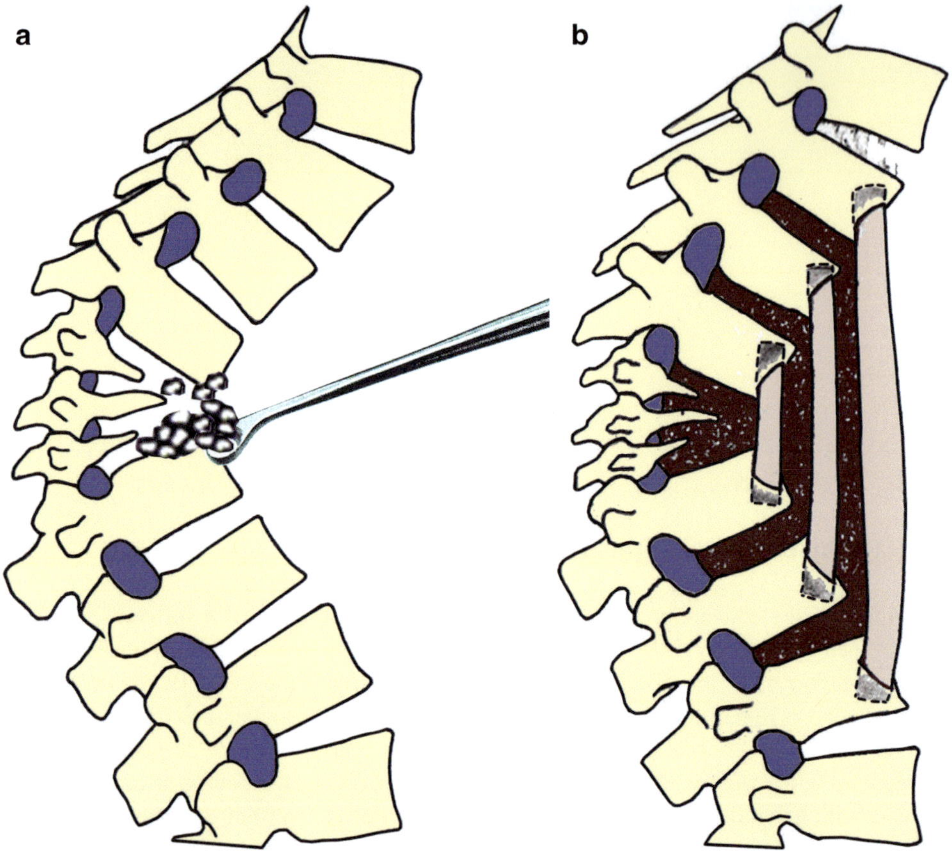

Fig. 11.1 The surgical treatment of spinal tuberculosis from 1950 to 1980 was limited to lesion clearance and bone grafting and fusion. (**a**) Lesion eradication, (**b**) anterior bone grafting and fusion

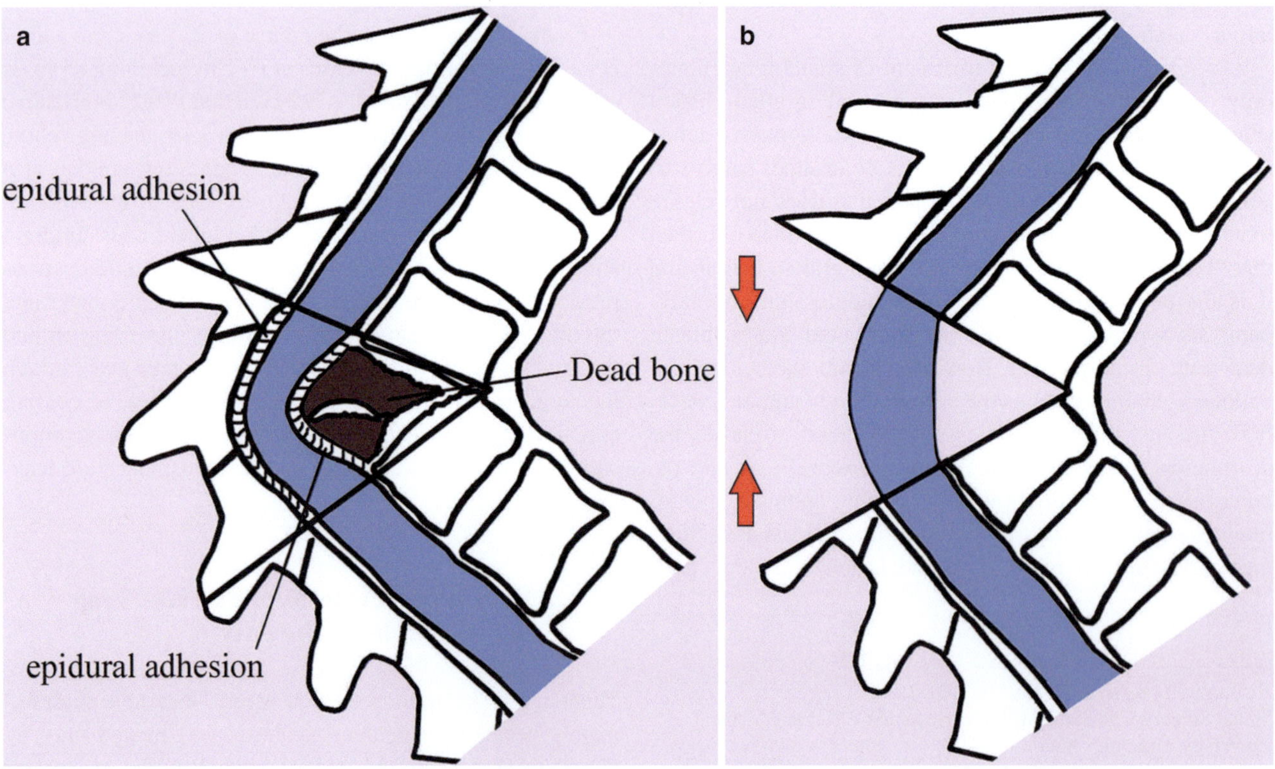

Fig. 11.2 PVCR is the effective method to correct tuberculous kyphosis. (**a**) Tuberculous kyphosis has a large curve and epidural adhesion. (**b**) PVCR corrects tuberculous kyphosis

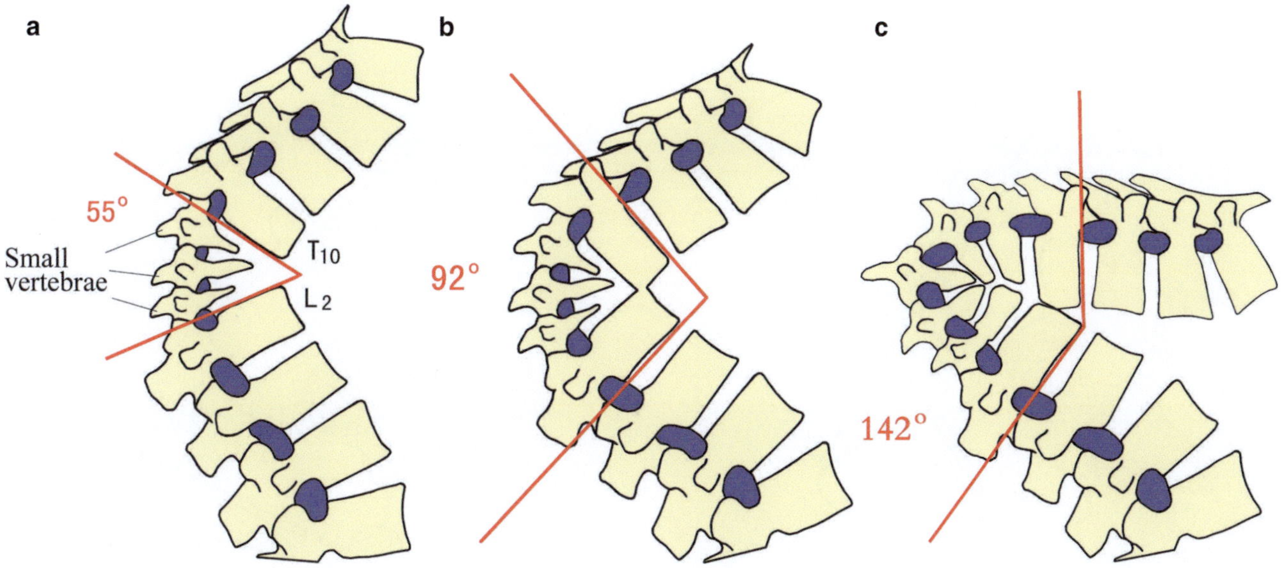

Fig. 11.3 Comparison of the difficulty of tuberculous kyphosis surgery. (**a**) Indication for PSO; (**b**) Indication for VCR; (**c**) contraindication

tuberculous kyphosis in 1980, this disease is now a "curable disease."

Due to the difficulty of this operation, special surgical instruments and special surgical techniques are required to complete this operation. It is also necessary to strictly select the surgical indications, such as the age of the patient, the degree of the curve, and the location of the apex. These are the keys to successful surgery. Xinjiang Institute of Spine Surgery treated 85 cases of tuberculous kyphosis with PVCR from 1980 to 2006 and achieved satisfactory treatment results. The definition of cure is extended to deformity correction with osteotomy for tuberculosis angular kyphosis on top of stabilization and grafted fusion.

As we are spinal deformity surgeons, it is our responsibility to eliminate the angular kyphosis of the patient, and we should work hard to solve it, rather than give up halfway.

11.1.3 The Pathological Evolution of Tuberculosis Kyphosis

There are an estimated 20 million people with spinal tuberculosis worldwide today. Early diagnosis and early treatment are undoubtedly important measures. Especially in patients with multi-segment involvement under 10 years of age, severe kyphosis is a common sequela. As spinal tuberculosis first invades the vertebral body and the intervertebral disc, the anterior column of the spine is damaged, forming abscesses, dead bones, and cheese-like substances. Once tuberculosis lesions of the vertebral body and intervertebral disc are stabilized after anterior debridement or pus drainage, the support of the anterior column of the vertebral body is significantly compromised. With the development of the posterior components of the spine (vertebral arch and posterior edge of the vertebral body) year by year, kyphosis will definitely increase year by year. As the patient grows toward maturity, tuberculosis kyphosis deformity will progress to a situation calling for hard work of surgery. The lateral X-rays show 3–4 vertebrae curled and coiled, and 2–3 vertebral bodies absent. The anterior edge of vertebral bodies up and down contacts each other to form a U-shaped loop. Two to three spinous processes, lamina, pedicles, and the posterior edge of the vertebral body form "small vertebra" (Fig. 11.3a, b) at the apex level of the kyphosis. By then spinal osteotomy becomes more technical demanding even a contraindication for surgical treatment (Fig. 11.3c).

The differential diagnosis of this disease is not a problem by asking whether history of tuberculosis, history of fever and night sweats and other venomous symptoms, the existence of cold abscess or skin sinus and pus drainage, X-rays of the spine or lung have, and history of surgical treatment. These medical histories are helpful in diagnosing tuberculosis kyphosis. Differential diagnosis with X-ray film: Thoracic and lumbar spine tuberculosis is often blurred on the X-ray film (PA position) due to the kyphosis of the spine, especially when the kyphosis is angular. The collapsed or eroded vertebral body can be clearly seen on the lateral X-ray film, leaving only the remaining posterior edge of the vertebral body and pedicles. Oftentimes two or more vertebral bodies are involved, and 2–3 intervertebral spaces are spontaneously fused. Due to the collapse of at least two vertebral bodies and the anterior edges of the upper and lower vertebral bodies close to each other, the vertebral arch portion of the damaged

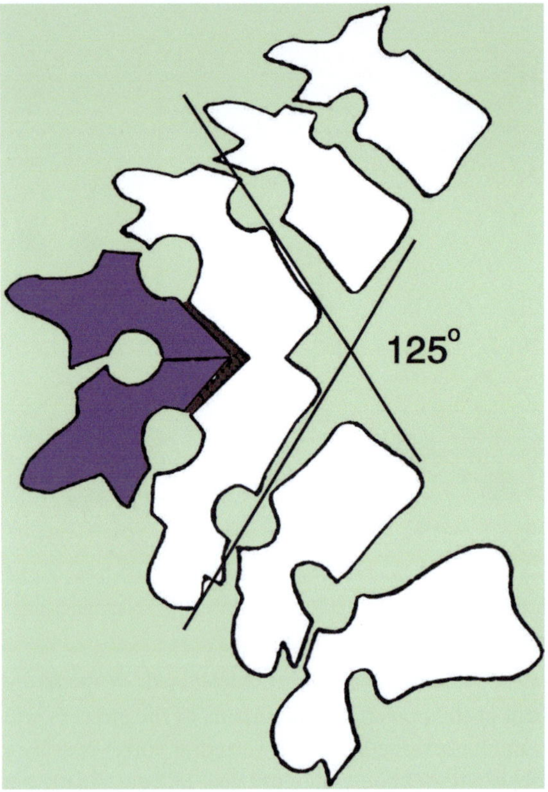

Fig. 11.4 Tuberculous kyphosis contains at least two vertebral bodies collapsed and destroyed

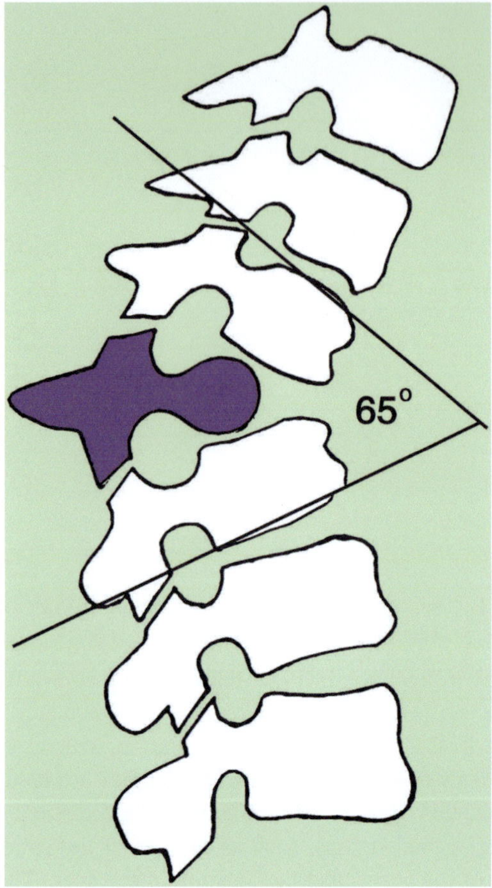

Fig. 11.5 Congenital kyphosis often involves only one vertebral body

vertebral body protrudes backward, forming a typical angular kyphosis deformity. Following further spontaneous fusion between the vertebral bodies, anteriorly bone growth is arrested. The posterior column including vertebral arch, lamina and spinous process continue to grow and develop. Therefore, children's kyphosis deformity increases year by year during development. The earlier the onset of spinal tuberculosis, the heavier the kyphosis is. Therefore, the timing of corrective surgery for tuberculosis kyphosis should not be toward the late end. It should be corrected ideally when the kyphosis angle is less than 90°, by then the best correction effect is expected.

Differentiation of tuberculosis angular kyphosis and congenital angular kyphosis: Tuberculosis angular kyphosis is often greater than 90°. Bone fusion often occurs between three and four vertebral bodies around the apex, and at least two vertebral bodies collapse and fail (Fig. 11.4). Congenital angular spine kyphosis is smaller than tuberculosis kyphosis, and there is no bony fusion in the intervertebral space. Oftentimes only one vertebra is involved (Fig. 11.5).

11.2 Indications and Contraindications

11.2.1 Surgical Indications

The surgical indication for tuberculosis kyphosis should firstly be described as a case where the tuberculosis lesion has stabilized after medical treatment or surgical intervention. Age should be between 5 and 25 years, the apex of kyphosis is in the range of T10 to L3. The kyphotic Cobb angle is within 100° (Fig. 11.6). For young patients with severe kyphosis above 100°, if the vertebrae adjacent to the apical vertebrae is not fused, halo-pelvic traction is firstly applied to check the response. If the kyphotic angle is reduced to about 90° after 3 weeks of traction, vertebral column resection with instrumentation can also be performed. In short, regardless of age, patients with severe kyphosis should be put on halo-pelvic traction first, and then receive surgery under this traction. The second is whether the patient's general health status and

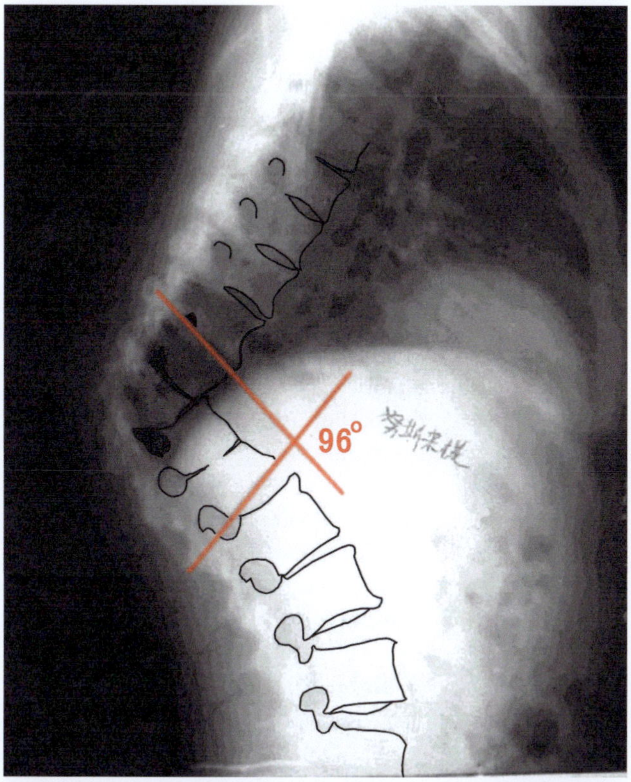

Fig. 11.6 The kyphosis within 100° is the indication for surgery

symptoms of tuberculosis venom have disappeared. Whether anti-tuberculosis drugs are used for enough time before surgery, and whether the symptoms of tuberculosis venom are controlled. Whether there is pulmonary or renal tuberculosis, patients should first be treated for comorbidities, and after all the symptoms of tuberculosis have disappeared, surgical correction for kyphosis is considered.

11.2.2 Contraindications

1. Kyphosis beyond 125°. The upper and lower segments of the angular kyphosis have formed a stiff thoracic lordosis and excessive lumbar lordosis, and several vertebrae around the apex curl into a parallel V-shaped loop (Fig. 11.7). This is a related contraindication to surgery.
2. The kyphotic apical vertebra is above T10. The higher the less suitable for surgical treatment.
3. Poor general condition and uncontrolled local or systemic tuberculosis symptoms. Surgical correction should be postponed against these situations. Anti-tuberculosis treatment or surgical debridement should be performed first and leaving deformity for further correction in the future.
4. Age beyond 30 years. The older, the less suitable for surgery.

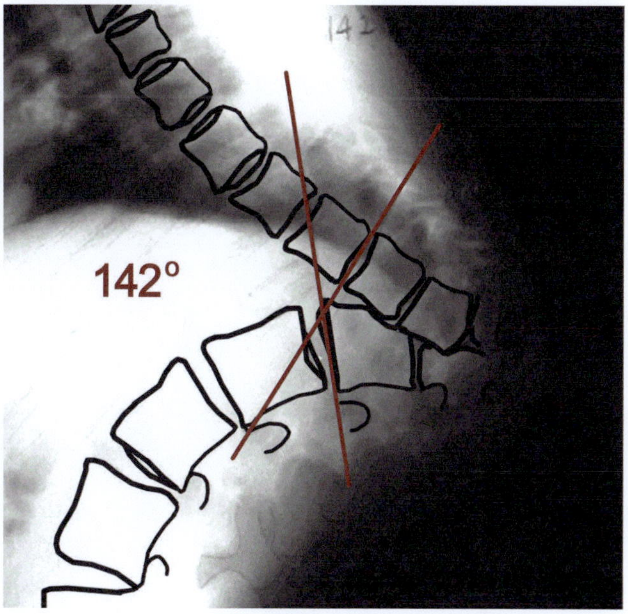

Fig. 11.7 V-shaped kyphotic angle is a contraindication for surgery

11.3 Preoperative Preparation

1. Anti-tuberculosis drug treatment before surgery.
2. Vertical suspension traction: Before surgery, the kyphosis below 80° should receive vertical suspension traction more than ten times a day, 5–25 min each time, keep both feet off the ground. After 2 weeks of traction, measure the distance from the spinous process of C2 to the sacrococcygeal joint under traction (Fig. 11.8). Compare with the length measured at the beginning of the traction to assess whether it is elongated. In addition, a lateral X-ray should be taken under vertical suspension traction to measure whether the Cobb angle has changed.
3. Halo-pelvic traction:
   Patients with kyphosis of more than 80° should undergo surgery after 3–4 weeks of halo-pelvic traction (Fig. 11.9a–c). Spinal osteotomy, correction of kyphosis and instrumentation under halo-pelvic traction, and local anesthesia are performed in one stage to treat the spinal deformity. If surgical instruments touch or compress the spinal cord during the operation, the patient is able to describe the discomfort or movement of the lower extremities to the surgeon, which is more reliable than any spinal cord monitoring and wake-up test.

   Adjustment and speed of distraction during traction: The halo-pelvic traction should be fast and then slow, initially 5–3 mm/day, then 2–1 mm/day, and finally no more than 1 mm/day. Avoid excessive distraction. It should be closely observed whether the patient has symptoms of

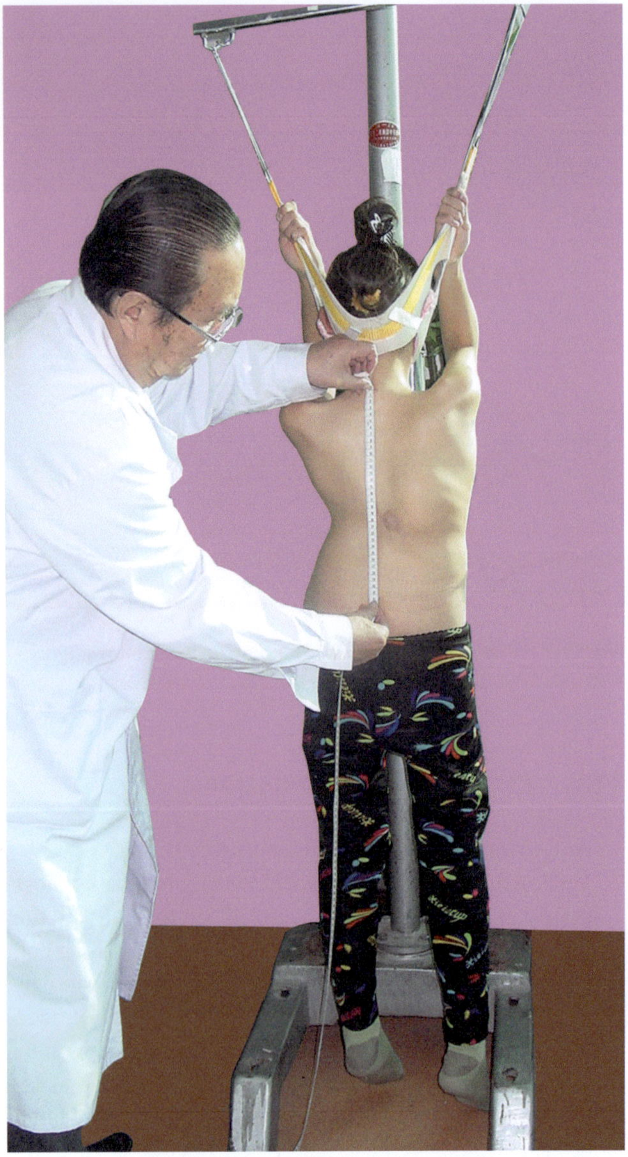

Fig. 11.8 Measure the distance between the spinous process of the axis and the sacrococcygeal joint

over-distraction. If there are difficulties in sticking out the tongue, slurred speech, salivation, etc., traction should be stopped immediately or released by 5 mm to observe whether the patient recovers. If there is no recovery, it should be further reduced by 5 mm, continue to observe. If necessary, the halo-pelvic traction should be removed to facilitate recovery. As the halo-pelvic traction must be gradually performed in a long process to be able to adapt to the prolongation of the change of bone and soft tissues, the entire halo-pelvic traction process should be completed within 4–8 weeks, and must not be rushed to achieve success. Avoid traction too fast to avoid irreversible spinal cord and nerve injury.

For the placement of pelvic pin, cranial halo, pelvic ring, and support rod, as well as the precautions during halo-pelvic traction, see Chap. 7 of the book for traction therapy of spinal deformity (Sect. 11.3, halo-pelvic traction).

4. Instrument preparation: Tian's spinal osteotome set is an indispensable instrument to facilitate operation from the posterior approach to the anterior side of the spinal column (Fig. 11.10). The various curvatures of this instrument are used to work around the dura mater and resect the vertebral body through the posterior approach to ensure that the spinal cord and nerve root are not damaged. However, the skill of using a thin-blade osteotome for surgery needs special training before it can be used freely.
5. Anesthesia and body positioning:
   (a) Anesthesia under halo-pelvic traction: Perform PVCR under halo-pelvic traction. (1) There are many advantages of using local infiltration anesthesia. As the anesthetic contains a small amount of epinephrine hydrochloride, the bleeding in the incision is reduced, the field is clear, to facilitate the operation. When operating near the dura mater and nerve root, the patient can remind the operator upon nerve root impingement. (2) Intubation of general anesthesia with a fiberoptic bronchoscope is also a good method. The disadvantage is that it is impossible to talk to the patient.
   (b) Anesthesia without halo-pelvic traction: General anesthesia with tracheal intubation.
   (c) Positioning: The lying position of the patient during surgery can be divided into two types. (1) Prone position without halo-pelvic traction (Fig. 11.11). (2) Prone position with halo-pelvic traction. The main thing is to talk about the prone position with halo-pelvic traction. The patient cannot be suspended on the traction frame for surgery. The patient should rest on the table with solid support of pads. The nuts on the four upright pins on the cranial ring are loosened by 3 cm up and down (Fig. 11.12) to avoid impact on anesthesia and breath.

11.4 Surgical Technique of PVCR

1. Operation steps:
   Tuberculosis kyphosis is a kind of angular kyphosis. The apex of the kyphotic angle protrudes to the back and is located under the skin of the back, and the surrounding soft tissue is thin. It is suitable for incision along the spinous process. First, expose the bilateral lamina, and then remove the transverse process, expose the pedicle and

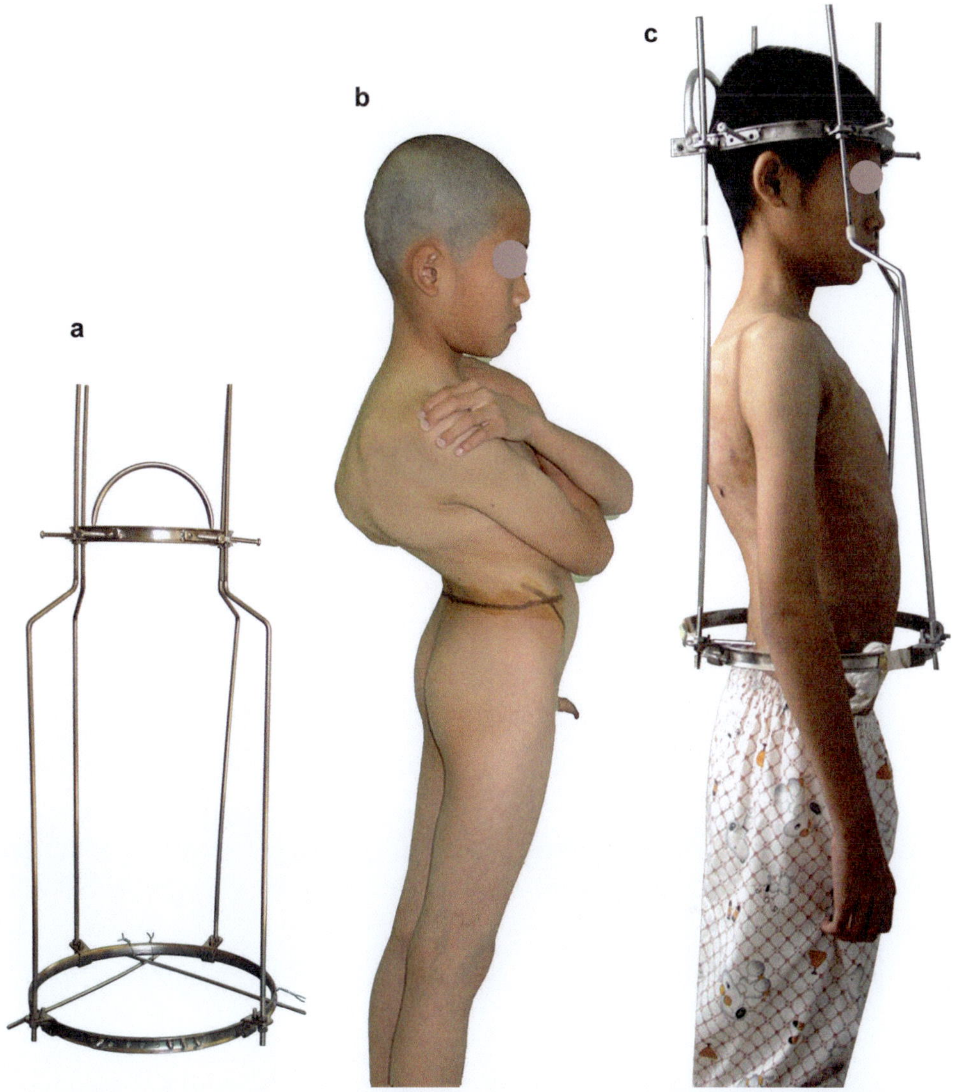

Fig. 11.9 Preoperative preparing for tuberculosis kyphosis correction using halo-pelvic traction for 3–4 weeks. (**a**) Halo-pelvic traction device required for preoperative traction. (**b**) Appearance before traction. (**c**) Appearance after traction

vertebral body from both sides, and perform PVCR. In particular, the application of Tian's spine osteotomes for wedge osteotomy to remove the vertebral body by bypassing the dura mater is the most convenient approach and surgical method.

Local infiltration anesthesia: After disinfection, the operator and assistant first perform local infiltration anesthesia along the spinous process. Infiltration injection should be performed in the predetermined incision by layers, generally in three layers: (1) Intradermal along the spinous process, slightly more than the full length of the incision. (2) The infiltration of the muscle layer behind the lamina of both sides should also exceed the range of the intended incision and dissection. (3) Blockage of nerve roots between the transverse processes and the intervertebral foramen. If local infiltration can be performed step by step, most patients can undergo surgery without pain. The biggest advantage of local anesthesia is that the patient can reflect the real situation to the surgeon at any time, especially when the dura mater is touched or pulled, the patient can give signals promptly. This is much more effective than any monitoring and wake-up test.

Step 1 Incision: Along the spinous process incision, about 15–25 cm long. The incision should not be too short so that it is easy to separate and expose to both sides (Fig. 11.13).

Step 2 Exposure: Separate and expose the spinous process, lamina, articular process, and transverse process to both sides. The exposure should be wide enough to work around the vertebral arch to remove the vertebral body (Fig. 11.14).

Step 3 Removal of Transverse Process and Lamina: Use a straight osteotome to resect the transverse process

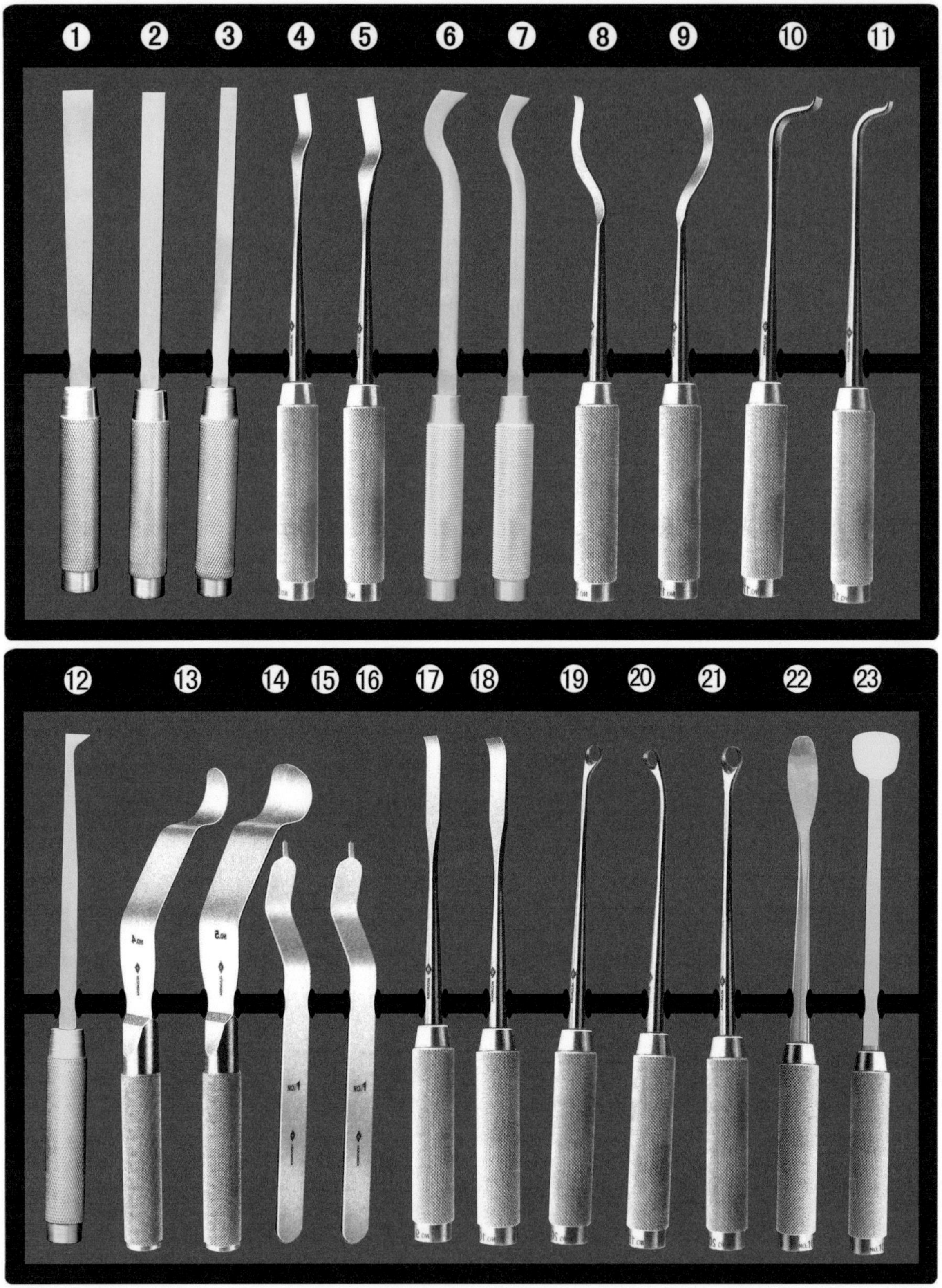

Fig. 11.10 A set of 23 Tian's spine osteotomes: No. 1–3 straight osteotomes (large, medium, and small); No. 4–5 shovel osteotomes (large and small); No. 6–7 crescent osteotomes (large and small); No. 8–9 left or right curved osteotomes; No. 10–11 push-down osteotomes (large and small); No. 12 oblique beveled osteotomes; No. 13–14 lever (wide and narrow); No. 15–16 nerve root retractor; No. 17–18 Anonymous elevator (large and small); No. 19–21 ring curette(left and right, straight); No. 22 Tian's small elevator; No. 23 Tian's large elevator.

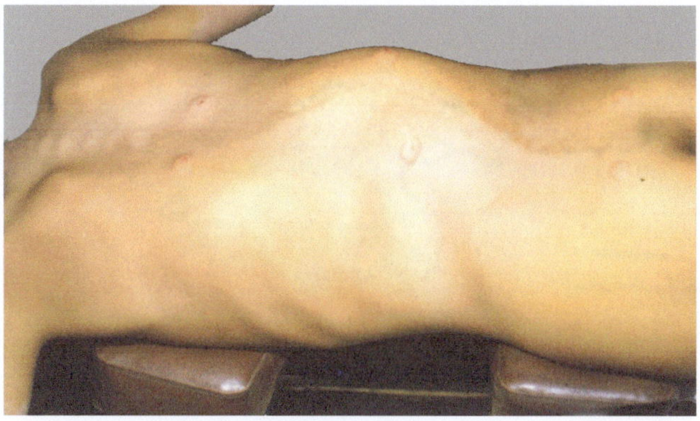

Fig. 11.11 Patients without halo-pelvic traction, prone to perform surgery on the Hall–Relton stand

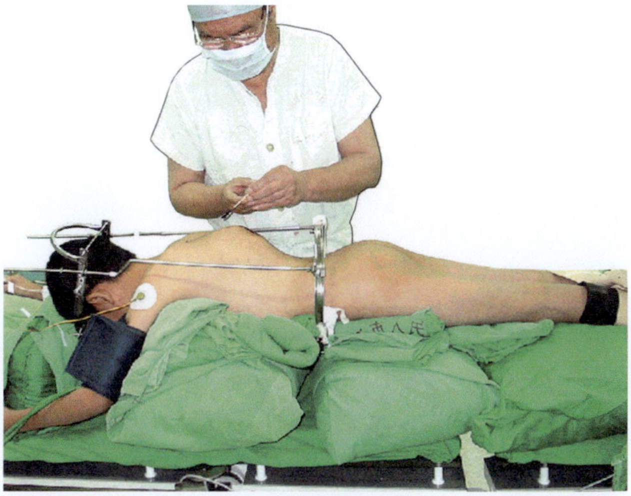

Fig. 11.12 A patient with a halo-pelvic traction lying prone on the operating table. The pad should be placed between the human body and the operating table. Do not allow the patient to hang on the shelf. Loosen the nuts on the four upright posts by 3 cm above and below each

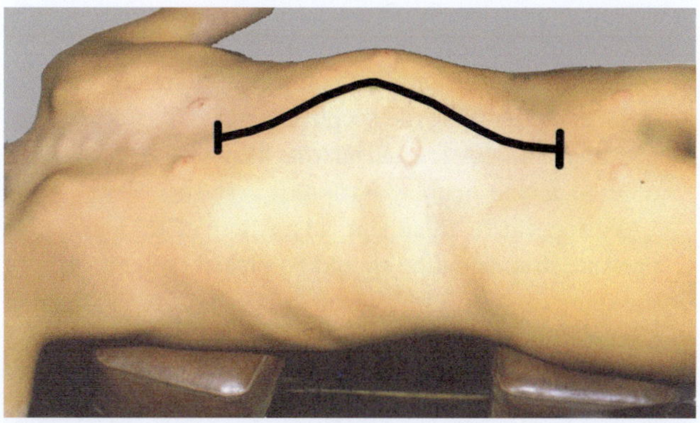

Fig. 11.13 The incision along the spinous process is 15–25 cm long

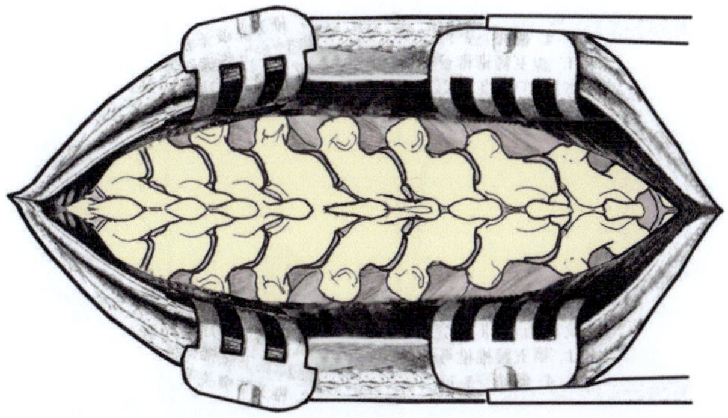

Fig. 11.14 Extensive exposure of the lamina and transverse processes through the posterior approach

along the outer edge of the pedicle. Use a shovel to remove the lamina cap, exposing the dural canal and spinal nerve root (Fig. 11.15a, b).

Step 4 Elevation and exposing the pedicle and vertebral body: Using a vertebral body elevator to strictly peel from the periosteum to expose the lateral surface of the pedicle and the lateral surface of the waist of the vertebral body directly under the anterior longitudinal ligament (Fig. 11.16). Then insert the lever to retract the soft tissue on both sides of the vertebral body and the segmental vessels from the anterior vertebrae (Fig. 11.17).

Step 5 Dissect the epidural adhesions, and remove the pedicles and the lateral part of the vertebral body: Use an anonymous elevator to dissect the epidural adhesions (Fig. 11.18). Use a straight bone knife to remove the pedicles and the lateral part of the vertebral body by layers (Fig. 11.19).

Step 6 Removal of the central part of the vertebral body: Use a spatula and crescent osteotome to remove the central part of the vertebral body (Fig. 11.20a, b).

Step 7 Dissect the posterior longitudinal ligament: Use the posterior longitudinal ligament elevator to carefully dissect the posterior longitudinal ligament (Fig. 11.21) to avoid rupture and bleeding of the anterior epidural plexus.

Step 8 Push down the thin layer of bone that is temporarily retained at the trailing edge of the vertebral body: Use a push-down osteotome to push down the thin layer of bone at the trailing edge of the vertebral body (Fig. 11.22).

Step 9 Palpation in front of the dura: The surgeon inserts the fingers of both hands into the osteotomy space to check whether there is residual bone fragment (Fig. 11.23). If it has been cleared, immediately close the osteotomy space and fixation.

Step 10 Close the osteotomy space to correct the kyphosis: After tensioning the temporarily fixed steel

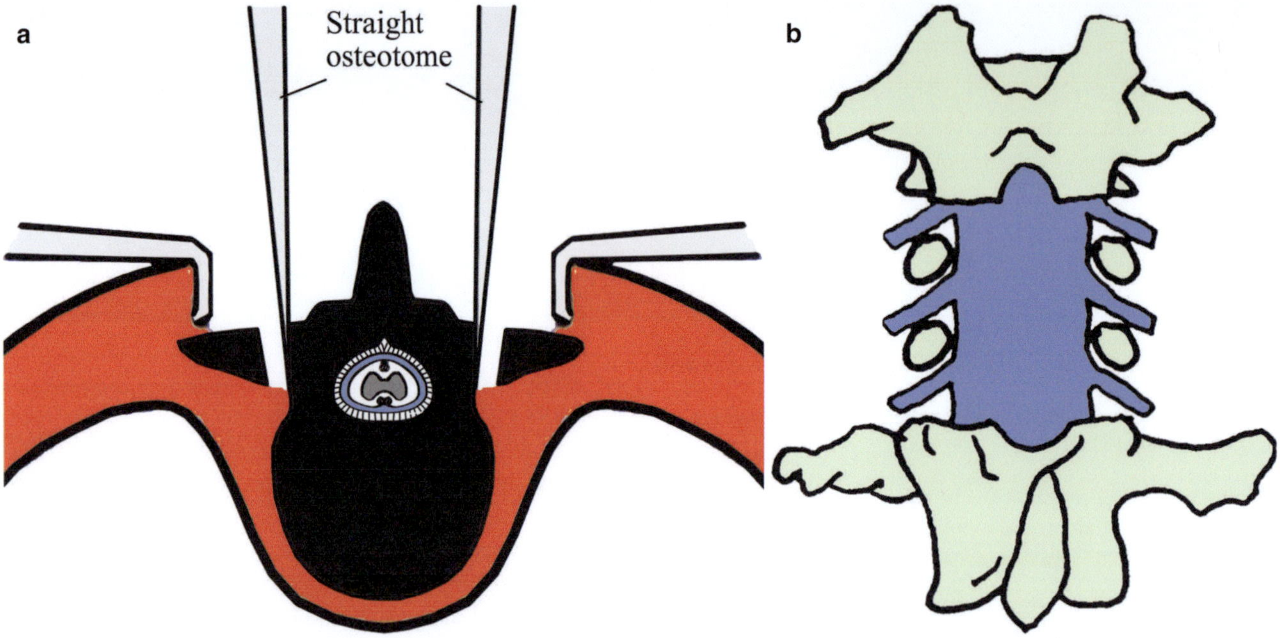

Fig. 11.15 Resection of transverse process and laminectomy. (**a**) Use a straight osteotome to resect both lateral transverse processes; (**b**) Resect two lamina covers

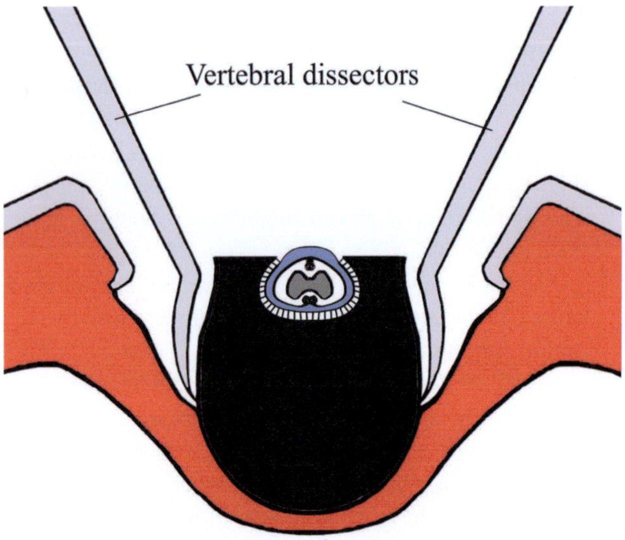

Fig. 11.16 Elevation forward along the pedicle and vertebral waist

wire to close the osteotomy space (Fig. 11.24), the kyphotic deformity of the spine has been partially corrected. Then, the screw–rod system is connected and tightened to achieve correction of kyphosis.

Step 11 Replace with permanent internal fixation: There are three commonly used internal fixation methods. (1) Simple posterior bone grafting on top of lamina after closing (Fig. 11.25). (2) Interbody struct grafting and screw–rod system (Fig. 11.26). (3) Fixation by distal distraction and proximal compression (Fig. 11.27a, b). Due to the length of the tuberculosis kyphotic segment, anterior distraction and

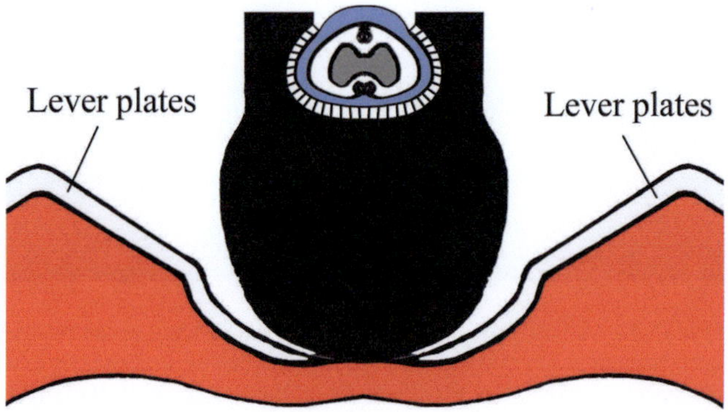

Fig. 11.17 Elevate the anterior longitudinal ligament to expose the vertebral body

posterior compression and fixation are normally adopted. For children during development, distal distraction and proximal compression and internal fixation are often used in order to distract on the growth rods in stages.

Postoperative treatment: (1) After VCR, a negative pressure drainage tube should be placed on both sides of the spine for 48–72 h. More than 100 ml of blood drained assures the patency of the tubing. (2) Anti-infection and anti-tuberculosis treatment must last for a certain period of time after surgery to prevent recurrence of tuberculosis after surgery. (3) According to the situation and reliability of intraoperative fixation, consider external immobilization with plaster vest or brace. (4) Follow up 3–6 months after the operation, including X-ray to decide to stop the anti-TB drug treatment or remove the external fixation.

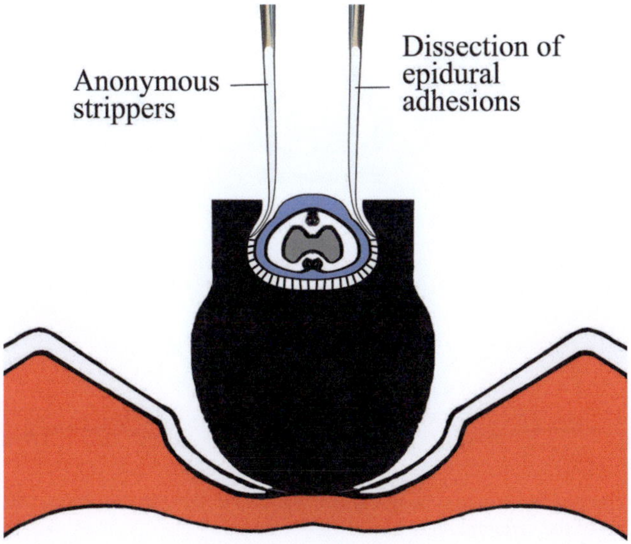

Fig. 11.18 Dissect the epidural adhesion with an anonymous elevator

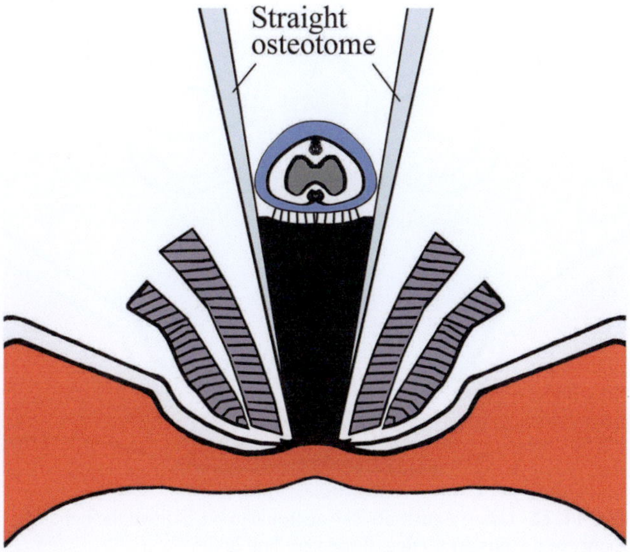

Fig. 11.19 The pedicle and lateral part of the vertebral body are removed layer by layer

11.5 Typical Case Study

Ms. Li, female, 19 years old. Her back had a bulging at the age of 14, with back pain, fatigue, sweating and low fever, and other tuberculosis symptoms. With X-ray, diagnosis of T11–T12 tuberculosis was established. The patient had tuberculosis debridement twice in other hospitals. Symptoms such as fever and back pain gradually disappeared after the operation, and the systemic condition recovered quickly, but the kyphosis of the spine progressed, leaving an ugly kyphosis progressing year by year. The patient was admitted to our hospital on May 5, 1988, for treatment of kyphosis. Examination showed that both sides of the waist had oblique incisions. Lateral X-ray showed a kyphosis of 88° Cobb with T11 as the apex, and anteroposterior X-ray showed bilateral proximal 11th–12th ribs were removed without paravertebral abscess and psoas abscess. The bone in the vertebral defect area was stable. The erythrocyte sedimentation rate was normal. Diagnosis: tuberculous angular kyphosis (stable lesion). After 33 days of halo-pelvic traction, PVCR was performed under local anesthesia to correct the deformity. The kyphotic Cobb angle was reduced to 11° after operation, the correction rate was 87.5%, the anteroposterior and lateral X-rays and the appearance returned to normal. The patient had plaster vest immobilization and was discharged on August 14 (Fig. 11.28a–h). She had follow-up for 22 years. The internal fixation has not been removed but there is no symptom. She is currently working in the post office of a company. She is in good health with no tuberculosis recurrence.

11.6 Precautions and Complications Prevention

11.6.1 Precautions

1. Tuberculosis kyphosis was previously considered as an "incurable disease": Spinal tuberculosis was regarded as a cure if the tuberculosis lesion was stable and the bone graft fusion was good after drug treatment and bone removal and fusion. As for the remaining tuberculosis kyphosis, it is considered an "incurable disease."
2. From 1980 to 2006, the author performed PVCR on tuberculosis kyphosis, which was considered an "incurable disease." This surgical technique of wedge osteotomy excises the lesion surrounding the dural sac and then closes the osteotomy space to correct the kyphosis. The anterior open and posterior closed internal fixation and bone graft fusion surgery eliminates the stenosis and compression of the spinal canal in one stage. And after the complete spinal osteotomy and wedge resection, the kyphosis of the angular spine was corrected, and the appearance of tuberculous kyphosis was improved.
3. However, the operation of tuberculosis kyphosis osteotomy is difficult and risky and requires special surgical instruments and surgical techniques. If the operation is not careful, it may cause serious surgical complications.
4. When performing PVCR to correct tuberculosis kyphosis, special surgical instruments and surgical techniques

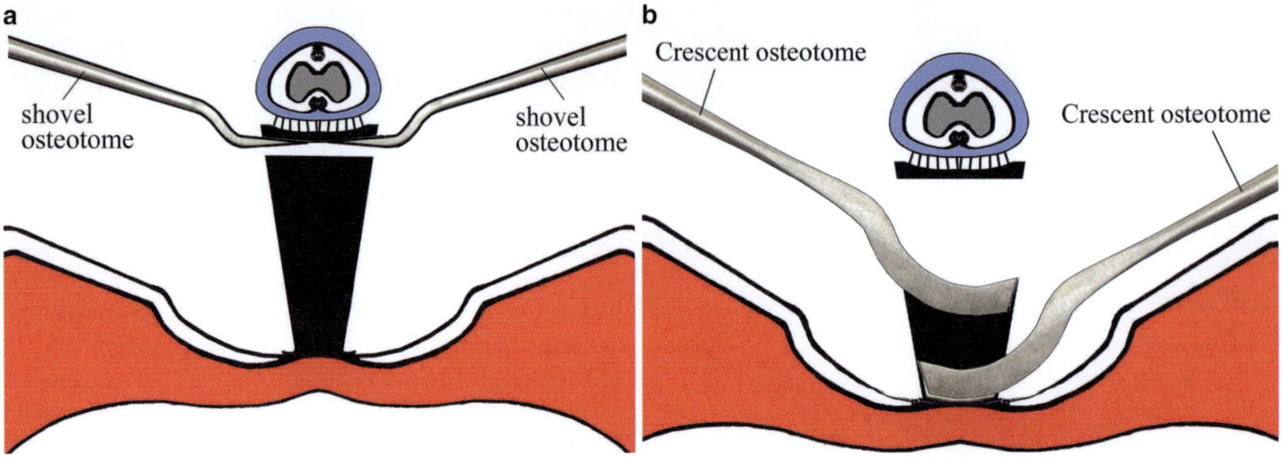

Fig. 11.20 Using a shovel and a crescent osteotome to remove the central part of the vertebral body. (**a**) Use a shovel to remove the central part of the vertebral body. (**b**) Use a crescent osteotome to remove the central part of the vertebral body

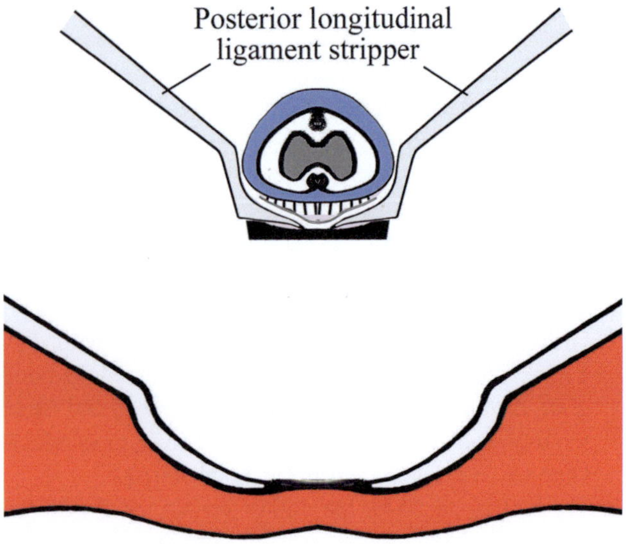

Fig. 11.21 The posterior longitudinal ligament is elevated from the subperiosteal with the posterior longitudinal ligament elevator

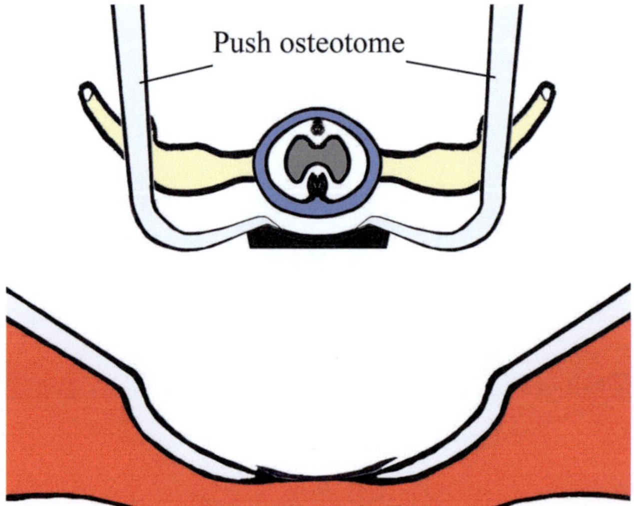

Fig. 11.22 Using a push-down osteotome to push down the bone fragments of the posterior edge of the vertebral body

are required, such as various curved thin-blade osteotomes, in order to work around the dura mater through the posterior approach for vertebral resection, you also need to train the surgical skills of using osteotome for surgery to complete the operation and prevent surgical complications.

5. It is necessary to make full use of the curvature of the device to work around the dura mater and absolutely avoid friction between the device and the dura mater to avoid spinal cord injury through the dura mater.
6. Absolutely avoid using an elevator or a retractor to pull off bone tissue anterior to the dural sac and spinal cord. The dura mater must not be touched; otherwise, it will easily cause neuro deficit.
7. Issues of bleeding and hemostasis:
   (a) For bleeding of segmental vessels, there is no need to ligate segmental arteries and veins. It is only necessary to strictly dissect toward the anterior from the lateral pedicle and the periosteum of the vertebral body to the anterior longitudinal ligament, and then use the lever to open the space and stop the segmental blood vessels from bleeding (Fig. 11.29a, b).
   (b) For the bleeding of the vertebral cancellous bone sinus, applying bone wax on the osteotomy surface is effective to stop the bleeding (Fig. 11.30a, b). But hard bone wax is needed to take effect.
   (c) For the bleeding of the anterior dural venous plexus, use the posterior longitudinal ligament elevator to

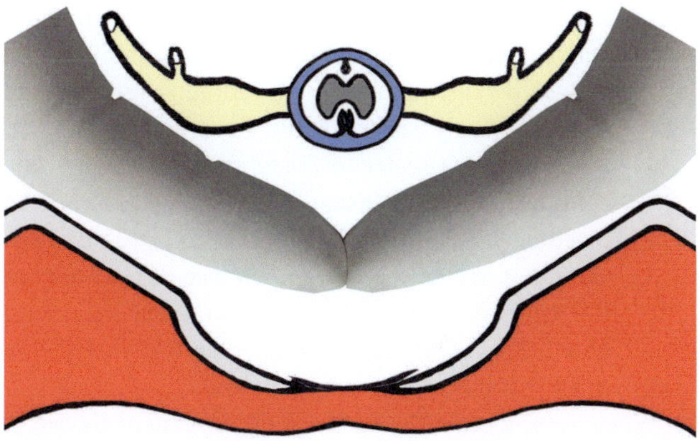

Fig. 11.23 Use the index finger to palpate the presence of bone fragments in the osteotomy space

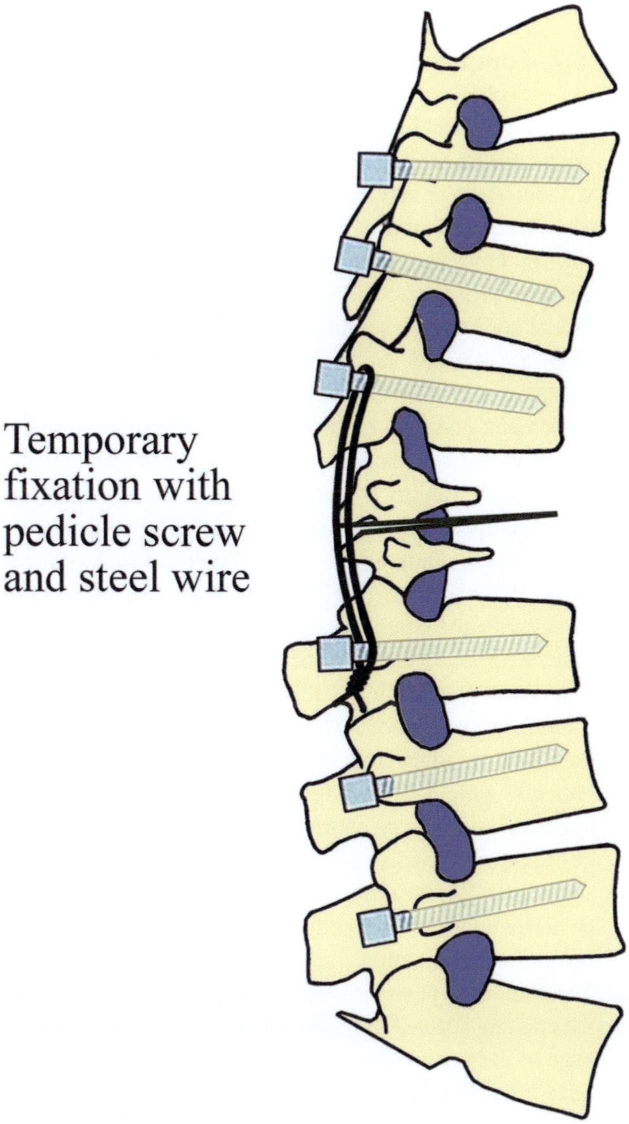

Fig. 11.24 Tension the temporarily fixed wire to close the osteotomy gap

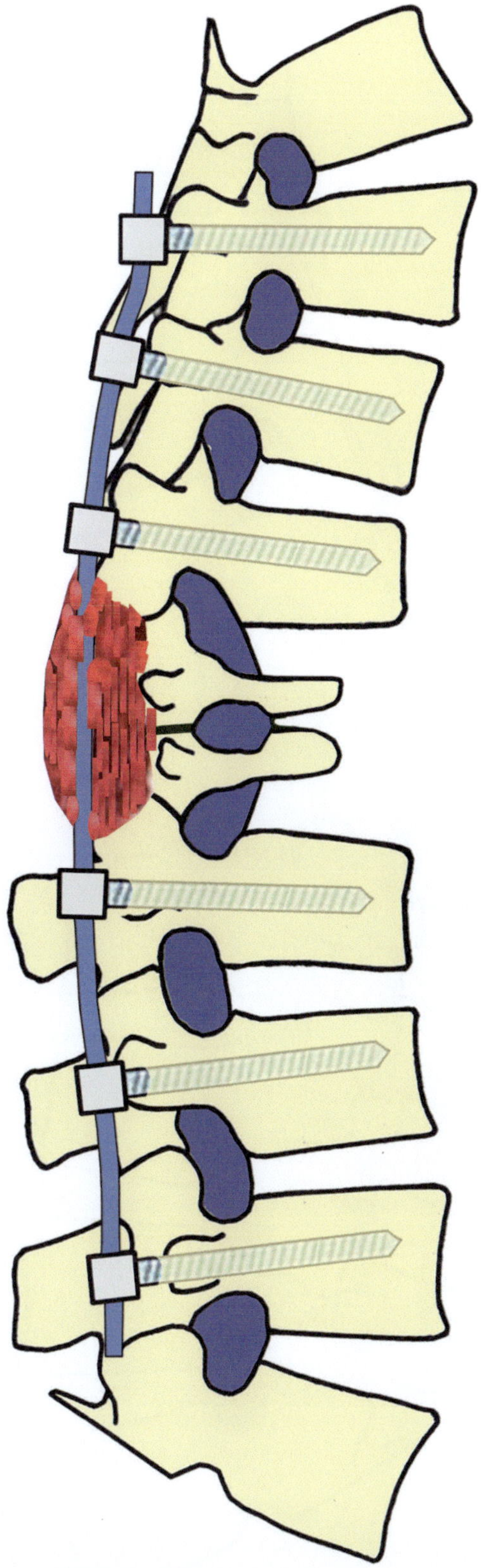

Fig. 11.25 Internal fixation and laminar bone grafting with screw–rod system after close of osteotome

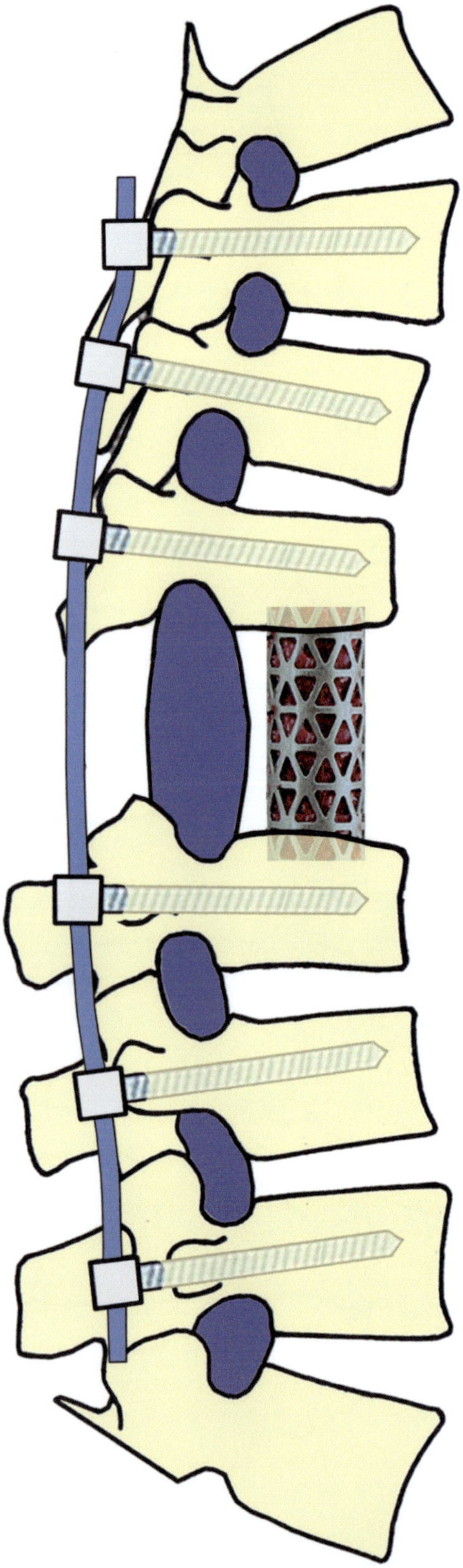

Fig. 11.26 Interbody strut fusion and screw–rod fixation

strictly elevate the posterior longitudinal ligament from the subperiosteal, so that the anterior dural venous plexus is not damaged. Once the epidural venous plexus ruptures, the bleeding is very violent. The osteotomy space should be closed quickly to allow the dura mater to dilate and widen. Then the epidural venous plexus is compressed, and the bleeding stops naturally (Fig. 11.31a, b). Forceps clamping or electrocautery is a waste of time to control epidural venous plexus bleeding and will cause blood loss. Only by closing the osteotomy gap quickly can hemostasis be achieved.

8. When the epidural adhesion is really difficult to elevate, it can be treated by "floating" methods. But the floating bone chip should not be large enough to cause compression on the spinal canal after reduction.

11.6.2 Complications Prevention

1. Shock: When an operation involves a large area, the operation time is long, and the amount of bleeding is large; without salvage actions, hemorrhagic shock may occur. Therefore, care must be taken to prevent shock during surgery. Once shock occurs, it should be treated promptly and actively.
2. Spinal cord and nerve injury: When the anterior vertebral body is released and the posterior vertebral arch is removed, the spine is extremely unstable, prone to displacement, and may cause paraplegia. Therefore, special attention must be paid to maintaining the stability of the spine during surgery to prevent spinal displacement. Once the spinal is displaced to cause spinal cord compression, the source of compression should be eliminated immediately. If the pedicles or facet joint are not adequately resected in the osteotomy area, nerve root compression may occur after correction of kyphosis, attenuated sensation of lower limbs, and reduced muscle strength. Therefore, the pedicles and facet joint in the osteotomy area must be adequately resected.
3. Patients with active vertebral tuberculosis and severe kyphosis can also be thoroughly implanted with a bone graft after the lesion has been completely removed at the same time. It is best to use fibula as a strut graft. From the posterior approach, the pedicle screw system was used for correction and fixation.
4. Tuberculous kyphosis is often accompanied by adhesion of the epidural space. Especially when resecting the posterior edge of the vertebral body, it is often encountered that the bone fragments of the posterior edge of the vertebral body

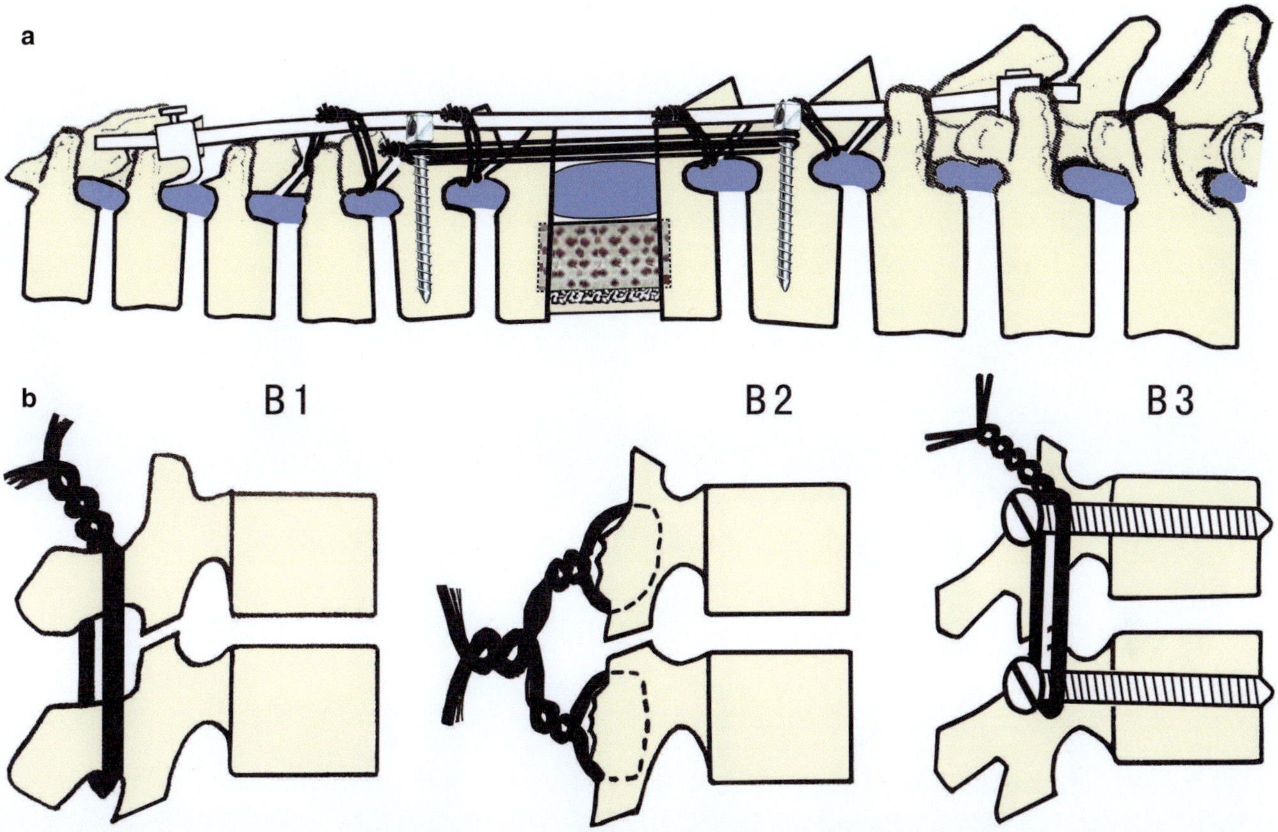

Fig. 11.27 Distal distraction and proximal compression internal fixation. (**a**) The distal distraction and proximal compression internal fixation can keep the spine straight. Prevent spine shortening and buckling of the spinal cord which cannot be accommodated in the spinal canal due to V-shaped osteotomy and posterior compression internal fixation. (**b**) There are three surgical methods for proximal compression: (1) interspinous wiring; (2) sublamina wiring; and (3) pedicle

are closely adhered to the dura mater and it is difficult to be elevated. Forced dissection for adhesions can sometimes cause damage to the spinal cord through the dura mater. Although the dura mater is not ruptured, the spinal cord has been injured by pulling and dissection, leaving the clinical manifestation of spinal cord injury after surgery. Therefore, in the case where it is really difficult to dissect, bone fragments floating can also be considered. In short, tuberculosis angular kyphosis is the most difficult operation in VCR. Its large angle, the U-shaped or V-shaped loop formed in serious cases cause problems for surgery.

5. Rongeurs should not be used to remove the bone tissue close to the dura mater, because there is often epidural adhesion in patients with tuberculosis kyphosis, which is prone to dura tear and thread pulling phenomenon. Once the dura mater is caught by the jaws of the rongeurs, dura tear occurs. The nerve fibers pulled out will be longer and longer, which is a destructive complication (Fig. 11.32a, b). Once it happens, it should be cut off and placed into the dura mater and sutured with one stitch. After the operation, mannitol is given for dehydration, prone position, and the head is placed at a lower position, and sandbag compression is applied locally. Three days later, if there is no extravasation of cerebrospinal fluid, the patient is jeopardized anymore. If the dura tear is too long, suture close is required.

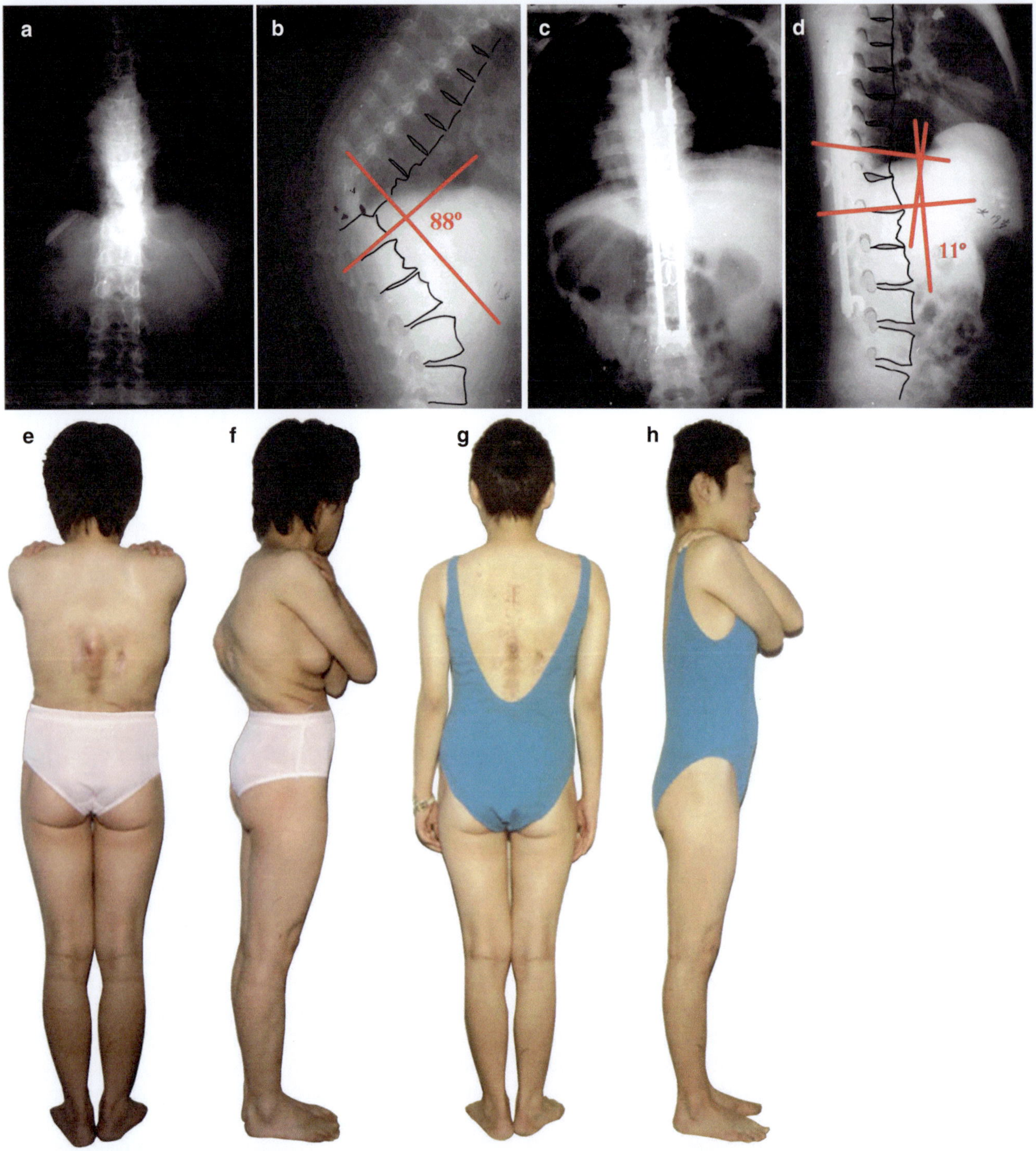

Fig. 11.28 Typical case: Patient Li X, female, 19 years old, has tuberculous angular kyphosis. (**a**) Preoperative X-ray (PA) shows that both sides of the ribs have been removed. (**b**) The preoperative lateral X-ray showed a kyphotic angle of 88°, and the bone fusion lesion was stable. (**c**) Postoperative X-ray (PA) showed good internal fixation. (**d**) After the PVCR, the Cobb angle changed from 88 to 11°, the spine straightened, and the angular kyphosis disappeared. (**e, f**) The angle of the spine before the operation was obvious in the anteroposterior and lateral position and there were scars on both sides for a history of debridement surgery. (**g, h**) Postoperative appearance of the anteroposterior and lateral position, the angular kyphosis disappeared, and the spine straightened

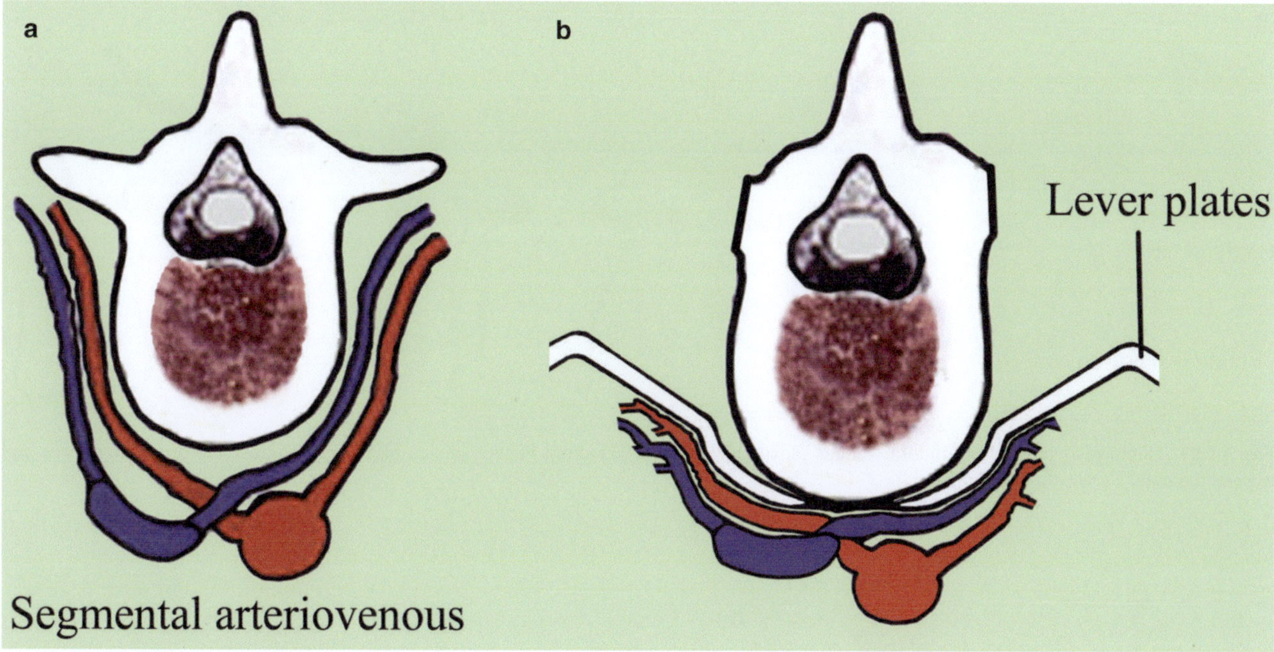

Fig. 11.29 Hemostasis of intercostal and lumbar blood vessels: (**a**) Hemorrhage of segmental arteriovenous veins; (**b**) strict subperiosteal dissection and blocking with a pry board

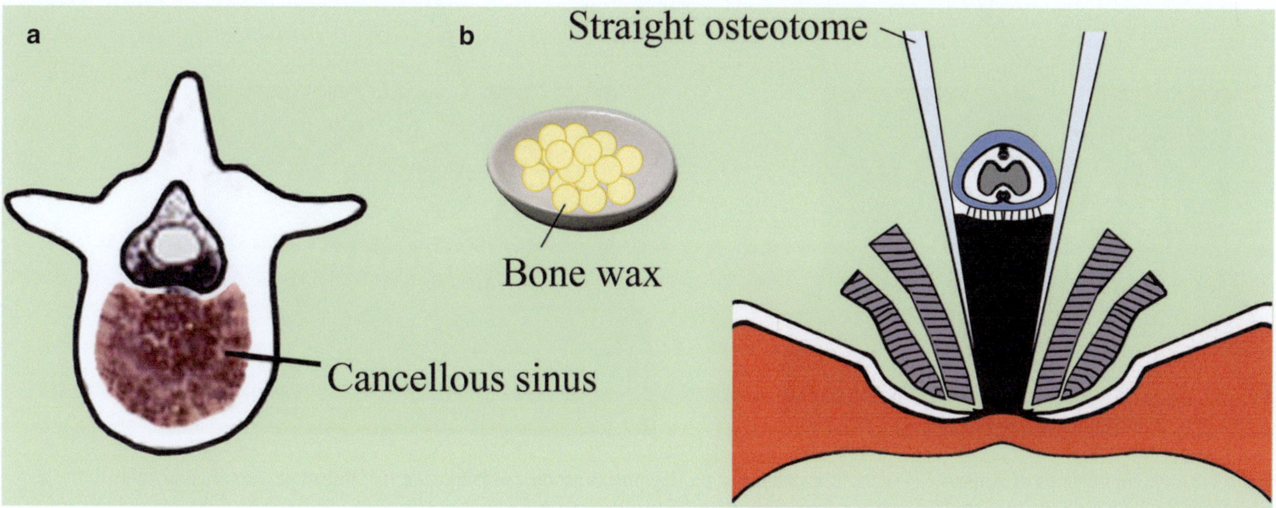

Fig. 11.30 Hemostasis method of cancellous bone sinus bleeding: (**a**) bleeding of cancellous bone sinus; (**b**) smooth cutting surface, bone wax application

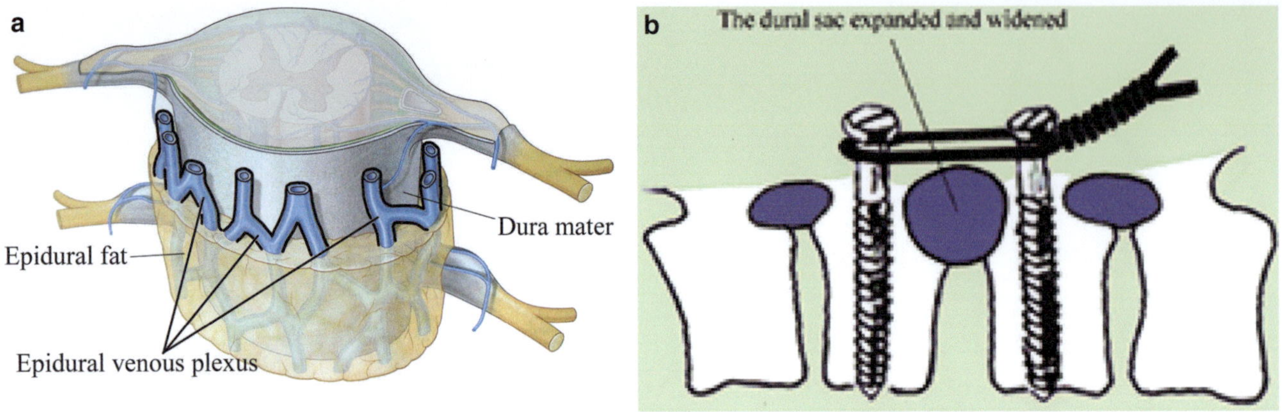

Fig. 11.31 Hemostasis method of epidural venous plexus bleeding. (**a**) Epidural venous plexus bleeding; (**b**) close the osteotomy space and expand the dural sac to stop bleeding

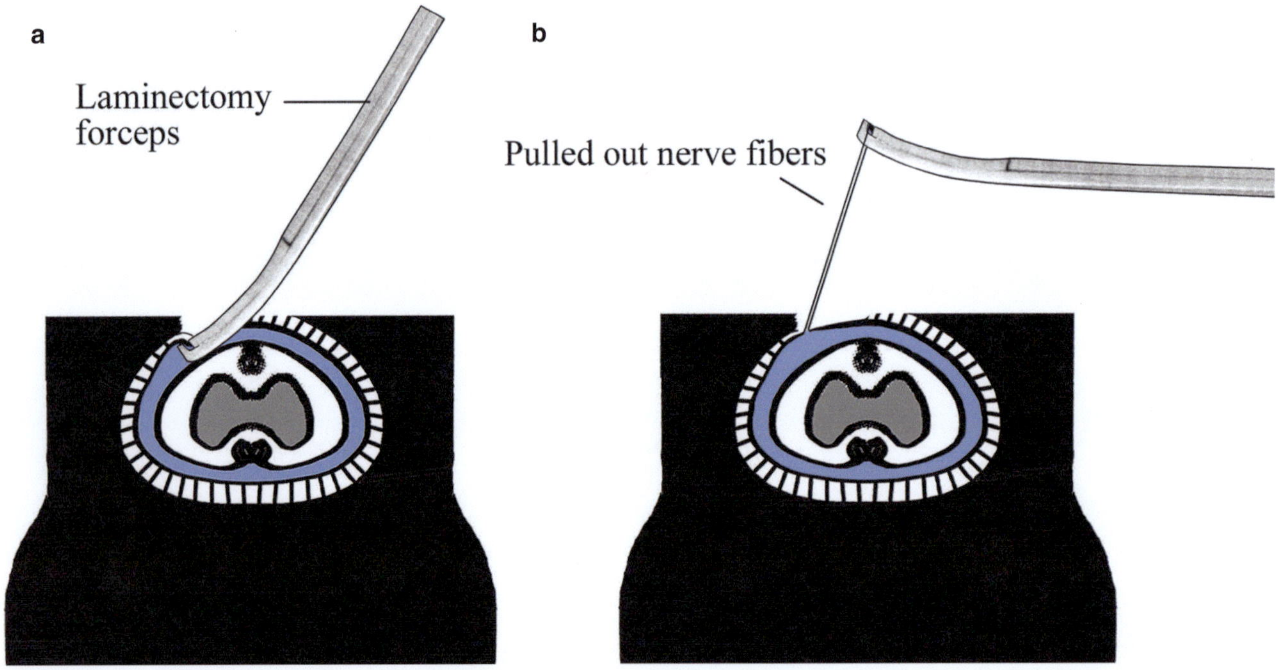

Fig. 11.32 Complications of rongeur—— dura tear and thread pulling phenomenon. (**a**) Dura tear. (**b**) Thread pulling phenomenon

Suggested Reading

1. Dove J, Hsu LC, Yau AC. The cervical spine after halo-pelvic traction. An analysis of the complications of 83 patients. J Bone Joint Surg Br. 1980;62-B(2):158–61.
2. Standring S. Gray's anatomy. Beijing: Peking University Medical Press; 2006. p. 14–98.
3. Tian H. Surgical treatment of kyphosis. Chin J Orthop. 1992;12(3):162–5.
4. Tian H. Corrective surgery for tuberculous kyphosis. Chin J Orthop. 1995;1:6.
5. Chen A, Xu W. Spinal surgery atlas. Beijing: People's Medical Publishing House; 2001. p. 77–233.
6. Tian H. Spinal surgeons should be good at using rongeurs and osteotome. Chin J Mod Oper Surg. 2002;6(1):67–8.
7. Tian H. Application of "Tian's spinal bone knife" in orthopaedic surgery. Chin J Orthop. 2003;11(15):1073–5.
8. Bradford DS, Zhang Y, Wang Y. The spine. Shenyang: Liaoning Science and Technology Press; 2003. p. 279–92.
9. Xu S, Ge B, Xu Y. Practice of orthopaedics. 2nd ed. Beijing: People's Military Medical Publishing House; 2003. p. 598–636.
10. Lei W, Li Q. Application guides for spinal implant system. Xi'an: The Fourth Military Medical University Press; 2004. p. 1–423.

11. Hou S. Spinal surgery. Beijing: People's Military Medical Publishing House; 2005. p. 444–610.
12. Tian H, Lv X, Ma Y. Treatment of severe spinal curvature with total spine osteotomy and internal fixation with head-sleeve ring. Chin J Orthop. 2007;15(3):167–72.
13. Tian H, Liu S, Ma Y. Practical spine surgery illustration. Beijing: People's Military Medical Press; 2008. p. 189–385.
14. Tian H, Liu S, Ma Y. Practical spine surgery. Guangzhou: Guangdong Science and Technology Press; 2008. p. 224–75.
15. Tian H, Wan Y, Li M. Halo-pelvic distraction techniques for the spinal deformity. Guangzhou: Guangdong Science and Technology Press; 2010. p. 1–305.
16. Tian H, Liang Y, Ma Y, et al. Treatment of ossification of thoracic ligamentum flavum with total osteotomy and decompression with Tian's bone knife. Chin J Orthop. 2010;18(20):1693–6.
17. Tian H, Alken A, Du P, et al. Posterior hemivertebrectomy for congenital horny kyphosis. Chin J Orthop. 2010;18(15):1250–3.
18. Tian H. Principles of diagnosis and treatment for scoliosis with diastematomyelia. Orthop J China. 2010;18(20):1753–5.
19. Tian H, Li M, Ma Y. Spinal deformity osteotomy orthopedics, vol. 5. Beijing: People's Medical Publishing House; 2011. p. 3–339.
20. Tian H. Pedicle lateral screw-rod system for the treatment of scoliosis. Orthop J China. 2011;19(13):1135–9.
21. Tian H. Tuberculous kyphosis osteotomy orthopedic surgery. Chin J Orthop. 2011;19(23):1937–40.
22. Tian H, Li M, Wang Z. Key points and diagrams of thoracolumbar surgery. Beijing: People's Medical Publishing House; 2012. p. 245–346.
23. Tian H, Zhang H, Liang Y. Surgical treatment of spinal deformity. Guangzhou: Guangdong Science and Technology Press; 2012. p. 1–483.
24. Huang W, Tian H, Lv X, et al. Lateral anterior decompression for late paralysis of thoracic tuberculosis. Orthop J China. 2012;20(7):647–9.
25. Zhang H, Tian H. Spinal tuberculosis surgery. Guangzhou: Guangdong Science and Technology Press; 2014. p. 3–439.
26. Tian H, Wang W. Surgical techniques for the treatment of spinal tuberculosis. Beijing: People's Military Medical Press; 2014. p. 3–412.
27. Tian H, Li F, Tan J. Children's spinal operative orthopaedics. Guangzhou: Guangdong Science and Technology Press; 2016. p. 1–443.

12 Posterior Vertebral Column Resection (PVCR) Correction for Severe Rigid Spinal Deformity

Jingming Xie

12.1 Objective and Clinical Relevance

Quite a few surgical options are available to manage spinal deformities. Common surgical techniques to treat scoliosis or kyphosis include correction with posterior pedicle screws and rods, anterior release and instrumented correction, or combined anterior and posterior correction. Considering that anterior instrumentation may not provide adequate corrective force while posing a threat of anterior thoracotomy to patients' respiratory function, more doctors tend to apply posterior instrumented correction. A large number of reports have emerged, addressing the good corrective effect of posterior spinal wedge osteotomy on patients with rigid and unbalanced sagittal deformity. With PSO, sagittal correction by 30–50° can be obtained in a single vertebral body. However, due to the limitation of pedicle height and the risk of nerve injury caused by dural buckling or bone impingement, PSO has a ceiling of corrective effect. For patients with severe, especially angular, rigid spinal deformity, posterior vertebral column resection (PVCR) may be the best choice.

Although MacLennan reported a case of vertebrectomy in 1922, Bradford et al. pioneered the treatment of rigid scoliosis (deformity) by using pedicle instruments in parallel with anterior and posterior vertebral column resection. He reported 24 cases of rigid decompensated scoliosis treated by this technique, with an average of 103° of scoliosis preoperatively. With a one-stage or two-stage anterior and posterior approach combined with vertebral column resection, postoperative scoliosis was reduced to 52°. Suk et al. and Lenke et al. reported the clinical application of PVCR in the correction of scoliosis or kyphosis caused by different causes. The first 70 cases reported by Suk were treated with PVCR to obtain the correction rate of 61.9% in the coronal plane and 45.2% in the sagittal plane; Lenke performed PVCR in 43 cases of severe spinal deformity in a group, with scoliosis from 11–150° to 3–76° after surgery, and kyphosis from 44–144° to 7–86° after surgery. Clinical comparative studies also suggest that, compared with combined anterior and posterior vertebral column resection, the posterior approach alone not only reduces respiratory complications but also significantly improves neuro safety.

Vertebral column resection completely removes all the anterior and posterior osseous structures of one or more vertebral segments, as well as the adjacent upper and lower disc structures, so that the spinal cord is the only structure connecting the two segments of the spine, creating a space for deformity correction and additional reconstruction. Through the role of temporary rods, maintenance of this reconstruction and corrective space allows three-dimensional correction of the spine without spinal cord tension and buckling. The main objective of its treatment is to lift the burden on the heart and lungs, relieve spinal cord compression, and take into account the overall balance by obtaining greater correction degrees, so that patients can gain the confidence toward a new life. PVCR reflects a unique correction concept and the most powerful corrective effect. In addition, due to its complicated operation procedures, long operation time, and a large amount of bleeding, it is also accompanied by a higher risk of complications.

12.2 Indications and Contraindications

1. Indications: The angle of the main curve beyond 100°, flexibility less than 10%; relatively large main curve with syringomyelia, Chiari deformity, or spinal cord tethering; complex spinal deformities which are not suitable for other corrective techniques such as conventional wedge osteotomy.
2. Contraindications:
   (a) Maldevelopment of the pedicles. No pedicle medullary cavity or extremely narrow canal of pedicles

J. Xie (✉)
Department of Orthopedics, The 2nd Affiliated Hospital of Kunming Medical University, Kunming, China
e-mail: xiejingming@vip.163.com

H. Tian et al. (eds.), *Spinal Osteotomy Orthopaedics*, https://doi.org/10.1007/978-981-16-1387-6_12

impeding pedicle screw placement, as shown by preoperative thin-slice CT.

(b) Severe respiratory and circulatory diseases, poor nutritional status, intolerance of surgery.

(c) Low risk appetite of family members of the patient and low cooperativeness, lack of awareness to confront the challenge with surgeons.

12.3 Operation Technique

1. Preoperative treatment:

   Before the operation, a full-length X-ray of the spine is routinely performed, and the Cobb angle of the scoliosis of the coronal plane and the Cobb angle of the sagittal plane are measured. Bending position and traction position to evaluate spinal flexibility; Spinal CT thin-slice scan and two-dimensional reconstructed image examination obtain the accurate measurement data of each pedicle. According to CT measurement of the pedicle medullary cavity diameter, the pedicle shape can be divided into three types, which can guide screw placement during the operation. Cervical, thoracic, and lumbar MRI examinations for intraspinal malformations.

   Pulmonary function, arterial blood gas analysis, and echocardiography are tested to evaluate respiratory and circulatory function in all patients before operation. Patients with moderate or severe ventilatory dysfunction are asked to do balloon blowing exercises, exhalation with lip retracted, and stair climbing before operation. Some patients are treated with intermittent positive airway pressure ventilation. Patients with malnutrition should be intervened with high nutrition meals before operation, and fed through a nasogastric tube if necessary. For severe malnutrition, parenteral nutrition is used before operation. In addition, for such patients, we should pay attention to their psychological status, strengthen communication and encouragement, strive to improve their fragile psychological state, increase patients' cooperation and psychological endurance, so that patients are confident to face the challenge of life together with doctors. We should strengthen the communication with patients' families and pay attention to their ability to bear the risk of operation.

   For extremely severe rigid spinal deformities with coronary and/or sagittal deformities>150°, angular deformities, flexibility <10%, continuous cranial-femoral traction can be accepted for 4 weeks before surgery. Gardner–Wells traction arch is used for the skull side, while bilateral supracondylar traction is used for the femur side. The initial total traction weight is 9 kg (the traction weight on the skull side and each femur is 3 kg). Increase the traction weight on the skull and bilateral femur by 1–2 kg each day. During traction, ask the patient for tolerance (eating, sleeping, pain, etc.) daily and check the nervous system function in detail.

2. Anesthesia and position:

   In the process of PVCR operation, good anesthesia cooperation is an important guarantee. Before the vertebral column resection, the anesthesiologist may use controlled hypotension to reduce the amount of bleeding. After the vertebral column resection and before correction, normal mean arterial pressure should be maintained to ensure spinal cord perfusion. In addition, due to the long operation time, the large amount of fluid exchange, the combined use of multiple anesthetics, and their interactions, wake-up tests will be difficult. Right before the wake-up test, anesthetic drugs should be tapered, combined with the use of faster metabolizing sedative drugs. The design of anesthesia protocols should give more consideration to reducing signal interference to intraoperative nerve evoked potential monitoring.

   The patient takes a prone position during the operation, ideally on the Jackson table. The operating table can also be adjusted according to the needs of the deformity and make necessary cushion at the point of force. The general principle is to reduce the compression of the chest and abdominal cavity and reduce the tension of the deformed trunk. Keep eye protection in mind during surgery.

3. Operation procedure: The whole operation is divided into four stages

   Stage 1: exposure and pedicle screw placement: According to the data of the shape of each pedicle and the diameter of the medullary cavity obtained before the operation, if the first attempt to prepare the screw pathway fails using the conventional technique, the "five step rescue screw placement technique" can be used in turn to carefully adjust and establish the pathway for the pedicle screws. For simple angular kyphosis, at least three segments of the upper and lower vertebra need to be covered in fixation to ensure the stability of the reconstructed spine; in the case of scoliosis, the upper and lower end vertebrae in the structural curve should be covered. No residue kyphosis or scoliosis is tolerated in the junction area; the principle is to fully consider the possibility of overall balance, disc degeneration, and reduction of loss of corrective effect.

   Stage 2: Vertebral column resection stage: After the posterior column structure is removed, the anterior and middle column structures of the spine are exposed and removed following removing transverse process and ribs on the convex and then the concave side. The temporary fixation rod should be placed before the vertebral column resection is completed to ensure the stability of the spine. Mind the protection of lumbar nerve roots.

Stage 3 Correction: After vertebral column resection, the spinal cord is the only structure connecting the ends of the spine, allowing a corrective space and 360° decompression around the spinal cord. Under direct vision of the dural sac, firstly, the space created by VCR allows some compression maneuver to shorten the spine, reduce the tension of the spinal cord, and increase the compliance of the spinal cord to correction. The technique of in-situ rod bending, alternative rod changing, distraction, compression, closing and opening are used for correction. The tension of the spinal cord must be checked at any time to indicate prompt adjustment. The correction must be advanced step by step. Avoid the attempt to do everything in one step.

Stage 4 Bone grafting for fusion: Titanium mesh is implanted into the intervertebral space if the gap >1 cm after correction. If the gap is <1 cm, impact grafting with autograft is the option. Additional grafts are applied in the posterior part of PVCR space and in between the facet joint and lamina. One dose of methylprednisolone is routinely administered at the beginning of correction procedure. Wake-up test is performed immediately after vertebral column resection and correction is complete.

4. Postoperative management:

   To maintain circulation stability, strengthen nutrition support and respiratory management. X-ray and CT are taken postoperatively. Patients are followed up for 3, 6, and 12 months after operation and afterward once a year.

12.4 Introduction of Typical Cases (Figs. 12.1, 12.2, and 12.3)

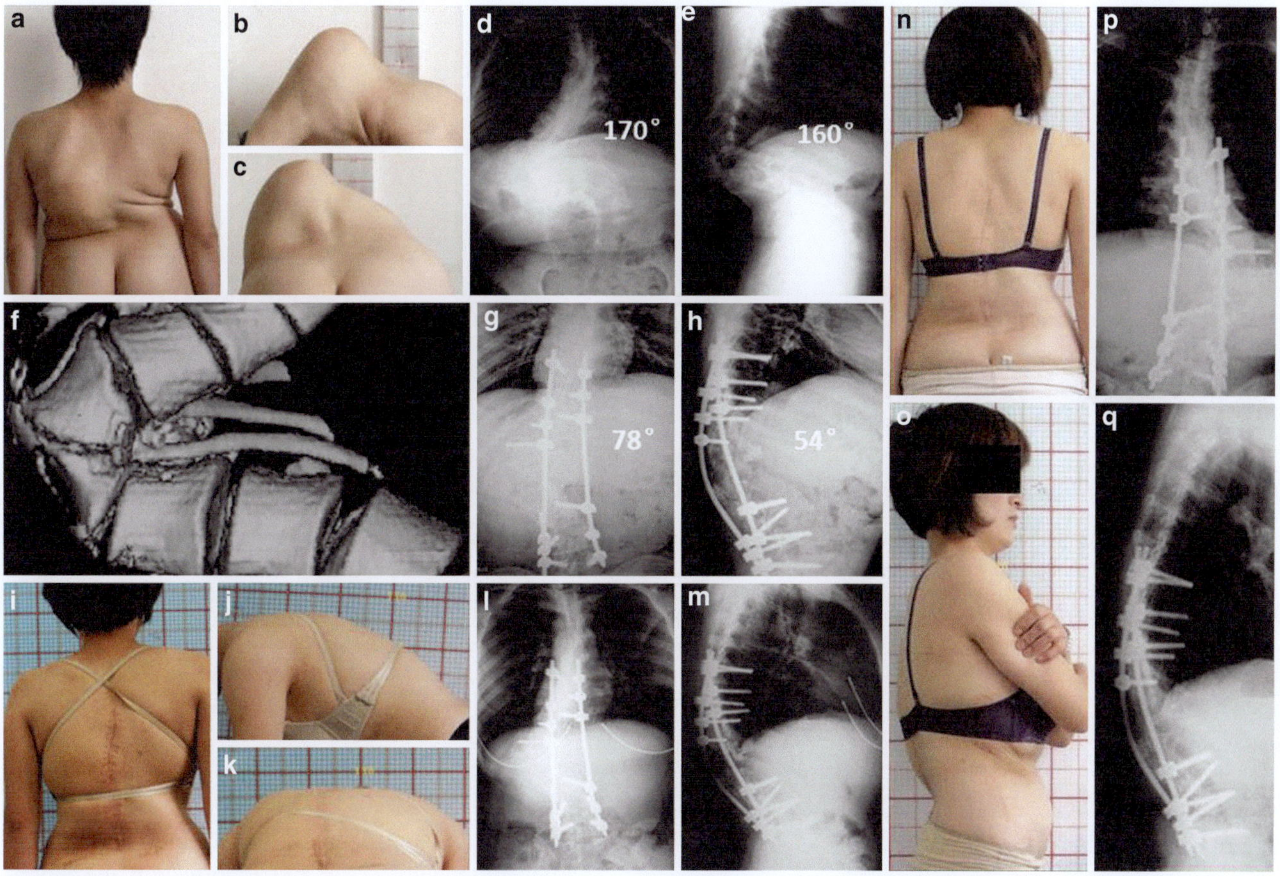

Fig. 12.1 Case 1: female, 25 years old, severe rigid spinal deformity (congenital), underwent one-stage posterior vertebral column correction (PVCR). Preoperative appearance (**a–c**) and X-ray films of the front and side of the patient showed severe angular and rigid scoliosis (**d**, **e**); Preoperative CT three-dimensional reconstruction showed the abnormal structure of the apical region (**f**); The corrective effect after operation (**g**, **h**). The appearance (**i–k**) and corrective effect (**l**, **m**) were followed up 36 months after operation. The appearance (**n**, **o**) and corrective effect (**p**, **q**) were followed up 72 months after operation (Xie JM, Wang YS, Zhao Z, et al. Posterior vertebral column resection for correction of rigid spinal deformity curves greater than 100°. J Neurosurg Spine,2012,17:540–551)

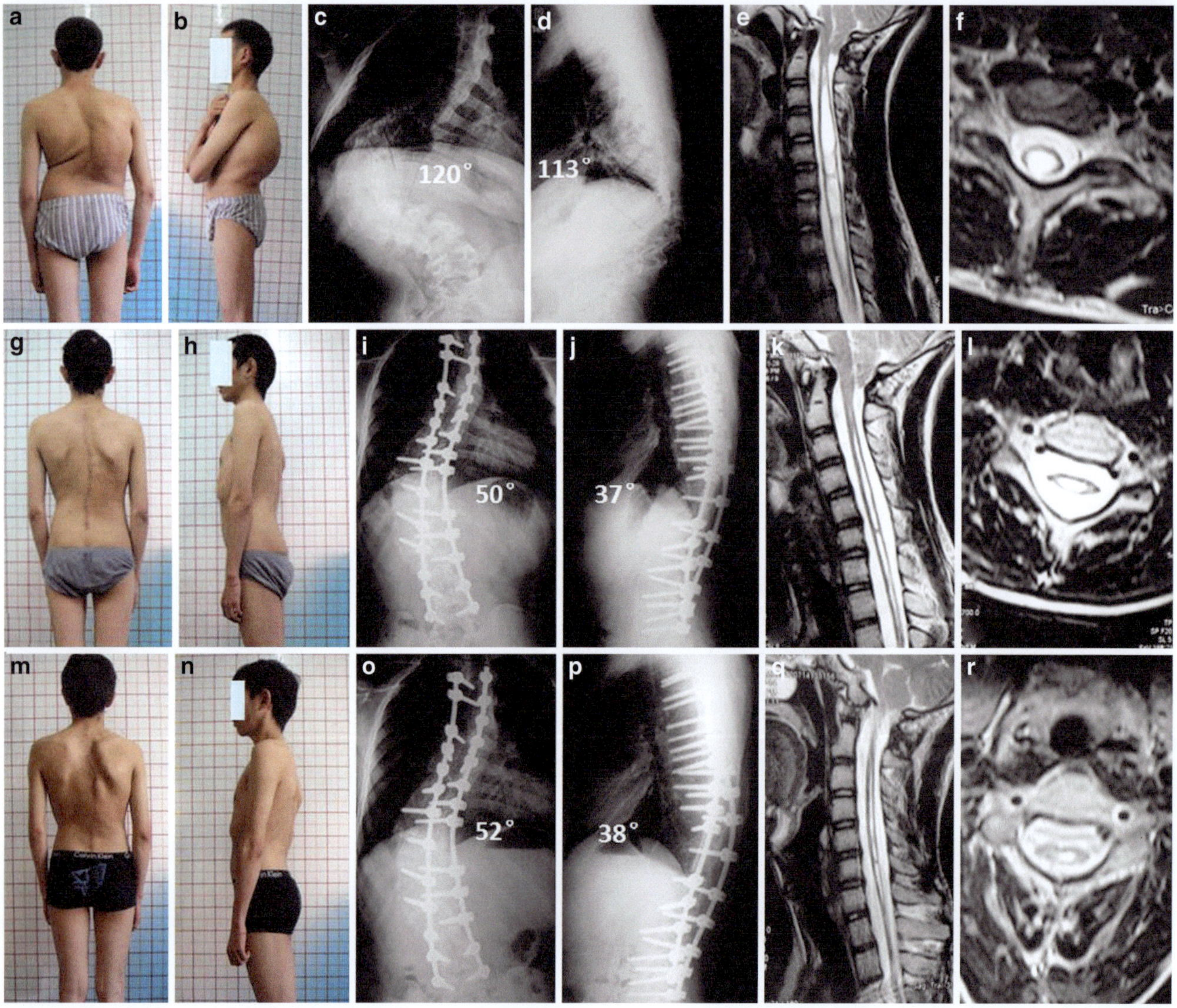

Fig. 12.2 Case 2: Male, 17 years old, severe spinal deformity with Chiari deformity and spinal syringomyelia, underwent one-stage PVCR surgery. The patient's preoperative appearance (**a**, **b**), positive and lateral X-ray films showed severe scoliosis of the spine (**c**, **d**); preoperative sagittal and horizontal MRI showed Type I Chiari deformity and the neck continued to the syringomyelia of the thoracic segment (**e**, **f**). Appearance (**g**, **h**) and corrective effect (**i**, **j**) at 3 months after operation, re-examination of MRI showed significant improvement in spinal cavity (**k**, **l**). The follow-up appearance (**m**, **n**) and corrective effect (**o**, **p**) were followed up for 36 months after operation. A review of MRI showed that the syringomyelia was further improved (**q**, **r**) (Wang Y, Xie J, Zhao Z, et al. Changes in CSF flow after one-stage posterior vertebral column resection in scoliosis patients with syringomyelia and Type I Chiari malformation. J Neurosurg Spine. 2013, 18: 456–64)

12.5 Key Points and Caveats

1. Spinal cord safety:

   For severe and rigid spinal deformity, PVCR divided the curved spine into two parts, and re-alignment the spine through three-dimensional maneuvers. Thus, spinal cord injury following spinal column displacement is the primary problem during operation. PVCR creates space with bone tissue-free movement but does not allow the spinal cord to move too much with the ends of the spine. Throughout the process of PVCR correction, the contradiction between dynamic and static changes of spine and cord are exist, with the progress of correction. Adjusting and obtaining the balance between dynamic and static at any time is the essence of PVCR correction. Keep correction with spinal cord hypotonic at any time, which is the most critical method to prevent spinal cord injury during surgery. The correction process of PVCR is based on the

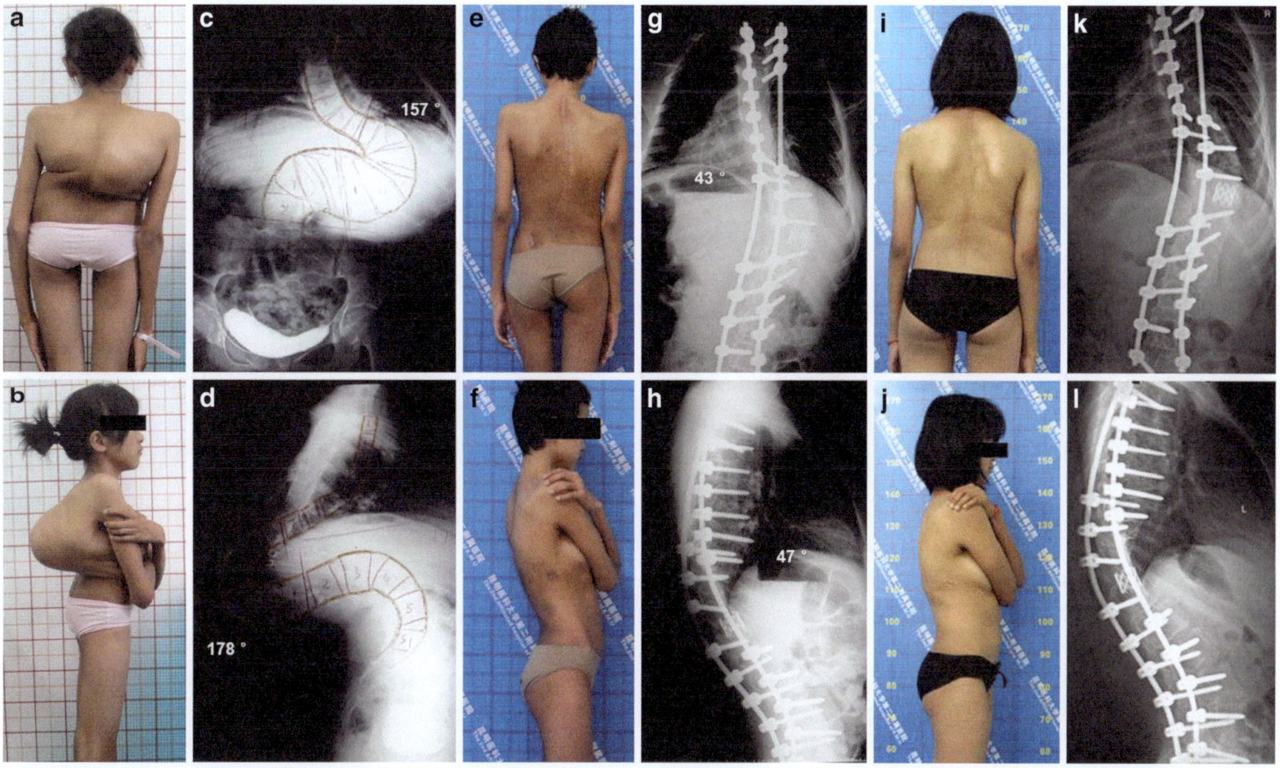

Fig. 12.3 Case 3: Female, 17 years old, severe rigid spinal deformity, underwent one-stage PVCR surgery. The patient's preoperative appearance (**a**, **b**) and positive and lateral X-ray films showed extremely severe rigid scoliosis (**c**, **d**). Appearance (**e**, **f**) and correction effect (**g**, **h**) were followed up at 3 months after operation. Appearance (**i**, **j**) and correction effect (**k**, **l**) were followed up for 24 months after operation (Wang Y, Xie J, Zhao Z, et al. Preoperative short-term traction prior to posterior vertebral column resection: procedure and role. Eur Spine J. 2015 Jan 1. DOI 10.1007/s00586-014-3752-6)

premise of shortening the spine, to ensure that the spinal cord tension is no higher than the beginning of the correction. The key to accurate and timely judgment of spinal cord tension is to continuously evaluate the dural sac with "vision" and "touch." Make full use of the space after vertebral resection to properly adjust the spine to reduce the spinal cord tension, pay attention not to cause excessive dural spinal cord buckling due to shortening. This important step can effectively increase the compliance of the spinal cord, for the displacement of angular or rotation of the spine, thereby effectively protecting the safety of the spinal cord during correction.

Spinal cord safety protection, in addition to mastery of corrective principles and techniques during operation, also depends on a comprehensive and reasonable surgical system: preoperative assessment of spinal cord high tension and surgical strategy forming; preoperative measurement and classification of pedicle diameter, intraoperative screw implantation technique; monitoring of nerve evoked potentials during operation and responding strategies. It must be clearly recognized that as an effective method for treating severe rigid spinal deformities, PVCR is also a very risky and challenging operation, which must be completed by an experienced treatment team.

2. Extreme deformity and preoperative traction:

   For those severe rigid and angular spinal deformities whose deformity angle is greater than 150° and the flexibility is less than 10%, it is extremely difficult and risky to directly perform corrective operation. A little carelessness will lead to disastrous consequences. Short-term preoperative, large-weight traction within the patient's tolerance range gradually improves the deformity to a certain extent. The task of aggressive surgical correction is done preoperatively, which reduces the risk of correction. It is expected that in the shortest time before operation, skull-femoral traction will achieve the greatest improvement in spinal deformity, which will effectively reduce the difficulties in the implementation of steps such as exposure, pedicle screw placement, and vertebral resection. Observe the spinal cord tolerability of patients by preoperative traction and evaluate the spinal cord safety during the operation. Reduce deformity before surgery to reduce spinal cord threats caused by rapid spinal displacement with rapid corrective; additionally, it is expected that during the traction process, effective respiratory function exercises and nutritional support treatments are conducted in parallel to increase the tolerance of the general physical condition to operation.

3. Control Bleeding:

   A large dose of tranexamic acid can be used. The loading dose is 100 mg/kg in 30 min before the operation, followed by maintenance of 10 mg/kg/h until the end of the operation. Ligation of one pair of segmental vessels can effectively reduce intraspinal hemorrhage without spinal cord ischemic damage.
4. Avoid nerve damage caused by pedicle screw placement.

12.6 Complication Prevention and Treatment

For patients receiving PVCR, severe rigid spinal deformity, cardiopulmonary dysfunction, poor overall nutritional status, spinal cord function is on the verge of decompensation, and spinal cord dysfunction has even occurred. These patients have less spinal tolerance to the changes of tension and blood supply during correction. Therefore, they face greater difficulties and risks in the effective correction of deformities, trunk reconstruction, spinal cord protection, and prevention of complications. The incidence of complications related to PVCR operation is up to 40–64.3%.

1. Neurological complications:

   The incidence of neuro deficit is high. It not only seriously affects the quality of life of patients, resulting in family and social burden, but also significantly increases the pressure of medical staff. The Scoliosis Research Society (SRS) reported that the incidence of spinal cord injury caused by operation in the most common adolescent idiopathic scoliosis patients is as high as 0.3–1.4%. Reports from just a few PVCR treatment centers worldwide in recent years indicated a high risk of neuro deficit. Suk reported some cases of severe spinal deformity treated with PVCR in three groups, with neurological complications occurring at 17.1%, 6.3%, and 8.0%, respectively. Lenke et al. reported that neurological complications were 26.5% (39/147). In the process of PVCR operation to correct severe rigid spinal deformity, many steps affect spinal cord safety. From the perspective of operation procedures, the risks come from: (1) Vertebral column resection; (2) deformity correction step. In terms of the characteristics of the disease, thoracic location of the apex, kyphoscoliosis, main curve greater than 100°, preoperative neurological abnormalities, and myelopathy leading to the high tension of the spinal cord (such as syringomyelia, spinal cord tethering, Chiari deformity, etc.) suggest higher risk of iatrogenic spinal cord injury. PVCR-related neurological complications are catastrophic once they occur, so prevention is in the first place. Spinal surgeons should fully consider the high-risk factors that lead to neurological complications when planning for surgery. At the same time, a variety of electrophysiological monitoring techniques should be used during the operation to detect and deal with potential neural damage in time.
2. Non-neurological complications:

   In 2012, Auerbach et al. reported that three-column osteotomy (87 cases of PSO, 18 cases of PVCR) was used to treat 105 patients with spinal deformity. The total complication rate was about 35% and the non-neurological complication rate was 15.2%. The incidence of non-neurological complications was 15.4% in adolescent idiopathic scoliosis cases reported by Carreon et al. In our case, the overall incidence of non-neurological complications was 22.6%. The most common complications occur in the respiratory system and the cardiovascular system. Our non-neurologic complications are higher than those in other literature, which are considered to be related to severe preoperative deformities, poor cardiopulmonary function, and more intraoperative bleeding.

   Long-term existence and development of deformities lead to: (1) impaired respiratory function; (2) the potential tendency of abnormal cardiac reserve function, the three-dimensional structural changes of spine and heart/large blood vessels in a short time during PVCR operation; (3) poor digestion and absorption, poor nutritional status; and (4) major bleeding. These factors post patients to extremely high risk of complications. The application of high-dose tranexamic acid, reasonable and effective ligation of segmental blood vessels, lung function exercise, detailed examination of the cardiovascular system, and the development of a detailed perioperative treatment plan will help reduce the incidence of non-neurological complications.

In summary, PVCR obtains good corrective effect and effective improvement of the overall appearance of spinal deformity in patients with severe rigid spinal deformity and is currently the most effective treatment method for patients with severe rigid spinal deformity. However, the complex pathophysiological characteristics of severe rigid spinal deformity and the unique nature of the PVCR procedure itself also determine the high risk during the treatment. The application of PVCR in the treatment of severe rigid spinal deformity needs to factor in these characteristics, comprehensively consider and implement the treatment plan from both perspectives of safeguarding life and safeguarding the spinal cord. This is the key to determining the success or failure of treatment.

Suggested Reading

1. Xie J, Wang Y, Zhang Y, et al. Initial clinical report of posterior total corpectomy for correction of rigid kyphosis or scoliosis. J Spine Surg. 2008;2(6):1–4.
2. Xie JM, Wang YS, Zhao Z, et al. Posterior vertebral column resection for correction of rigid spinal deformity curves more than 100 degrees. J Neurosurg Spine. 2012;17(6):540–51.
3. Lenke LG, O'Leary PT, Bridwell KH, et al. Posterior vertebral column resection for severe pediatric deformity: minimum 2-year follow-up of thirty-five consecutive patients. Spine. 2009;34(20):2213–21.
4. Lenke LG, Newton PO, Sucato DJ, et al. Complications after 147 consecutive vertebral column resections for severe pediatric spinal deformity: A multicenter analysis. Spine. 2013;38(2):119–32.
5. Kim SS, Cho BC, Kim JH, et al. Complications of posterior vertebral resection for spinal deformity. Asian Spine J. 2012;6(4):257–65.
6. Xie JM, Zhang Y, Wang YS, et al. The risk factors of neurologic deficits of one-stage posterior vertebral column resection for patients with severe and rigid spinal deformities. Eur Spine J. 2014;23(1):149–56.
7. Xie J, Lenke LG, Li T, et al. Preliminary investigation of high-dose tranexamic acid for controlling intraoperative blood loss in patients undergoing spine correction surgery. Spine J. 2015;15(4):647–54.
8. Wang YS, Xie JM, Zhao Z, et al. Perioperative major non-neurologic complications in 105 patients undergoing posterior vertebral column resection (PVCR) procedures for severe rigid deformities. Spine. 2015;40(16):1289–96.
9. Auerbach JD, Lenke LG, Bridwell KH, et al. Major complications and comparison between 3-column osteotomy techniques in 105 consecutive spinal deformity procedures. Spine. 2012;37(14):1198–2.
10. Wang Y, Xie J, Zhao Z, et al. Changes in CSF flow after one-stage posterior vertebral column resection in scoliosis patients with syringomyelia and Chiari malformation type I. J Neurosurg Spine. 2013;18:456–64.
11. Wang Y, Xie J, Zhao Z, et al. Preoperative short-term traction prior to posterior vertebral column resection: procedure and role. Eur Spine J. 2015; https://doi.org/10.1007/s00586-014-3752-6.

13 Osteotomy for Traumatic Spinal Deformity

Huizhong Tian, Yuan Ma, Yingsong Wang, and Li Li

13.1 Overview

13.1.1 Biomechanics of Traumatic Kyphosis

The most common region of spinal fracture is the thoracolumbar (T11–12), mainly due to the characteristics of anatomical position and biomechanical of thoracolumbar segment. The thoracic spine has thoracic cage support, with a smaller vertebral body, narrow intervertebral space, long and overlapping spinous processes, and short interspinous ligaments. The articular processes of the thoracic spine are on the coronal plane. All these factors limit the activity of the thoracic spine, so the fracture rarely occurs in the T1–T10 vertebral body. T11–T12 vertebrae are similar to the lumbar vertebrae in structure. Ribs have little stabilizing effect on the corresponding vertebrae due to their free ends. These vertebrae are located in the transition zone of the thoracic spine with less activity and the lumbar spine with more activity. When the spine is subjected to hyperextension or axial compression violence, it is easy to cause compression or burst fracture of the vertebral body. As the complex structure of the posterior vertebral ligament is relatively intact, local kyphosis with fracture vertebral body as the center often occurs after the injury, which is the main reason that traumatic kyphosis is commonly found in the thoracolumbar levels.

13.1.2 Effect of Traumatic Kyphosis on Cardiopulmonary Function

If the thoracic deformity limits the free expansion and shrinkage of the lung, and causes respiratory system diseases, especially in patients with severe kyphosis, the chest and abdomen are not in a straight line, which results in the limitation of diaphragm movement, significant reduction of lung function, patients are prone to lung infection, and even pulmonary heart disease, leading to cardiovascular failure. Clinically, some patients with kyphosis may have heart enlargement and heart murmur, and most of them have palpitation and shortness of breath even when they do mild physical exercises. The results of the preoperative pulmonary function test show that most patients have restrictive ventilation disorder, which hinders airway clearance function and easily induces airway obstruction and mixed ventilation disorder. After deformity correction, the above symptoms can be relieved to a certain extent. Therefore, the objective of deformity correction surgery is not only to correct deformity and improve appearance but also to control and improve cardiopulmonary function. Owing to the improvement of cardiopulmonary function, the cardiac output and vital capacity are increased. When the activity is increased, the symptoms such as palpitation and shortness of breath are obviously relieved.

Kyphosis deformity causes the volume of the abdominal cavity to decrease, causing gastrointestinal pressure and gastrointestinal peristalsis to slow down, leading to poor digestion and absorption, lack of appetite, loss of body weight, etc. After the operation, the digestive function of most patients can be improved, appetite and weight will increase.

13.1.3 Imbalance and Compensation of Gravity Line

Kyphosis leads to the displacement of the spinal gravity line and the anterior inclination of the trunk. In order to overcome the anterior inclination, the cervical and lumbar must increase their lordosis to maintain the global balance. When the kyphosis is severe, the cervical and lumbar lordosis is not fully compensated, hip and knee joint will be flex to compensate. As a result of long-term flexion compensation,

H. Tian · Y. Ma (✉) · L. Li
Spinal Surgery, The Sixth Affiliated Hospital of Xinjiang Medical University, Urumqi, China

Y. Wang
Department of Orthopedics, The 2nd Affiliated Hospital of Kunming Medical University, Kunming, China

H. Tian et al. (eds.), *Spinal Osteotomy Orthopaedics*, https://doi.org/10.1007/978-981-16-1387-6_13

the cervical and lumbar vertebrae appear early degenerative changes and flexion contracture deformity of hip and knee joints. After deformity correction, the hyperlordosis of the cervical and lumbar vertebrae will be significantly improved, and the flexion of the hip and knee joints can also be corrected. When kyphosis causes the gravity line of the spine to move forward, the abdominal muscles and soft tissues will also experience wide contracture. These changes can further aggravate kyphosis, which is also the main reason for the dynamic instability of the spine. These patients often feel pain and fatigue in the back, and their symptoms increase with the aggravation of deformity. The main causes of low back pain include segmental instability of the spine, stenosis of the intervertebral foramen, angular deformity of spine, and compression of fracture block in the spinal canal.

13.1.4 Neuro Symptoms

Some patients already have underlying compression of the spinal canal in the early stage of injury, and then with the aggravation of local kyphosis and instability of the spine, the proliferation of scar tissue in and around the spinal canal, it further aggravates the stenosis of the spinal canal and causing compression symptoms of spinal cord or nerve root.

13.2 Surgical Approaches

13.2.1 Surgical Indication

No matter acute or late posttraumatic kyphosis, surgical correction should be considered when the kyphosis angle of the thoracolumbar segment is more than 30° and the anterior kyphosis angle is less than 10°. Among patients with thoracolumbar fractures with complete or partial neurological impairment, more than 50% of the patients with spinal canal compression need spinal fusion because of progressive spinal instability or kyphosis. It is suggested that the spine fracture with severe bone destruction and kyphosis angle >30° may have facet joint subluxation and damage of the posterior column, which may lead to late spinal instability. Therefore, it is suggested that rotated displacement, lateral displacement, spinal fractures with more than 50% of spinal canal compression, and kyphosis deformity >30° are all indications for surgical treatment.

13.2.2 Surgical Technique

The operation is mainly aimed at patients with severe old thoracolumbar fracture and dislocation, severe kyphosis, complete or incomplete paraplegia, and nerve root compression. The best timing of operation is before the incomplete fusion of dislocated vertebral body and inferior vertebral body. Due to the high potential of bleeding in this operation, 2000 ml of blood should be prepared before operation.

1. Preoperative preparation: blood type, skin preparation, preparation of a set of Tian's spine osteotome, and implant-specific instruments.
2. Anesthesia: general anesthesia with tracheal intubation or local infiltration anesthesia.
3. Position: prone or lateral.
4. Operation procedure:

    The first step: incision and exposure. The midline incision should be made along the spinous processes, about 20–30 cm long. A total of 5–6 laminae are exposed in the upper 2 and lower 3 lamina centered on the displacement level. The lower vertebra of displaced level is often the vertebrae with compressed fracture. It is necessary to expose the bilateral lamina, articular process, and the tip of the transverse process. This vertebrae is the posterior process and the most superficial in the operation field. It is the vertebrae to be resected (Fig. 13.1).

    The second step: laminectomy and articular process resection. First, the spinous process and lamina of the lower vertebrae to the displaced space are removed (Fig. 13.2a, b). Then the upper and lower articular processes and the bilateral pedicles are removed (Fig. 13.3a, b). So far, the posterior and lateral sides of the spinal cord and the nerve root are exposed. The spinal cord and the nerve root are usually in a state of kinking and tension. The operator may feel the existence of compression from the anterior by palpating on the dura. The scope and angle of wedge resection of the total spine from the spinous process to the anterior longitudinal ligament should be determined according to the needs. Generally, the scope of resection for traumatic kyphosis is usually wedge resection of the total spine including one intervertebral disc (Fig. 13.4).

    The third step: to expose the vertebral body. The transverse process is resected from the root of the bilateral trans-

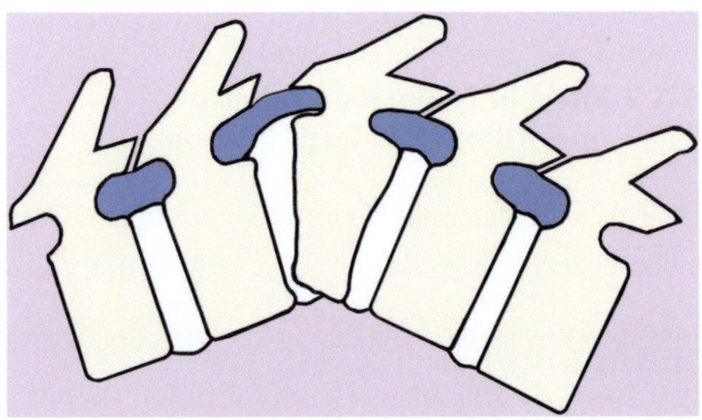

Fig. 13.1 Thoracolumbar compression-dislocation fracture lead to more than 30° of angular kyphosis, compression fracture makes upper vertebral displaces anteriorly

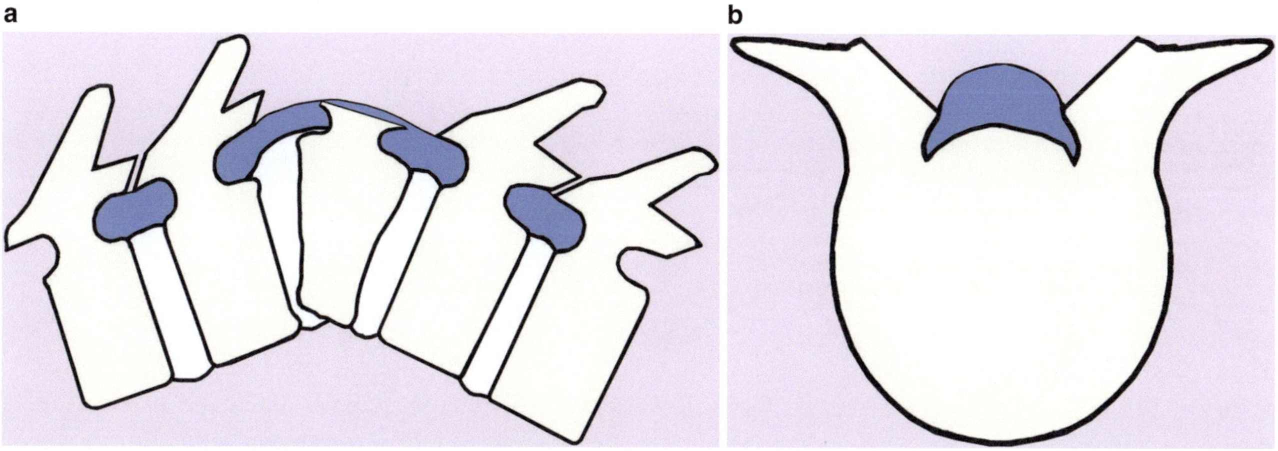

Fig. 13.2 Laminae and spinous process have been resected, leaving only part of the articular process and pedicle. (**a**) Lateral view; (**b**) axial view

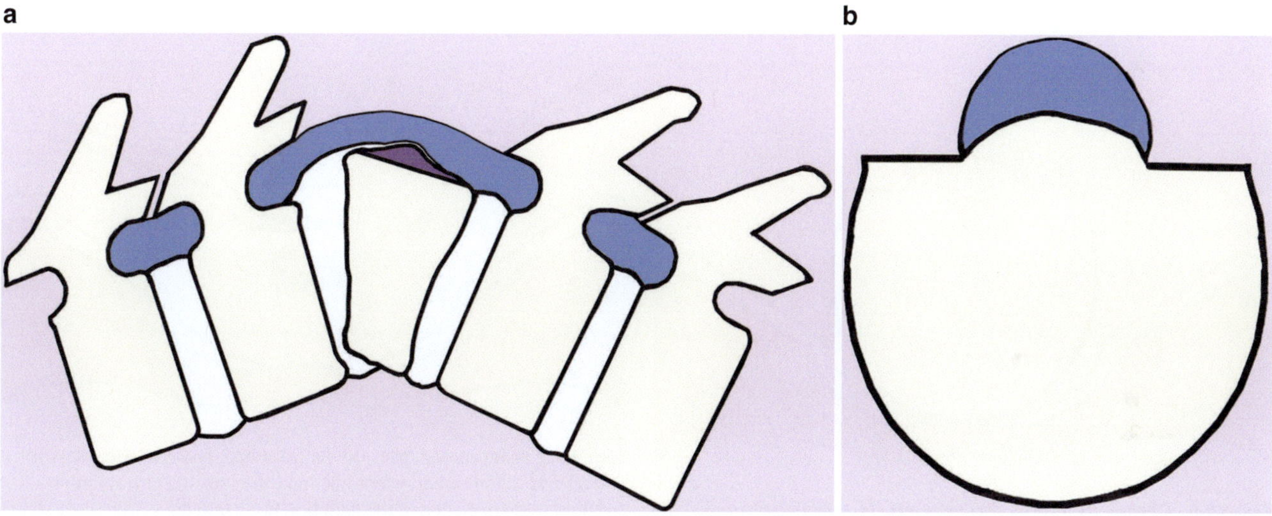

Fig. 13.3 Pedicle has been removed, and it can be seen that the posterior edge of the vertebral body protrudes into the spinal canal and compresses the dural canal. (**a**) Lateral view; (**b**) axial view

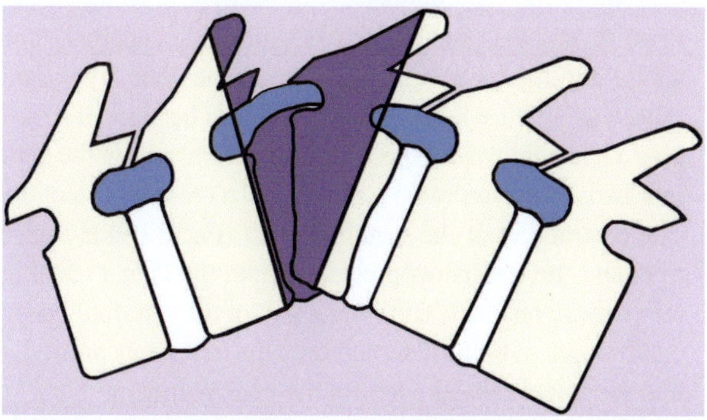

Fig. 13.4. Wedge resection includes the posterior arch and upper 3/4 of the vertebral body of the compression fracture level and the lower 1/5 of the upper vertebra and the disc involved in the fracture-dislocation of the spine.

verse processes, and the anterior lateral edge of the exposed vertebral body is exposed to the anterior along the lateral edge of the vertebral body with Anonymous osteotome (an instrument in the Tian's osteotome set) (Fig. 13.5). It must be strictly carried out under the periosteum, especially when the vertebral body is exposed, the elevator should advance along the waist of the vertebral body to avoid damaging the segmental blood vessels. Then change to the lever and lever off the soft tissue around the vertebral body and segment blood vessels, and expose the whole vertebral body (Fig. 13.6). Scope of vertebral body expose: including the whole wedge vertebral body with compression fracture and the inferior edge of the upper vertebral body and disc of the upper vertebral body (see Fig. 13.4).

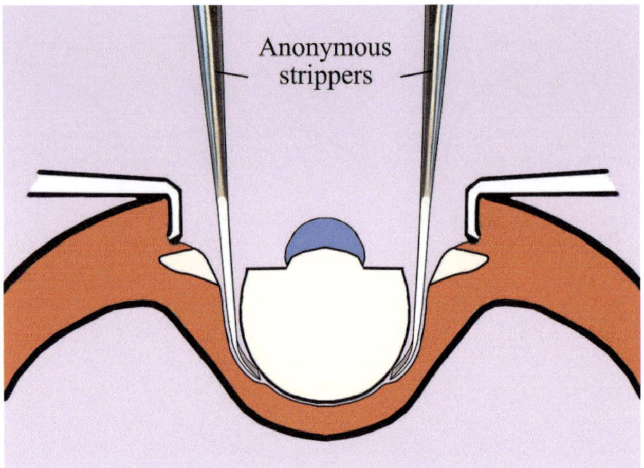

Fig. 13.5 Use the anonymous elevator to elevate along the waist of the vertebral body, strictly under the periosteum, directly to the anterior edge of the vertebral body, so as to avoid damaging the segmental blood vessels

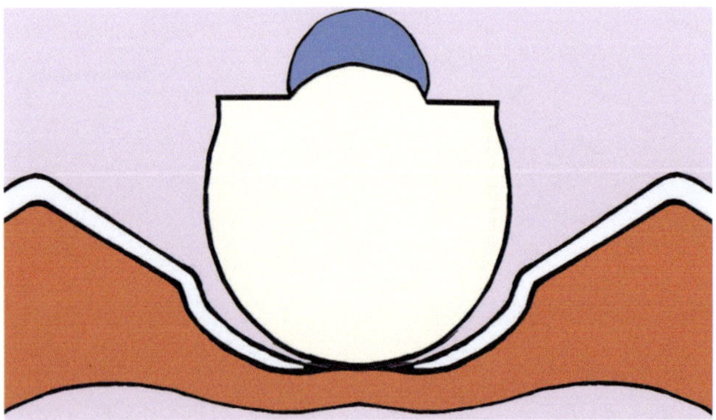

Fig. 13.6 Change to the lever to lever off the soft tissue around the vertebral body and segment blood vessels, exposing the whole vertebral body

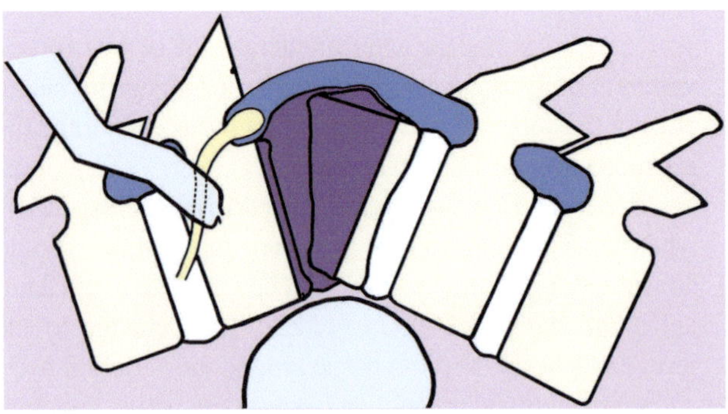

Fig. 13.7 Protect the spinal nerve roots of the superior level outside the operation field with a nerve root retractor to facilitate corpectomy

The fourth step: retract the spinal nerve root. The spinal nerve roots exiting through the upper intervertebral foramen are retracted and protected outside the operation field with the nerve root retractor (Fig. 13.7).

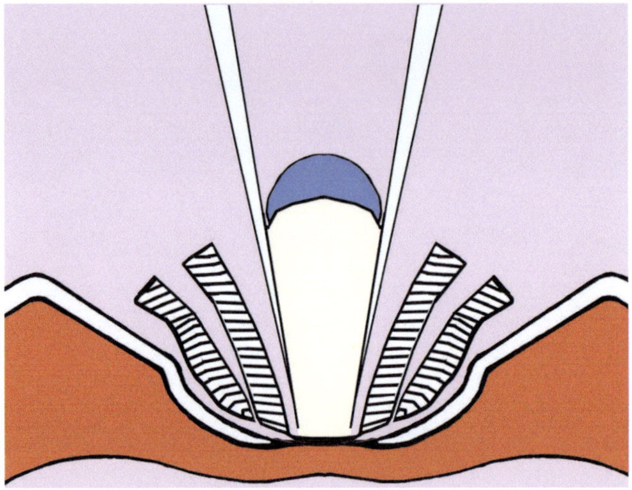

Fig. 13.8 The lateral part of the vertebral body is excised with straight osteotome in layers, hemostasis with bone wax

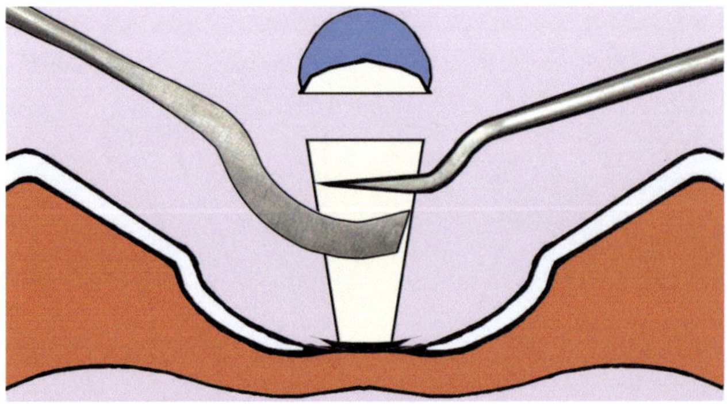

Fig. 13.9 The central part of the vertebral body is excised with a shovel and the crescent osteotome, and the bone fragments protruding from the posterior edge of the vertebral body into the vertebral canal are reserved for the final step

The fifth step: vertebral osteotomy. First, remove the lateral part of the vertebral body (Fig. 13.8) with straight osteotome layer by layer. For the bleeding of cancellous bone sinus, stop the bleeding by applying bone wax. Apply hard bone wax after each cut. The surface must be smooth so as to play a real hemostasis role. Then, the central part of the vertebral body is excised with a shovel and a crescent osteotome. The central part of the vertebral body (Fig. 13.9) is excised first, and the fragments protruding into the spinal canal are temporarily retained. The central part of the vertebral body is cut through on both sides, and only the fragments protruding into the spinal canal are left for the final treatment.

The sixth step: posterior edge resection. The posterior edge of the vertebral body and the bone fragments protruding into the vertebral canal are left for final treatment until most of the vertebral bodies are excised. The methods of resection of posterior edge of vertebral body and fragments protruding into vertebral canal are as follows. First, use the posterior longitudinal ligament elevator to separate a gap

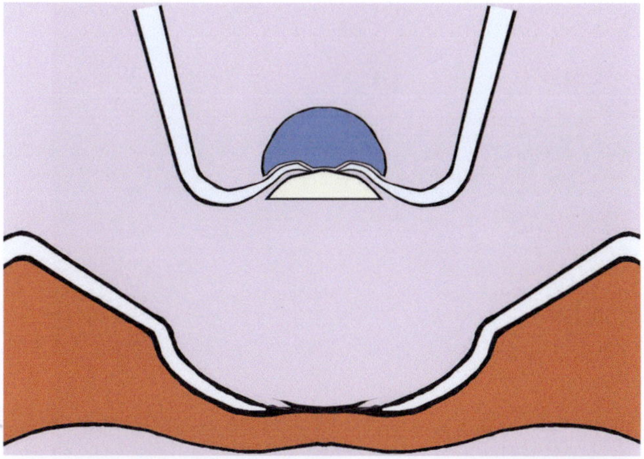

Fig. 13.10 Use the pusher to pull down the posterior edge of the vertebral body and the bone fragments protruding into the vertebral canal

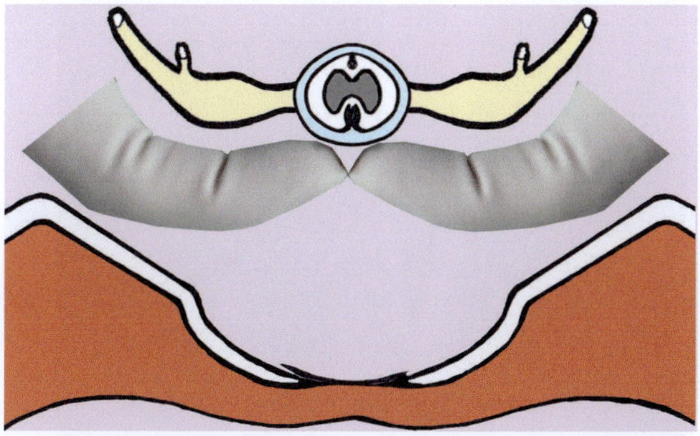

Fig. 13.11 Fingers palpation to check whether the bone fragments in front of the dura mater has been completely removed, and whether the dural sac has been relaxed and expanded, so as to check before closing the osteotomy space

from the posterior bone sheet, then use the pusher to push down the posterior bone sheet of the vertebral body and the fragments protruding into the spinal canal (Fig. 13.10). Remove the bone fragments with the nucleus pulposus forceps. Pay attention to protect the integrity of the dural canal, prevent dural tear and CSF leakage. After resection of the posterior edge of the vertebral body and the fragments protruding into the spinal canal, if there are no residual fragments in the osteotomy space by palpation (Fig. 13.11), the osteotomy space shall be closed immediately.

The seventh step: reduction and internal fixation. Generally, the osteotomy space of traumatic kyphosis is not wide, and the commonly used instrumentation is by screw–rod fixation. Generally, 2–3 screws on each side above and below the osteotomy space are adequate, or, 8–12 screws and 2 rods in total (Fig. 13.12). In some cases, distal extension and proximal compression may be performed as required.

The eighth step: place the drainage tube and close the incision. Place T-shaped drainage tube, close the incision by layers to complete the operation.

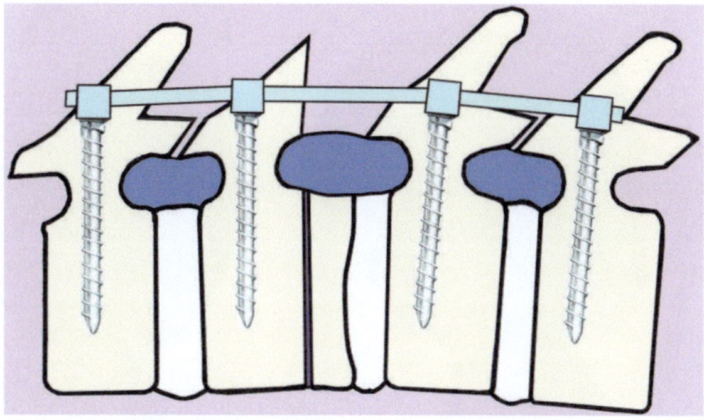

Fig. 13.12 Reduction and internal fixation have been completed. The cancellous bone of the vertebral body is facing the cancellous bone surface, so no interbody bone grafting is needed. Only grafting with bone chips on top of the lamina is needed

5. Postoperative management:

   The patient should lie in a flatbed when returned to the ward. The drainage tube is connected with a negative pressure drainage bottle, the drainage tube is removed 24–48 h later, and the suture was removed 10 days later. After removing the suture, the patient is allowed to ambulate. A plaster vest is applied with traction by occipital-mandible belt suspending on a vertical frame.

13.2.3 Typical Cases

- Case 1. A 16-year-old female, traumatic kyphosis. She was treated with a U-shaped rod and wiring internal fixation in other hospitals. The wire broke after the operation and the correction failed. The patient came to our hospital for a revision surgery. A thorough examination was done after admission. The preoperative Cobb angle was 75°. Vertebral column resection plus proximal compression and distal distraction and internal fixation were performed. The operation went smoothly. After the operation, the Cobb angle of X-ray film became 1°, the height increased by 3 cm, and the body shape improved significantly (Fig. 13.13a–f).
- Case 2. A 36-year-old male was admitted to the emergency department because of a lumbar and back injury in a traffic accident. After X-ray and CT examination, he was diagnosed with an L1 flexion compression fracture with kyphosis deformity, with a Cobb angle of 33°. On the 5th day after admission, T12-L1 kyphosis osteotomy under general anesthesia with endotracheal intubation and internal fixation with screw–rod system was performed. The operation went smoothly. Postoperative kyphosis was corrected, Cobb angle was 2° (Fig. 13.14a–i), and the patient was discharged after 10 days when the suture was removed.

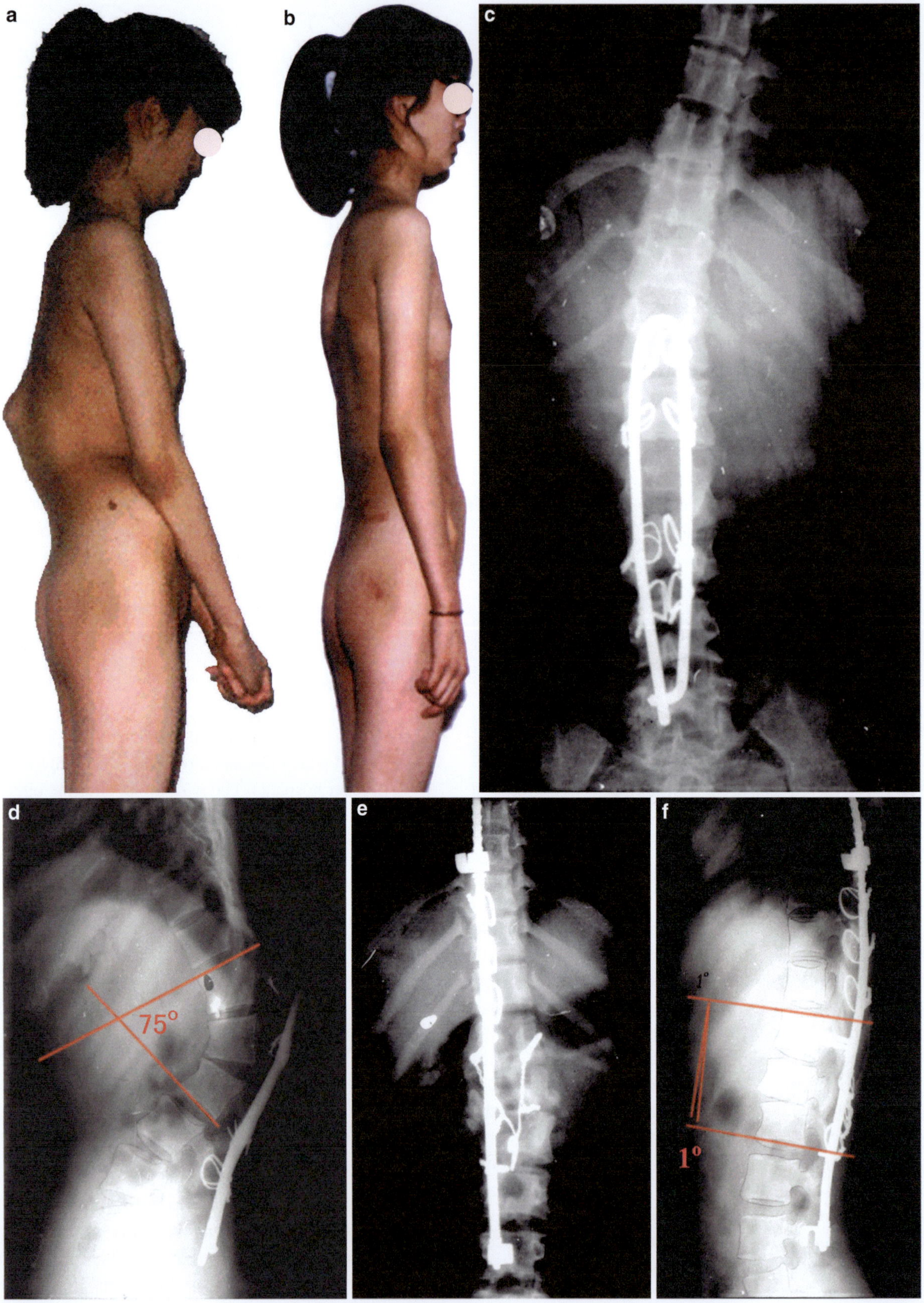

Fig. 13.13 Traumatic angular kyphosis. (**a**) Angular kyphosis was evident before operation. (**b**) Kyphosis was corrected after surgery. (**c**) Preoperative anteroposterior X-ray, (**d**) Kyphosis was 75° in the preoperative lateral X-ray, (**e**) posterior X-ray films after total spinal osteotomy, (**f**) postoperative lateral X-ray showed Cobb angle changed to 1°

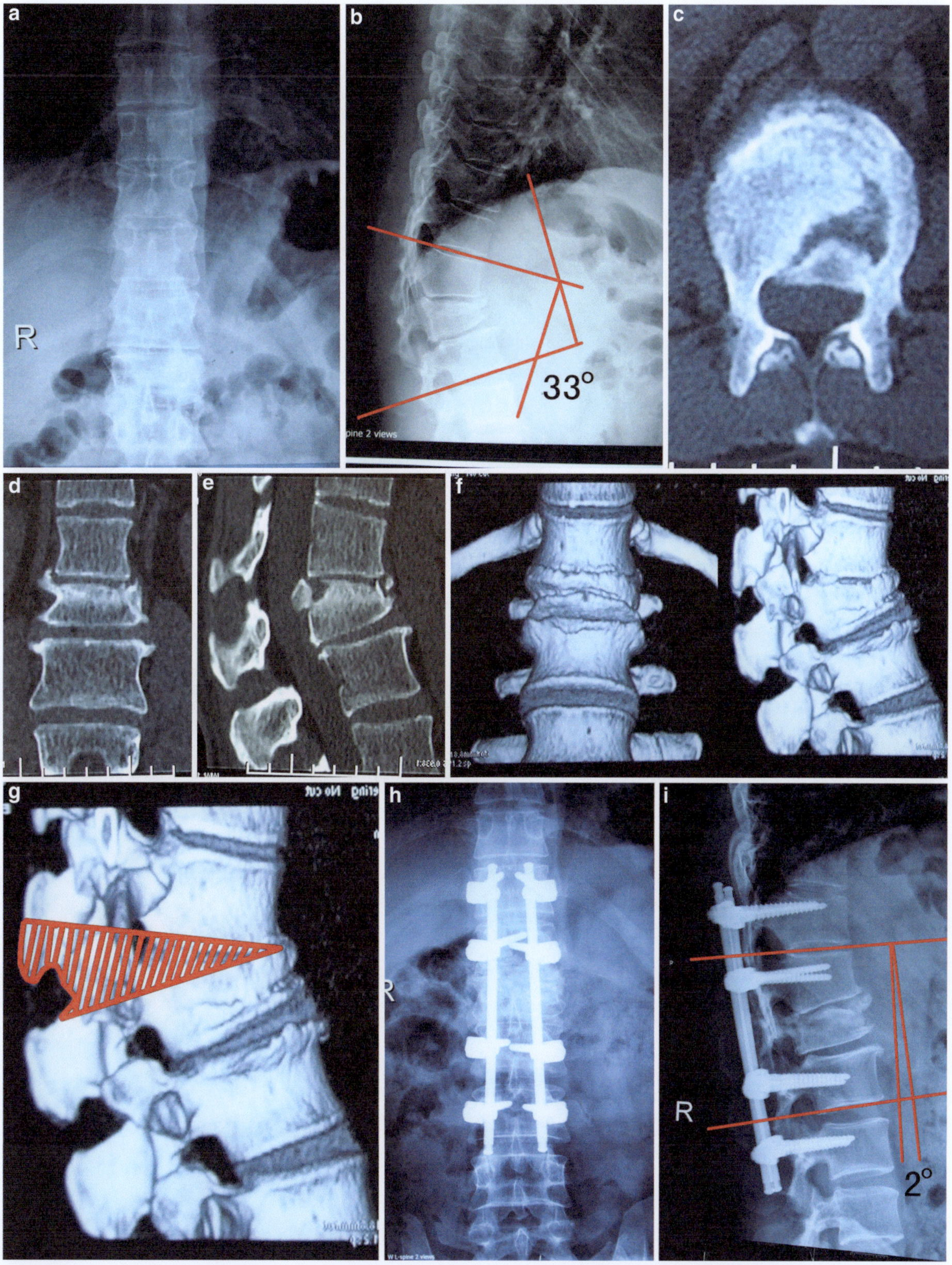

Fig. 13.14 Typical cases 2: (**a**) L1 compression fracture in the anteroposterior radiograph; (**b**) lateral radiograph kyphosis deformity Cobb angle 33°; (**c**) posterior vertebral fracture seen on preoperative CT. The fragment protruded slightly back into the spinal canal without neurological symptoms; (**d**) CT coronal showed a comminuted fracture at the upper edge of L1 vertebra; (**e**) CT sagittal showed a comminuted fracture at the upper edge of L1 vertebra. Posterior fragments protruded into the spinal canal, compression of anterior vertebral body, kyphosis deformity Cobb angle 33°; (**f**) preoperative CT three-dimensional reconstruction; (**g**) scope of vertebral column resection. (**h**) Orthotopic radiograph of screw–rod system internal fixation; (**i**) Cobb angle changed to 2° after total spinal osteotomy

Suggested Reading

1. Tian H. Surgical treatment of kyphosis kyphosis. Chin J Orthop. 1992;12(3):162–5.
2. Tian H, Yuan T, Tian S. Posterior invasion and vertebral osteotomy. Spinal Deformation. 1992;7(1):4–11.
3. Tian H, Li F. Spinal deformity and osteotomy. Xi'an: World Book; 2001. p. 377–735.
4. Tian H. Spinal surgeons should be good at using rongeurs and osteotome. Chin J Mod Oper Surg. 2002;6(1):67–8.
5. Tian H. Application of "Tian's spinal bone knife" in orthopaedic surgery. Chin J Orthop. 2003;11(15):1073–5.
6. Tian H. Report of 25 cases of traumatic paraplegia treated with posterior spinal decompression by posterior approach. Chin J Orthop. 2006;07:549–50.
7. Tian H, Lv X, Ma Y. Treatment of severe spinal curvature with total spine osteotomy and internal fixation with head-sleeve ring. Chin J Orthop. 2007;15(3):167–72.
8. Tian H, Liu S, Ma Y. Practical spine surgery. Guangzhou: Guangdong Science and Technology Press; 2008. p. 87–409.
9. Tian H, Liu S, Ma Y. Practical spine surgery illustration. Beijing: People's Military Medical Press; 2008. p. 152–675.
10. Tian H. History of treatment of spinal deformity in China. Chin J Orthop. 2009;17(9):706–7.
11. Tian H, Li M, Ma Y. Spinal deformity osteotomy orthopedics, vol. 5. Beijing: People's Medical Publishing House; 2011. p. 3–339.
12. Tian H. A brief history and popularization of spinal osteotomy with thin blade bone knife. Chin J Orthop. 2012;20(23):2207–8.
13. Tian H, Zhang H, Liang Y. Surgical treatment of spinal deformity. Guangzhou: Guangdong Science and Technology Press; 2012. p. 1–483.
14. Tian H, Li M, Wang Z. Key points and diagrams of thoracolumbar surgery. Beijing: People's Medical Publishing House; 2012. p. 1–470.
15. Tian H, Ma Y, Xie J. Spinal osteotomy orthopedics. Guangzhou: Guangdong Science and Technology Press; 2018. p. 2–541.

MIX
Papier aus verantwortungsvollen Quellen
Paper from responsible sources
FSC® C105338

If you have any concerns about our products,
you can contact us on
ProductSafety@springernature.com

In case Publisher is established outside the EU,
the EU authorized representative is:
Springer Nature Customer Service Center GmbH
Europaplatz 3, 69115 Heidelberg, Germany

Printed by Libri Plureos GmbH
in Hamburg, Germany